# Promising Cancer Therapeutic Drug Targets: Recent Advancements

Edited by

**Ashok Kumar Pandurangan**
*School of Life Sciences*
*B.S. Abdur Rahman Crescent Institute of Science and Technology*
*Chennai-600048, India*

**Promising Cancer Therapeutic Drug Targets: Recent Advancements**

Editor: Ashok Kumar Pandurangan

ISBN (Online): 978-981-5238-57-0

ISBN (Print): 978-981-5238-58-7

ISBN (Paperback): 978-981-5238-59-4

First published in 2025.

need for a court order if at any point you breach any terms of this License Agreement. In no event will any delay or failure by Bentham Science Publishers in enforcing your compliance with this License Agreement constitute a waiver of any of its rights.

3. You acknowledge that you have read this License Agreement, and agree to be bound by its terms and conditions. To the extent that any other terms and conditions presented on any website of Bentham Science Publishers conflict with, or are inconsistent with, the terms and conditions set out in this License Agreement, you acknowledge that the terms and conditions set out in this License Agreement shall prevail.

**Bentham Science Publishers Pte. Ltd.**
80 Robinson Road #02-00
Singapore 068898
Singapore
Email: subscriptions@benthamscience.net

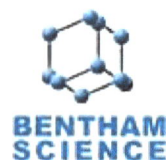

# CONTENTS

PREFACE ............................................................................................................ i

LIST OF CONTRIBUTORS ............................................................................ ii

**CHAPTER 1 EXOSOMAL DELIVERY OF CRISPR/CAS9 ASSEMBLY: APPROACH TOWARDS CANCER THERAPEUTICS** ......................................... 1
*Kaumudi Pande, PP Mubthasima, Rajalakshmi Prakash and Anbarasu Kannan*
    **INTRODUCTION** ................................................................................... 1
    **CRISPR AS A POTENTIAL THERAPEUTIC AGENT FOR METASTASIS** ....................... 4
        Molecules Involved in Metastasis ........................................... 4
        Metastatic Molecules Targeted by CRISPR/Cas9 System .............. 7
    **EXOSOMES AS A POTENTIAL CARRIER (THERAPEUTIC CARRIER): EXOSOMES-BASED DELIVERY OF SMALL MOLECULES, BIOACTIVE MOLECULES, SIRNA** ..... 9
    **GREAT BEGINNING OF THE CRISPR/CAS SYSTEM IN HUMAN TRIALS** ................ 13
    **DIFFERENT DELIVERY SYSTEMS FOR CRISPR/CAS** ................................. 14
    **EXOSOMAL-BASED DELIVERY FOR CRISPR** .......................................... 18
    **CONCLUSION** .................................................................................... 19
    **FUTURE PERSPECTIVE** ....................................................................... 19
    **REFERENCES** ..................................................................................... 20

**CHAPTER 2 CANCER STEM CELLS AND THEIR ROLE IN CHEMO-RESISTANCE** ........ 27
*Vaishali Ji, Chandra Kishore and Krishna Prakash*
    **INTRODUCTION** ................................................................................... 27
        Normal Stem Cells and Cancer Stem Cells Linked to Carcinogenesis ........... 28
        Transporter Proteins in Stem Cells and Cancer .................................. 29
        Chemotherapy Resistance in Cancer and Cancer Stem Cells .................. 29
        Controlling Drug-Resistant Cancer Cells ......................................... 30
        Cell Signaling in Cancer Stem Cells Cancer Therapy ......................... 32
    **CONCLUSION** .................................................................................... 35
    **REFERENCES** ..................................................................................... 35

**CHAPTER 3 IMPORTANCE OF NATURAL COMPOUNDS TARGETING THE MITOPHAGIC PROCESS IN BREAST CANCER TREATMENT** ..................... 41
*Prathibha Sivaprakasam, Karthikeyan Chandrabose, Sureshkumar Anandasadagopan, Hariprasth Lakshmanan and Ashok Kumar Pandurangan*
    **INTRODUCTION** ................................................................................... 42
        Breast Cancer Statistics ............................................................. 43
        Breast Cancer and Indian Scenario ................................................ 44
        Mitophagy .............................................................................. 45
        Mitophagy and Cancer ............................................................... 46
            *Mutations in PARK2 (Parkin)* .............................................. 46
        Mitophagy Mediated by HIF1α - BNIP3, NIX, and FUNDC1 ................ 47
            *HIF1α and the Tumor Microenvironment* ................................. 47
            *BNIP3 and NIX in Cancer Mitophagy* .................................... 47
            *FUNDC1 in Cancer Mitophagy* ............................................. 48
        KRAS Mutations and Cancer Mitophagy ........................................ 48
        Biological Role of Mitophagy ...................................................... 49
        Manipulating Mitophagy as a Potential Target for Cancer Therapy ......... 50
        Induction of Mitophagy Increases Cancer Cell Death and Chemotherapy Sensitivity ......... 51
        Inhibition of Mitophagy Enhances Drug Sensitivity ........................... 51

Classical Inhibitors of Mitophagy ................................................ 52
Novel Inhibitors of Mitophagy ................................................ 53
Role of Natural Compounds in Mitophagy ................................................ 53
    *Withaferin* ................................................ 53
    *Curcumin* ................................................ 54
    *Gingerol* ................................................ 54
    *Thymoquinone* ................................................ 55
    *Artepillin C* ................................................ 55
    *Cucurbitacin B* ................................................ 55
    *Triptolide* ................................................ 55
    *Allicin* ................................................ 56
    *Jolkinolide B* ................................................ 56
    *Chalocomoracin* ................................................ 56
**CONCLUSION** ................................................ 57
**AUTHOR'S CONTRIBUTION** ................................................ 57
**REFERENCES** ................................................ 57

**CHAPTER 4  BIOACTIVE NATURAL COMPOUNDS AS INHIBITORS OF SIGNAL TRANSDUCER AND ACTIVATOR OF TRANSCRIPTION 3: PROSPECTS IN ANTI-CANCER THERAPEUTICS** ................................................ 66
*Praveen Deepak*
**INTRODUCTION** ................................................ 66
**THERAPEUTIC TARGETING OF STAT3 SIGNALING IN CANCER** ................................................ 68
Targeting of STAT3 to Prevent Activation ................................................ 69
Targeting Protein-Protein Interactions in the STAT3 Signaling Pathway ................................................ 70
Targeting Nuclear Translocation of STAT3 ................................................ 71
Targeting Binding of STAT3 to the Promoter Region of DNA ................................................ 71
**TARGETING STAT3 BY NATURAL BIOACTIVE COMPOUNDS** ................................................ 72
Polyphenols as Inhibitors of STAT3 ................................................ 72
    *Flavonoids as STAT3 Inhibitors* ................................................ 73
Flavones in the Regulation of STAT3 ................................................ 75
Flavanones in the Regulation of STAT3 ................................................ 76
Flavanol in the Regulation of STAT3 ................................................ 77
Flavonol in the Regulation of STAT3 ................................................ 77
Anthocyanidin in the Regulation of STAT3 ................................................ 78
Isoflavonone as STAT3 Inhibitors ................................................ 78
Chalcones as STAT3 Inhibitors ................................................ 79
Other Polyphenols Targeting STAT3 ................................................ 79
Non-Polyphenolic Compounds as Inhibitors of STAT3 ................................................ 81
**CONCLUSION** ................................................ 81
**ACKNOWLEDGEMENTS** ................................................ 82
**REFERENCES** ................................................ 82

**CHAPTER 5  TARGETING CANCER STEMNESS BY EXOSOMES AS A THERAPEUTIC APPROACH AGAINST OVARIAN CANCER** ................................................ 94
*Kaumudi Pande* and *Anbarasu Kannan*
**INTRODUCTION** ................................................ 94
**MECHANISM OF CANCER STEM CELLS LEADING TO OVARIAN CANCER AND ITS METASTATIC SITES** ................................................ 97
**MITOCHONDRIAL & EMT MECHANISMS ON OVARIAN CANCER AND ITS METASTATIC SITES** ................................................ 100
**NATURAL AND SMALL MOLECULES TARGETING OVARIAN CANCER** ................................................ 102

EXOSOMES-BASED DELIVERY OF DRUGS AND OTHER MOLECULES
TARGETING OVARIAN ........................................................................................... 105
CONCLUSION ....................................................................................................... 106
LIST OF ABBREVIATIONS ................................................................................. 107
REFERENCES ........................................................................................................ 107

**CHAPTER 6 SPHINGOSINE KINASE AS A TARGET TO TREAT GASTROINTESTINAL
CANCERS** ..................................................................................................... 113
*Mit Joshi* and *Bhoomika M. Patel*
INTRODUCTION ................................................................................................... 114
    Currently Available Therapies to Treat Gastrointestinal Cancer ......................... 115
    Sphingolipid Metabolism .................................................................................. 115
    Sphingolipid Enzymes ...................................................................................... 117
        *Sphingosine Kinases* ................................................................................... 117
        *Ceramidase* ................................................................................................ 118
        *Glucosylceramide Synthase* ...................................................................... 118
        *Ceramide Synthase* ................................................................................... 118
    Importance of Ceramide .................................................................................... 118
    Role of S1P in the Growth of Cancer and Metastasis ....................................... 119
    S1P Receptors .................................................................................................. 120
    Presence of Sphingolipids in the Digestive System .......................................... 122
        *Metabolism of Sphingolipids in the Gastrointestinal Tract* ........................ 122
        *Sphingolipids and Colorectal Tumorigenesis* ............................................ 123
    Sphingolipids and Intestinal Inflammation ...................................................... 124
    Sphingolipids in Liver Cancer .......................................................................... 125
CONCLUSION ....................................................................................................... 125
REFERENCES ........................................................................................................ 125

**CHAPTER 7 HIPPO SIGNALING AND ITS REGULATION IN LIVER CANCER** ................. 133
*Naveen Kumar Perumal, Vasudevan Sekar, Annapoorna Bangalore Ramachandra,
Nivya Vijayan, Vani Vijay, Venkat Prashanth* and *Madan Kumar Perumal*
INTRODUCTION ................................................................................................... 133
    Hippo Pathway ................................................................................................. 134
    The Mammalian Hippo Pathway ....................................................................... 134
    Hippo Pathway in Cancer ................................................................................. 135
    Hippo Pathway in Liver Cancer ........................................................................ 136
    Association of Hippo and Tumor-Related Pathways .......................................... 136
        *Hippo and Wnt Pathway* ............................................................................ 136
        *Hippo and TGF-β Pathway* ........................................................................ 137
    Hippo and other Pathways ................................................................................ 138
    Role of Hippo Signaling in Liver Cancer Development ..................................... 138
    Role of Key Proteins in Regulating Hippo Pathway ......................................... 140
    Role of Mst1 in Liver Cancer ........................................................................... 141
    Effects of Targeting Mst1 Protein During Liver Carcinogenesis ....................... 141
    Role of YAP in Liver Cancer ............................................................................ 142
    Effect of Targeting Yap Protein During Liver Carcinogenesis .......................... 144
    Role of LATS 1/2 in Liver Cancer .................................................................... 144
    Effects of Targeting LATS1 and LATS2 Protein During Liver Carcinogenesis ............. 145
CONCLUSION ....................................................................................................... 146
REFERENCES ........................................................................................................ 147

**CHAPTER 8  IMMUNOTOXIN: A NEW GENERATION AGENT FOR CANCER TREATMENT** ................................................................................................ 156

*Subha Ranjan Das, Dibyendu Giri, Tamanna Roy, Surya Kanta Dey, Rumi Mahata Angsuman Das Chaudhuri, Suman Mondal* and *Sujata Maiti Choudhury*

INTRODUCTION ................................................................................................ 156

Mechanism of Action ................................................................................ 158

*Diptheria Toxin (DT)* ...................................................................... 158

*Pseudomonas Exotoxin A* ............................................................... 159

*Immunoconjugates for Cancer Therapy* ......................................... 159

*Antibody-drug Conjugates* .............................................................. 160

*Radioimmunoconjugates (RICs)* ..................................................... 162

*The Antibody as a Targeting Moiety* .............................................. 163

Ligand as a Target and Cytokine Receptor as a Targeting Moiety ............ 164

Growth Factor Receptors as Targets ......................................................... 164

Targeting Antigens Associated with Tumors ............................................. 164

*The Antibody as a Targeting Moiety* .............................................. 165

*HER2 Specific Immunotoxins* ......................................................... 165

*Immunotoxins Against Hepatocellular Carcinoma (HCC)* ............. 169

*Immunotoxin Therapy for Lung Cancer* ......................................... 170

*Immunotoxins for Leukemia* ........................................................... 171

*Immunotoxins for Colorectal Cancer Therapy* .............................. 171

*Immunotoxin Therapy of Glioblastoma* ......................................... 173

CONCLUSION ................................................................................................... 174

REFERENCES ................................................................................................... 175

**CHAPTER 9  MULTIFACTORIAL DRUG - A REVOLUTION IN THE TREATMENT OF CANCER BY INHIBITING HEDGEHOG PATHWAY** ............................................. 184

*M. Santosh Kumar, Poornima D. Vijendra, Pratap G. Kenchappa* and *A. Gowtami*

INTRODUCTION ................................................................................................ 185

CANCER AND Hh PATHWAY ......................................................................... 186

HEDGEHOG SIGNALING AND HUMAN DISEASES ................................... 188

Type I- Ligand-Independent Hedgehog Signaling .................................... 190

Type II- Ligand-Dependent Autocrine/Juxtacrine Signalling ................... 190

Type IIIa/b: Ligand-Dependent Hh Signaling in Paracrine Manner ......... 191

HH SIGNALING PATHWAY TARGETS AND MULTIFACTORIAL DRUGS ..... 191

Inhibitors of Hedgehog Pathway .............................................................. 195

CONCLUSION ................................................................................................... 197

REFERENCES ................................................................................................... 197

**CHAPTER 10  PROMISING NATURAL AGENTS FOR TARGETING MICRO-RNAS IN CANCER** ........................................................................................................... 201

*Rumi Mahata, Subhabrata Das, Suman Mondal, Surya Kanta Dey, Anirban Majumder* and *Sujata Maiti Choudhury*

INTRODUCTION ................................................................................................ 201

miRNA Synthesis ...................................................................................... 203

MicroRNA (miRNAs) in the Development of Tumorigenesis and Carcinogenesis ............. 203

Modulation of miRNA Expression in Cancer Using Phytocompounds ...... 205

Resveratrol ................................................................................................ 206

Berberine ................................................................................................... 207

Indole-3-Carbinol (I3C) ............................................................................ 208

Quercetin ................................................................................................... 208

    Epigallocatechin-3-Gallate (EGCG) ................................................................... 209
    Curcumin ................................................................................................... 209
    Genistein ................................................................................................... 210
    Paclitaxel ................................................................................................... 211
    Betulinic Acid (BA) ................................................................................... 212
    Cucurbitacin B ........................................................................................... 213
    Oleanolic Acid ........................................................................................... 213
    Camptothecin ............................................................................................. 214
    Vincristine ................................................................................................. 214
  **CONCLUSION** .................................................................................................. 214
  **LIST OF ABBREVIATIONS** ............................................................................. 215
  **REFERENCES** ................................................................................................... 216

**CHAPTER 11 UNDERSTANDING THE MECHANISM OF TARGETED THERAPY- THE NEXT GENERATION FOR CANCER TREATMENT** ............................................... 223
*K.R. Padma, K.R. Don* and *P. Josthna*
  **INTRODUCTION** ............................................................................................. 224
  **ROLE OF NATURAL PRODUCTS IN CHEMOTHERAPY** ............................. 224
  **NEW CANCER THERAPIES BASED ON BIO-TARGETS** .............................. 226
  **UNDERSTANDING THE MECHANISM OF REPURPOSED DRUGS IN THE TREATMENT OF CANCER** ............................................................................... 229
  **IMMUNOGENICITY OF MONOCLONAL ANTIBODIES** ............................. 231
  **CUTTING-EDGE IN CANCER THERAPY** ..................................................... 232
  **CONCLUSION** .................................................................................................. 232
  **CONTRIBUTIONS** ............................................................................................ 232
  **REFERENCES** ................................................................................................... 233

**CHAPTER 12 CELL DEATH APOPTOTIC PATHWAYS AND TARGETED THERAPEUTIC RESEARCH IN CANCER** ................................................................. 238
*Jutishna Bora, Richismita Hazra* and *Sumira Malik*
  **INTRODUCTION** ............................................................................................. 238
  **MECHANISM OF CELL DEATH** .................................................................... 241
  **APOPTOSIS AND CANCER** ............................................................................ 242
  **APOPTOSIS AND CANCER THERAPY** ......................................................... 243
  **PLANT-DERIVED COMPOUNDS EXHIBITING ANTI-CANCEROUS ACTIVITY** ......... 243
  **CONCLUSION** .................................................................................................. 247
  **ACKNOWLEDGEMENTS** ................................................................................ 247
  **REFERENCES** ................................................................................................... 247

**CHAPTER 13 APOPTOSIS DEFECTS IN CANCER AND ITS THERAPEUTIC IMPLICATIONS** ..................................................................................................... 253
*Jutishna Bora, Sayak Banerjee, Indrani Barman, Sarvesh Rustagi, Richa Mishra* and *Sumira Malik*
  **INTRODUCTION** ............................................................................................. 254
  **APOPTOTIC DEFECTS AND CANCER** ......................................................... 254
    Defects in Caspase Signaling .................................................................... 254
    Defects in Intrinsic Pathways .................................................................... 255
    Defects in Extrinsic Pathways ................................................................... 256
  **POTENTIAL LIMITED ROLE OF APOPTOTIC CELL DEATH** .................... 257
  **TARGETED THERAPIES AND CANCER** ...................................................... 259
    Targeting Anti-apoptotic Bcl-2 Family Members ..................................... 259
    Mcl-1 Inhibitors ........................................................................................ 259

　　　XIAP Inhibitors ........................................................................................ 260
　　　Caspase Activators in Cancer Therapy ..................................................... 260
**CONCLUSION** .......................................................................................... 260
**ACKNOWLEDGEMENTS** ......................................................................... 261
**REFERENCES** .......................................................................................... 261

**SUBJECT INDEX** ................................................................................. 266

# PREFACE

The development of a population of cells that can invade tissues and spread to distant sites, resulting in significant morbidity, is what is known as cancer. Cancer is an abnormal growth of cells brought on by multiple changes in the gene expression, which result in a dysregulated balance of cell proliferation and cell death. A group of illnesses affecting higher multicellular organisms include cancer. The capacities to invade locally, disseminate to nearby lymph nodes, and metastasize to distant organs in the body distinguish malignant cancer from benign tumors. The acquisition of multidrug resistance and relapse pose the biggest challenge in the development of anticancer drugs. Traditional cancer treatments directly affect the DNA of the cell, but modern anticancer medications use molecularly focused therapy, such as focusing on proteins that have an aberrant expression in cancer cells. Conventional methods for completely eliminating cancer cells were found to be ineffective. Although targeted chemotherapy has been beneficial in treating some cancers, its efficacy has frequently been constrained by drug resistance and adverse effects on healthy tissues and cells. The aberrant tumor signaling, however, involves pathways for phosphoinositide 3-kinase (PI3K)/Akt, mammalian target of rapamycin (mTOR), Wnt/-catenin, mitogen-activated protein kinase (MAPK), signal transducer and activator of transcription 3 (STAT3), and notch signaling. Targeted chemotherapy has been beneficial in some cases of cancer, but its efficacy has frequently been constrained by drug resistance and adverse effects on healthy tissues and cells. On the other hand, the majority of researchers are interested in the promising field of immunotherapy. Targeting cancer stem cells and microRNAs generally play a vital role in cancer medication development together with aberrant tumor signaling pathways. The main cause of medication resistance and tumor recurrence is recognized to be cancer stem cells. MicroRNAs are brief non-coding molecules that are 20-22 nucleotides long. It has the propensity to control a number of important signaling pathways that encourage cancer. Therefore, the current book discusses several of these important anticancer targets, such as cancer stem cells, microRNAs, (PI3K)/Akt, mTOR, Wnt/-Catenin, MAPK, STAT3, and notch signaling pathways. Additionally, numerous clinical trial phases for promising natural and synthetic medication candidates are outlined.

**Ashok Kumar Pandurangan**
School of Life Sciences
B.S. Abdur Rahman Crescent Institute of Science and Technology
Chennai-600048, India

# List of Contributors

**Anbarasu Kannan**
Department of Biochemistry, CSIR-Central Food Technological Research Institute, Mysuru-570020, India
Academy of Scientific and Innovative Research (AcSIR), Ghaziabad-201002, India

**Ashok Kumar Pandurangan**
School of Life Sciences, B.S. Abdur Rahman Crescent Institute of Science and Technology, Seethakathi Estate, GST road, Vandalur-600048, Chennai, Tamil Nadu, India

**Annapoorna Bangalore Ramachandra**
Department of Biochemistry, CSIR-Central Food Technological Research Institute, Mysuru-570020, India
Academy of Scientific and Innovative Research (AcSIR), Ghaziabad-201002, India

**Angsuman Das Chaudhuri**
Department of Human Physiology, Vidyasagar University, Midnapore 721102, West Bengal, Pin-721102, India

**A. Gowtami**
Department of Studies in Biochemistry, Davangere University Shivagangothri, Davangere-577007, Karnataka, India

**Anirban Majumder**
Biochemistry, Molecular Endocrinology and Reproductive Physiology Laboratory, Department of Human Physiology, Vidyasagar University, Midnapore, West Bengal, Pin-721102, India

**Bhoomika M. Patel**
National Forensic Science University, Gujarat, India

**Chandra Kishore**
Department of Pulmonary, Critical Care and Sleep Medicine, Icahn School of Medicine at Mount Sinai, New York, USA

**Dibyendu Giri**
Department of Human Physiology, Vidyasagar University, Midnapore 721102, West Bengal, Pin-721102, India

**Hariprasth Lakshmanan**
Department of Biochemistry, School of Life Sciences - Ooty Campus, JSS Academy of Higher Education and Research, Mysuru, Karnataka, India

**Indrani Barman**
Program of Biotechnology, Faculty of Science, Assam Down Town University, Guwahati, Assam, India

**Jutishna Bora**
Amity Institute of Biotechnology, Amity University, Jharkhand, Ranchi, Jharkhand-834002, India

**Kaumudi Pande**
Department of Biochemistry, CSIR-Central Food Technological Research Institute, Mysuru-570020, India
Academy of Scientific and Innovative Research (AcSIR), Ghaziabad-201002, India

**Krishna Prakash**
ICAR-Indian Agricultural Research Institute (IARI), Hazaribagh, Jharkhand, India

**Karthikeyan Chandrabose**
Department of Pharmacy, Indira Gandhi National Tribal University, Amarkantak, Madhya Pradesh, India

**K.R. Padma**
Department of Biotechnology, Sri Padmavati Mahila Visvavidyalayam (Women's University), Tirupati, AP, India

| | |
|---|---|
| **K.R. Don** | Department of Oral Pathology and Microbiology, Sree Balaji Dental College and Hospital, Bharath Institute of Higher Education and Research (BIHER) Bharath University, Chennai, Tamil Nadu, India |
| **Mit Joshi** | Institute of Pharmacy, Nirma University, Ahmedabad, India |
| **Madan Kumar Perumal** | Department of Biochemistry, CSIR-Central Food Technological Research Institute, Mysuru-570020, India<br>Academy of Scientific and Innovative Research (AcSIR), Ghaziabad-201002, India |
| **M. Santosh Kumar** | Department of Studies in Biochemistry, Davangere University Shivagangothri, Davangere-577007, Karnataka, India |
| **Naveen Kumar Perumal** | Department of Bio-Medical Sciences, School of Biosciences and Technology, Vellore Institute of Technology, Vellore-632014, Tamil Nadu, India |
| **Nivya Vijayan** | Department of Biochemistry, CSIR-Central Food Technological Research Institute, Mysuru-570020, India<br>Academy of Scientific and Innovative Research (AcSIR), Ghaziabad-201002, India |
| **PP Mubthasima** | Department of Biochemistry, CSIR-Central Food Technological Research Institute, Mysuru-570020, India<br>Academy of Scientific and Innovative Research (AcSIR), Ghaziabad-201002, India |
| **Prathibha Sivaprakasam** | School of Life Sciences, B.S. Abdur Rahman Crescent Institute of Science and Technology, Seethakathi Estate, GST road, Vandalur-600048, Chennai, Tamil Nadu, India |
| **Praveen Deepak** | PG Department of Zoology, Swami Sahajanand College, Jehanabad-804417, Bihar, India |
| **Poornima D. Vijendra** | Department of Studies in Biochemistry and Food Technology, Davangere University Shivagangothri, Davangere – 577007, Karnataka, India |
| **Pratap G. Kenchappa** | Department of Studies in Biochemistry, Davangere University Shivagangothri, Davangere-577007, Karnataka, India |
| **P. Josthna** | Department of Biotechnology, Sri Padmavati Mahila Visvavidyalayam (Women's University), Tirupati, AP, India |
| **Richismita Hazra** | Amity Institute of Biotechnology, Amity University Kolkata, Kolkata, West Bengal-700135, India |
| **Rajalakshmi Prakash** | Department of Biochemistry, CSIR-Central Food Technological Research Institute, Mysuru-570020, India<br>Academy of Scientific and Innovative Research (AcSIR), Ghaziabad-201002, India |
| **Rumi Mahata** | Department of Human Physiology, Vidyasagar University, Midnapore 721102, West Bengal, Pin-721102, India |
| **Richa Mishra** | Department of Computer Engineering, Parul University, Ta. Waghodia, Vadodara, Gujarat, 391760, India |
| **Sureshkumar Anandasadagopan** | Department of Biochemistry and Biotechnology Lab, CSIR-Central Leather Research Institute (CLRI), Adyar, Chennai, India |

**Subha Ranjan Das** Department of Human Physiology, Vidyasagar University, Midnapore 721102, West Bengal, Pin-721102, India

**Surya Kanta Dey** Department of Human Physiology, Vidyasagar University, Midnapore 721102, West Bengal, Pin-721102, India

**Suman Mondal** Department of Human Physiology, Vidyasagar University, Midnapore 721102, West Bengal, Pin-721102, India

**Sujata Maiti Choudhury** Department of Human Physiology, Vidyasagar University, Midnapore 721102, West Bengal, Pin-721102, India

**Subhabrata Das** Biochemistry, Molecular Endocrinology and Reproductive Physiology Laboratory, Department of Human Physiology, Vidyasagar University, Midnapore, West Bengal, Pin-721102, India

**Sayak Banerjee** Amity Institute of Biotechnology, Amity University Kolkata, Kolkata, West Bengal-700135, India

**Sarvesh Rustagi** School of Applied and Life Sciences, Uttaranchal University, Dehradun, 248007 Uttarakhand, India

**Sumira Malik** Amity Institute of Biotechnology, Amity University, Jharkhand, Ranchi, Jharkhand-834002, India

**Tamanna Roy** Department of Human Physiology, Vidyasagar University, Midnapore 721102, West Bengal, Pin-721102, India

**Vaishali Ji** Department of Botany, Patna Science College, Patna, Bihar, India

**Vasudevan Sekar** Department of Biochemistry, CSIR-Central Food Technological Research Institute, Mysuru-570020, India

**Vani Vijay** Department of Biochemistry, CSIR-Central Food Technological Research Institute, Mysuru-570020, India
Academy of Scientific and Innovative Research (AcSIR), Ghaziabad-201002, India

**Venkat Prashanth** Department of Biochemistry, CSIR-Central Food Technological Research Institute, Mysuru-570020, India
Academy of Scientific and Innovative Research (AcSIR), Ghaziabad-201002, India

CHAPTER 1

# Exosomal Delivery of CRISPR/CAS9 Assembly: Approach towards Cancer Therapeutics

**Kaumudi Pande[1,2,#], PP Mubthasima[1,2,#], Rajalakshmi Prakash[1,2,#]** and **Anbarasu Kannan[1,2,*]**

[1] *Department of Biochemistry, CSIR-Central Food Technological Research Institute, Mysuru-570020, India*

[2] *Academy of Scientific and Innovative Research (AcSIR), Ghaziabad-201002, India*

**Abstract:** Exorbitant cancer malignancy is at the helm of multiple organ malfunction in humans and is considered a cause of increased cancer mortality worldwide. Clustered regularly interspaced short palindromic repeats (CRISPR) are powerful machinery for the therapeutic approach to tumors because of their substantial peculiarity, focusing on modulatory molecules, both oncogenes and tumor suppressors, to preclude tumor metastasis and enable apoptosis. Exosomes are considered an ideal delivery system because of their specificity and ability to prevent premature release of cargo. Exosomes are accessed as an effective conveyance of CRISPR/Cas9 elements and other attractive biomolecules to recipient cancer cells. The CRISPR/Cas9 loaded exosomes are endocytosed for further alteration of cellular metabolic pathways, either by knock-in or knock-out of the designed destined gene using sgRNA and Cas9 protein. The current study provides a platform to address the alliance between the CRISPR/Cas9 model and exosomes, depicting a remarkable therapeutic approach against cancer and other fatal diseases.

**Keywords:** CRISPR Clustered regularly interspaced short palindromic repeats, Cas - CRISPR-associated protein, CrRNA - CRISPR RNA, EMT - Epithelial to mesenchymal transition, gRNA - Guide RNA, MHC - Major histocompatibility complex, TracrRNA - trans-activating CRISPR RNA.

## INTRODUCTION

Cancer can be defined as the ungoverned multiplication of cells that propagate far and wide through discrete organs. The unbeatable accumulation of aggressive

* **Corresponding author Anbarasu Kannan:** Department of Biochemistry, CSIR-Central Food Technological Research Institute, Mysuru-570020, India and Academy of Scientific and Innovative Research (AcSIR), Ghaziabad-201002, India; Tel: +91-8870795252; E-mail: anbarasu@cftri.res.in
# Contributed equally

**Ashok Kumar Pandurangan (Ed.)**

cells creates an aching mass called "Tumor" that is benign in the preliminary phase, however, it undergoes extension in later phases. The characteristics of cancer cells include evasion of cell cycle regulatory checkpoints, chromosomal aberrations leading to a gain of function of specific oncogenes influencing conventional splitting of cells, subjugation of tumor suppressors by mutation or its related molecules, blocking of the body's immune system and its regular functions, prevention of caspase-mediated cell death, acquisition of mesenchymal cellular attributes, and blood vessel organization.

As reported by GLOBOCAN 2020, there are 19.3 million unprecedented cases of cancer with a survival rate of 9.3 million for the early detection of the disease [1]. The understanding of the occurrence of cancer can be extrinsic components, for instance, consumption of excessive nicotine present in cigarettes [2], consumption promoting foodstuffs such as processed meat, alcohol, junk food, and drinks, exposure to deadly radiation [3], and viral infections [4, 5]. Intrinsic abiogenetic records increase vulnerability to tumorigenesis [6]. By employing diagnostic tools corresponding to national databases, doctors can reveal different stages of cancer and advance further. The tumor of stage 0 is benign and exists at the place of its origin, and its early recognition can be remediable by eliminating the tumor through surgery. Stage I tumor is a minor protuberance that is settled at one site and neither augmented intensively in adjacent tissues nor stretched in another place towards lymph nodes. Stages II and III are regarded as the initiation of the migratory ability of cancer cells within easy-to-reach tissues along with lymph nodes. Treatment options for stages I-III include surgery, chemotherapy, and radiation therapy. Stage IV exhibits a highly precarious patient condition with a weakly favorable medicament since the tumor circulated rapidly to distant organs and recommended Targeted Immunotherapy in addition to the mentioned ones.

Cancer examinations can be performed through imaging trials, Endoscopy, Bioscopy, and discrete body fluid tests. Cancer metastasis is related to the expansion of unregulated cells that disrupt their prevailing morphology and attain locomotion efficiency in various parts of the human body (Fig. **1**). These metastatic cells breached the epithelial tissue lining and entered the biological fluids, such as blood, milk, saliva, semen, vaginal fluid, and urine, and further interfaced with healthy cells for their transition into tumor cells. This evolution of genes favors the synthesis of growth-promoting proteins, whereas it obstructs programmed cell death molecules [7]. Portments of metastatic carcinoma include pain, vomiting, body weight reduction, exhaustion, feverishness, infrequent excretion, and hemorrhage [8]. Therapeutic options for cancer that are currently used worldwide include chemotherapy, radiation therapy, and surgical removal of solid tumors coupled with either one of the aforementioned therapies. Targeted therapeutic interventions are of prime focus these days in order to avoid any cytotoxicity exerted by chemotherapy on adjacent normal cells.

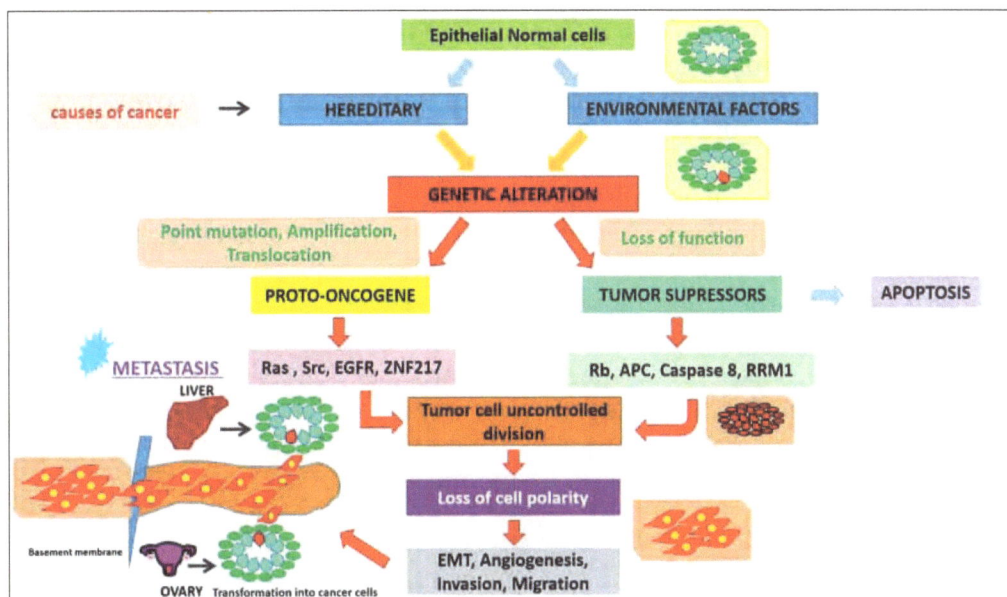

**Fig. (1).** Cancer metastasis.

Exosomes are nanovesicles of approximately 30-150 nm liberated by all types of living cells under natural as well as pathological conditions. The breakthrough in the discipline of extracellular vesicles emerged in the year 1983 searched out in Reticulocytes for endocytosis of iron [9] and it is composed of transferrin receptors, sphingomyelin, amino acid and glucose transporters liberated apart from the cell, therefore, designated as "Exosomes" [10]. Exosomes are produced by cellular machinery and further move out and mobilize in the extracellular space, interacting with other cells for the purpose of conveying specific molecules, consequently influencing the cellular metabolism of recipient cells. They are an exemplary means of proteins (CD63, CD81/82, Alix, TSG101, Rab) [11], nucleic acid family [12], and fatty acids (ATP-binding cassette transporter A1, low-density lipoprotein receptor, low-density lipoprotein receptor) [13], which are involved in immune response, modulate the tumor microenvironment, cancer infiltration, and evade cell death. Further studies have demonstrated that exosomes serve as clusters of biomarkers for the preliminary identification of malignancy.

Exosomes perform their function in cancer therapeutics by impeding the activity of constitutively expressed growth-promoting genes at former neoplastic spots, controlling their cellular habitat, and preventing affinity to different organs and tissues. Exosomes obtained from natural sources, such as milk- or plant-derived exosomes, have many qualities that can assist in directing **man-made therapeutic medicines [14].** Macrophage-derived exosomes are effective in reducing the number of tumor cells. Exosomes carry the Major Histocompatibility Complex and Heat shock proteins, which generate innate and adaptive immunity in recipient cells. Thus, exosomes can be employed in novel cancer therapies to destroy tumor cells [15].

CRISPR/Cas system is an adaptive immune system in bacteria. Single-guide RNA (gRNA) and CRISPR-associated endonucleases (Cas) are the main components of the CRISPR/Cas system. Cas9 is an endonuclease that functions as a pair of molecular scissors to cleave the target DNA sequence. Single-guide RNA is the combination of tracrRNA and crRNA. crRNA contains two main parts: a region that binds to tracrRNA and a spacer sequence that directs the complex to the target DNA. When tracrRNA binds to a crRNA, a functional guide RNA is formed for Cas9 recognition. Multiple crRNAs can be incorporated into a crRNA array and then packaged with tracrRNA to form sgRNA [16].

**There were no sources of data in the current study.** Systems use different RNP complexes and further distinguish themselves by the presence of a specific "signature protein" responsible for DNA degradation, namely, Cas3, Cas9, and Cas10 for types I, II, and III, respectively [17]. CRISPR triggers DNA repair by creating a double-strand break in the DNA. This break results in two types of genome modifications: knock-ins (KI) through homologous recombination and constitutive knockout (KO) through non-homologous end-joining [18].

CRISPR/Cas9 system is used in various applications, including genome editing, screening, chromatin immunoprecipitation, transcriptional activation and repression, epigenetic editing with live imaging of DNA/mRNA, and therapeutic applications [19]. Simplicity and high efficiency are the main advantages of the CRISPR/Cas9 system over other gene-editing systems. The main disadvantage of the CRISPR system is its off-target effects [20]. In this chapter, we discuss the role of the CRISPR/Cas9 system in cancer therapeutics and exosomes as a potential delivery system for CRISPR.

## CRISPR AS A POTENTIAL THERAPEUTIC AGENT FOR METASTASIS

### Molecules Involved in Metastasis

The expanded knowledge associated with the anomalous evolution of growth-promoting molecules has enabled the identification of novel indicators for cancer metastasis (Table 1). The hallmarks of tumor malignancy include disruption of DNA integrity by depletion of the tumor suppressor phosphoprotein p53 due to mutations in the coding region (2–11) in high-grade pelvic serous carcinoma [21]. The overexpression of mouse double minute 2 homolog (MDM2) in ductal carcinoma causes nuclear interaction with p53, leading to its aggregation, and has been reported as an additional channel for cancer development [22]. The establishment of cancer metastasis implicated the genesis of fresh blood vessels at the metastatic niche to obtain nourishment from the primitive veins. Angiogenesis encouraging C–C chemokine ligand 2 is a marker for advanced-stage breast cancer by causing the admission of C-C chemokine receptor type 2, resulting in inflammation and high vesicular compactness. The role of interleukin 6 in the initiation of angiogenesis is boosted by C–C chemokine ligand 2, which has a lower number of cancer victims [23]. The δ-catenin enciphered by the CTNND2 gene on chromosome 5 is involved in the attachment of cells to adjacent cells, and its expression increases in prostate cancer for the renewal of cell division by influencing cyclin D1 and phosphorylation of Histone3, therefore, maintaining cell viability. Its participation in lowering epithelial molecule E-cadherin results in the loss of surface attachment and cell migration *in vitro* and a two-fold increase in tumor measurement in mice depicting gene sequence modification at the 5' untranslated site in δ-catenin, enabling rapid growth of tumor cells [24].

**Table 1. Metastatic cancer molecules focused by CRISPR/Cas9 system.**

| Sl. No | Molecules | Type of Cancer | Metastatic Function | Role of CRISPR | References |
|---|---|---|---|---|---|
| 1 | Mutant p53 | Breast cancer | Interact with MDM2 and alter p53 towards cancer growth | Allow G1/S cell cycle arrest, restrict ZEB1, SLUG and TWIST1 | [22, 42] |
| 2 | δ-Catenin | Prostate cancer, Lung cancer | Stimulates cyclin D cell cycle progression, mutation G>A mutation at 5'-UTR of δ-Catenin impacts Wnt signalling. | Knockdown of CTNND2 gene prevents assemblage of β-catenin. | [24, 39] |
| 3 | Focal adhesion kinase | Non-small cell lung cancer | Overexpression in patients' tissue section, elevates cancer cell viability. | Inhibits the rate of proliferation, growth arrest, rescue cell cycle checkpoints. | [26, 41] |
| 4 | WAVE3 | Breast cancer | Maintain cancer stem cell microhabitat, EMT | Suppresses cancer cell motility and PI3K, TGF-β, and EGF signaling. | [44, 45] |
| 5 | CD133 | Colon cancer | Actuate AKT, β-catenin and NFkB molecules for commencement of tumorigenesis | Counteracts cell viability and migration by depletion of vimentin and survivin expression. | [36, 40] |

*(Table 1) cont.....*

| Sl. No | Molecules | Type of Cancer | Metastatic Function | Role of CRISPR | References |
|---|---|---|---|---|---|
| 6 | PTGS2 | Melanoma | Lymph node metastasis | Represses cell multiplication, colony formation and cell invasion. | [32, 43] |

PTK2 protein tyrosine kinase 2 (FAK) is a cytoplasmic protein that is confined to focal adhesions and undergoes phosphorylation at the tyrosine 397 region for its activation in response to growth factors and unclasps from the NH2-terminal Protein4.1-ezrin-radixin-moesin (FERM) domain for interaction with Phosphoinositide-3-Kinase Regulatory Subunit 2 to instigate AKT inclined towards multiple intracellular oncogenic pathways. Further studies have shown that nearly 92% of small-cell lung cancer tissue sections express FAK at varied intensities, and FAK mRNA is expressed in 23% of lung carcinomas [25]. The intervention of FAK in metastatic cascade was found to be examined in 38.6% of Nonsmall cell lung cancers with greater immune-reactivity in lymph nodal tissue specimens and 18% of 5-year life expectancy, subsequently accelerating cancer metastasis [26].

Wiskott-Aldrich syndrome verprolin-homologous 3 (WAVE3) is an actin cytoskeleton restructuring protein formed by gene sequence present on chromosome 13 of q arm region 12, comprised of 502-amino acids polypeptide sequence [27]. WAVE3 combines with the Arp2/3 complex for actin polymerization for cell mobility and has three times greater expression at the final stages of breast cancer. Conquering the farther body organs, for instance, the lungs by MDA-MB-231 adenocarcinoma cells, WAVE3 encourages tumor initiation in the lungs; however, the infusion of MDA-MB-231 cells with inactivated WAVE3 leads to the severe immunodeficient mice detected with a lower rate of cancer metastatic cells, thereby, inert WAVE3 declines the migratory potential of cancerous cells [28]. Surprisingly, we found that WAVE3 was immensely present in the metastatic grade of prostate cancer cells, mainly in the cytoplasmic compartment, and its silencing prevented the disruption of basement membrane curbing invasion [29].

Prostaglandin-endoperoxide synthase-2 (PTGS2) is an inflammatory agent of 70 kDa molecular weight that catalyzes the processing of arachidonic acid into prostaglandin H2. Recent studies have suggested that PTGS2 escalates Prostaglandin E2, fostering malignancies in a variety of cancer types, particularly colorectal, breast, head, and neck cancer [30], prostate cancer [31], and melanoma [32]. The crucial activity of PGE2 enables Src in the presence of cytosolic β-arrestin to stimulate the epidermal growth factor receptor to phosphorylate AKT on Serine -473 residue to trigger the PI 3-kinase/AKT mechanism in colorectal cancer [33].

Cyclooxygenase (COX-2) emerged as a predicted marker for breast cancer, ascertained mostly in post-menopause advanced stage in 83 patients and exhibiting lymph node metastasis in 92.6% of COX-2 positive patients, influenced by the RAS-MAPK schematic approach [34]. Prominin-1 (CD133) located in chromosome 4 is a glycoprotein often overexpressed in brain cancer confirmed by the histological glioma sections in the second and third grades [35]. CD133 is sufficient for the automatic regeneration of cancer stem cells, facilitating tumor initiation in ovarian and colon cancers. Its multipurpose regulation of cell proliferation molecules boosts cancer metastasis, notably observed in Wnt signaling engaged in the complex formation of C133 with β-catenin and NF-κB signalling influenced by CD133 in epithelial to mesenchymal transition (EMT), further advancing cancer metastasis [36].

Matrix metallopeptidase 9 (MMP-9) is a proteolytic enzyme that provides cell mobility by deteriorating the extracellular matrix, attaining mesenchymal characteristics in tumor cells. The prevalence of metastasis in the brain (p=0.0062) was reported to be evoked by breast carcinoma cells in the presence of MMP-9 in the serum, which describes colonization in other organs [37]. The fraction of MMP-9/MMP-2 in serum samples of hepatocellular carcinoma cases also increased significantly with respect to further staging of cancer [38]. Numerous tumor accretion molecules contribute to genetic modification, and cellular transformation, surpass physical barriers, diffuse in body fluids, and invade different body parts; therefore, there is a requirement for an effective technique that specifically targets oncogenes to stop cancer metastasis.

**Metastatic Molecules Targeted by CRISPR/Cas9 System**

CRISPR/Cas9 is a promising gene editing tool. CRISPR can precisely edit genes in both model organisms and humans and can act as a potential agent in cancer therapeutics. Metastasis is an important issue in cancer treatment. Targeting metastatic molecules using the CRISPR/Cas9 system can be used as a novel therapeutic agent in cancer treatment (Table **1**).

Several oncogenes that are modulated using CRISPR are discussed here; δ-catenin is overexpressed in many cancers, including prostate, breast, lung, and ovarian cancers. It acts as an oncogene that promotes the malignancy of lung adenocarcinoma. In lung adenocarcinoma, β-catenin enhances invasion and colonization *via* maintenance of cancer stem cells. δ-Catenin is encoded by the CTNND2 gene, the knockdown of which in an animal model by the CRISPR/Cas9 system leads to the loss of tumorigenicity and metastatic ability

[39]. Another study focused on CD133 as a stem cell marker and revealed that CD133 plays an essential role in the invasion and proliferation of colon cancer cells. Knockout of CD133 encoding gene using the CRISPR/Cas9 system in colon cancer has remarkable inhibitory effects on cell migration and invasion. In addition, CD133 knockout cells show decreased expression of the EMT marker vimentin [40].

Yet another molecule, Focal adhesion kinase (FAK) is a non-receptor tyrosine kinase that integrates mitogenic signaling, cell survival, and cytoskeleton remodeling. FAK1 localizes to nuclease during cell migration. Ablation of FAK by CRISPR/ Cas9 editing results in susceptibility to ionizing radiation, impaired oxidative phosphorylation, and basal DNA damage [41].

In addition to oncogenes, tumor suppressor genes such as p53 are mutated in many cancers. They respond to many cellular stressors, including DNA damage, hypoxia, oncogene activation, and reactive oxygen species (ROS). Upon activation, this leads to cell cycle arrest to restore genetic integrity, apoptosis, senescence, or ferroptosis to eliminate unrecoverable cells. Mutations in p53 facilitate cancer progression by accelerating cell proliferation, promoting cancer metastasis, inducing chemoresistance and radio resistance, and facilitating a pro-oncogenic tumor microenvironment. The use of CRISPR/Cas9 gene editing machinery will replace the mutant p53 gene with a functional gene that restores the normal functioning of p53. CRISPR/Cas9 can also be employed in a p53 genetic sensor system, which precisely and efficiently kills p53-deficient cancer cells [42].

Prostaglandin-end peroxide synthase 2 (PTGS2) plays an essential role in melanoma development and progression. PTGS2 is frequently expressed in malignant melanoma. Knockdown of PTGS2 using the CRISPR/Cas9 system in melanoma cells leads to inhibition of cancer cell migration, proliferation, and invasiveness. It also reduces tumor development and metastasis *in vivo* [43]. In addition to WAVE3, a member of the WASP/WAVE family of actin-cytoskeleton remodeling proteins plays a vital role in cancer cell invasion and migration in triple-negative breast cancer (TNBC). In addition, WAVE3 plays an essential role in cancer stem cell (CSC) maintenance and further leads to chemo resistance in cancer. Knockout of WAVE3 *via* CRISPR/Cas9 significantly attenuates CSC subpopulation and inhibits the transcription of CSC transcription factors [44]. Thus, CRISPR/Cas9 gene editing machinery can act as a potential cancer therapeutic agent to prevent cancer metastasis. The list of oncogenic molecules whose expression levels are modulated using CRISPR/Cas9 is depicted in Table **1**.

## EXOSOMES AS A POTENTIAL CARRIER (THERAPEUTIC CARRIER): EXOSOMES-BASED DELIVERY OF SMALL MOLECULES, BIOACTIVE MOLECULES, SIRNA

Exosomes are extracellular vesicles produced by all cell lines and play a vital role in intercellular communication. Exosomes are present in various body fluids, including blood, saliva, and urine. These are also present within the tissue matrix, known as matrix-bound nanovesicles (MBV). Exosomes originate in multivesicular bodies and are released into the extracellular space by the fusion of multivesicular bodies to the lipid bilayer [46]. Exosomes accommodate complex cargo, such as proteins, RNA, DNA, and lipids, and are delivered to specific target cells that reprogram the recipient cell. Exosome cargo can vary based on its origin. Exosomes represent the metabolic state of the cell line from which they get originated [47]. Exosomes deliver their cargo to recipient cells through receptor-ligand interactions, direct fusion of membranes, or internalization *via* endocytosis. Once internalized into the recipient cell, it fuses with the limiting membrane of the endosome, leading to horizontal genetic transfer by releasing cargo to the cytoplasmic space of the target cell [48]. Exosomes play an essential role in cancer progression. They carry pro-tumorigenic signals from cancerous cells and deliver them to non-cancerous cells, causing reprogramming of recipient cells [49].

Differential Centrifugation/Ultracentrifugation, chromatography, density gradient centrifugation, kit-based methods, and magnetic beads can be used to isolate exosomes from various sources [50]. The isolated exosomes were characterized by transmission electron microscopy (TEM), nano-sight, and western blotting [51]. Using TEM and Nano sight, the size of the exosome is estimated, and by using western blotting for exosome-specific markers such as CD9, CD81, and CD64, expression levels are estimated [52].

Numerous nano-based drug formulations have been developed to improve the therapeutic efficacy of molecular and chemical drugs (Table **2**). However, the cytotoxicity of materials and rapid clearance by the reticuloendothelial system (RES) or mononuclear phagocyte system (MPS) are major problems encountered in the clinical translation of these nano-based systems [53]. Exosomes have an advantage over other nano-based drug formulations owing to their natural biocompatibility. In addition, they have high stability, low immunogenicity, and a long circulation time. Some exosomes can even have a high capacity to escape from degradation or clearance by the immune system [54]. Exosomes of different origins have been used in cancer therapeutic applications. Cancer cell line-derived exosomes, normal cell line-derived exosomes, bovine milk-derived exosomes, and macrophage-derived exosomes are examples of the exosomes used in cancer therapeutics [14, 55 - 60]. Various plants and vegetables release exosome-like nanoparticles. They also contain lipids, proteins, and miRNAs, and because of their absence of toxicity and easy internalization by mammalian cells, they act as a good delivery system for cancer therapeutics. Plant-derived nanovesicles (PDNVs) can be used as effective delivery systems for small molecule agents and nucleic acids with therapeutic effects (siRNAs, miRNAs, and DNAs). Plant-derived nanovesicles alone have immunomodulatory, anti-inflammatory, and regenerative properties to treat liver diseases, inflammatory bowel disease (IBD), and cancer. PDNVs are stable in the gastrointestinal tract; therefore, drugs incorporated into PDNVs can be administered orally [61].

**Table 2. Various exosomes-based drug formulations for the delivery.**

| Sl.no | Type of Exosomes | Cargo/Drug | Method of Encapsulation | Efficacy of Modified Exosomes | References |
|---|---|---|---|---|---|
| 1 | Macrophage cell-derived exosomes | Paclitaxel | Sonication | Increase the drug delivery efficiency by 50 times compared to free drug. | [74] |
| 2 | EL4 cell-derived exosomes | Curcumin | Simple incubation | Increase curcumin's solubility and stability *in vitro* and bioavailability *in vivo*. | [55] |
| 3 | Bovine milk derived exosomes | Doxorubicin and Paclitaxel | Simple incubation | Increased tumor targetability compared to the free drug. | [14] |
| 4 | Mesenchymal cell derived exosomes | Doxorubicin | Electroporation | Higher tumor accumulation and faster liver clearance than free DOX. | [56] |
| 5 | HLF1 derived exosomes | Erastin | Sonication | EXO-erastin has a better inhibitory effect on proliferation and migration compared to free erastin. | [57] |
| 6 | Mouse immature dendritic cells (imDCs) derived exosomes tagged with Irgd | Doxorubicin | Electroporation | Highly efficient targeting and Dox delivery to αv integrin-positive breast cancer cells. | [58] |
| 7 | MDA-MB-231 derived exosomes | miRNA-126 | Kit method | Strongly suppressed A549 lung cancer cell proliferation and migration through the interruption of the PTEN/PI3K/AKT signaling pathway. | [59] |

*(Table 2) cont.....*

| Sl.no | Type of Exosomes | Cargo/Drug | Method of Encapsulation | Efficacy of Modified Exosomes | References |
|-------|------------------|------------|-------------------------|-------------------------------|------------|
| 8 | HEK293T derived exosomes | miRNA inhibitor oligonucleotide (miRNA 21i) and 5-FU | Electroporation | Reverse the chemoresistance in colon cancer cell. | [60] |
| 9 | iRGD tagged HEK293T cells derived exosomes | KRAS siRNA | Plasmid that simultaneously expressed KRAS siRNA and the Lamp2b protein in fusion with an iRGD peptide. | Potent tumor growth inhibition in a mouse model by intravenous administration. | [72] |
| 10 | HEK293T cell derived exosomes | TRPP2 siRNA | Electroporation | Inhibit EMT in FaDu cell | [73] |

Exosomes are modified to improve drug delivery by incorporating penetrating peptides such as iRGD, RGD, and RVG. These peptides are incorporated into exosomes in various ways. The plasmid contains an exosomal membrane protein Lamp2b gene fused with the targeting peptide RVG (rabies viral glycoprotein peptide) that has to be expressed in cells. The exosomes produced by the cell line have Lamp2b linked with RGV; RVG directs exosomes to organs that express the acetylcholine receptor [62]. Similarly, both iRGD- and RGD-tagged exosomes can be created [63, 64]. This penetrating peptide can be incorporated into the surface of exosomes by a chemical method, directly conjugating the peptide to the exosome surface using chemicals.

Therapeutic agents are incorporated into exosomes using both passive and active encapsulation methods. Passive encapsulation includes the incubation of the drug with exosomes or donor cells. Exosomes are incubated with the drug, and the drug moves passively based on its concentration gradient, hydrophobicity, and the efficiency of encapsulation changes [65]. The drug is incubated with donor cells to allow the incorporation of the drug into its derived exosomes, which is the principle behind the passive encapsulation method [66]. Active cargo loading includes sonication, extrusion, freeze-thaw cycles, electroporation, incubation with membrane permeabilizers, and the click chemistry method for direct conjugation. When the sonication mechanical shear force is compromised, the integrity of the membrane allows the diffusion of drugs through the membrane. Exosomes from donor cells were mixed with a drug using the extrusion method, and the mixture was loaded into a syringe-based lipid extruder with 100-400 nm porous membranes under controlled temperature. During extrusion, the exosome membrane is disrupted and vigorously mixed with the drug [67]. In the electroporation method, an electric field creates tiny pores in the exosome membrane, allowing drug diffusion through the membrane [68]. In the freeze-thaw method, the drug was incubated at room temperature and then kept at -80 °C, and the process was repeated for 3-4 cycles. This cycle increases the membrane permeability [69]. The use of permeabilizers, such as saponin, increases the permeability of the exosome membrane, allowing the diffusion of drugs through the membrane [70]. The drug can be directly conjugated to the surface of exosomes using the click chemistry method [71].

Several previously published studies have highlighted the incorporation of various bioactive molecules into exosomes of different origins. Paclitaxel is a potent chemotherapeutic agent incorporated into macrophage cell-derived exosomes *via* sonication that increases drug delivery efficiency by 50 times in drug-resistant MDCK-MDR1 (P-gp+) cells [12]. Curcumin is an anti-inflammatory molecule that can target inflammatory cell lines. Curcumin was incorporated into EL4 (mouse lymphoma cell line) exosomes by simple incubation and delivered to the cell line. Exosomes can increase the solubility and stability of curcumin *in vitro* and its bioavailability *in vivo*. It also increases the anti-inflammatory activity of curcumin by accumulating high levels of curcumin in cellular targets [55]. Bovine milk can act as a carrier for chemotherapeutic/chemopreventive agents and can serve as a scalable source of exosomes. Milk exosomes exhibited cross-species tolerance with no adverse immune or inflammatory responses. Doxorubicin and Paclitaxel are two different types of chemotherapeutic agents incorporated into bovine milk exosomes *via* simple incubation, which showed significantly higher efficacy than free drugs and increased tumor targetability [14]. Doxorubicin encapsulates in MCS (mesenchymal cell) derived exosomes *via* electroporation and delivers them to colorectal cancer, exhibiting higher tumor accumulation and faster liver clearance than free DOX. In addition, it showed increased inhibition of tumor growth [56]. Erastin is a ferroptosis (lipid peroxide-driven cell death caused by inhibition of the cystine/glutamate transporter) inducer; its low water solubility and renal toxicity have limited its application in therapeutics. Incorporating erastin into HLF1 cell-derived exosomes *via* sonication increases the uptake efficiency of erastin into MDA-MB-231 (breast cancer) cells compared with free erastin. EXO-erastin has a stronger inhibitory effect on proliferation and migration than free erastin [57]. Exosomes derived from mouse immature dendritic cells (imDCs) were engineered by incorporating iRGD peptides to increase the efficiency of drug delivery. iRGD peptides are specific to integrins; cells expressing integrin take up more exosomes and increase delivery efficiency. Doxorubicin is incorporated into iRGD-tagged exosomes, showing an increased inhibitory effect compared to imDC-derived exosomes [58].

Exosomes can also be used as delivery vehicles for miRNAs, to prevent cancer progression. miRNA-126 targets CXCR4 and suppresses its expression, thereby inhibiting tumor cell proliferation, migration, and invasion. miRNA-126 loaded in MDA-MB-231 exosomes (miRNA-231-Exo) and delivered to lung cancer cells strongly suppressed migration and cell proliferation through interruption of the PTEN/PI3K/AKT signaling pathway [59]. miRNA-21 induced resistance to 5-FU by downregulating human DNA MutS homolog 2 (hMSH2) in colorectal cancer. In combination therapy, miRNA inhibitor oligonucleotide (miRNA 21i) and 5-FU are incorporated into HEK293T (derived from the HEK 293 cell line)-derived exosomes *via* electroporation and delivered to colon cancer cells, which reverses chemoresistance [60]. siRNA has also been incorporated into exosomes for cancer therapy. KRAS siRNA inhibits KRAS miRNA translation. KRAS contained in iRGD-tagged exosomes derived from HEK293T cells increased the efficiency of siRNA delivery. Intravenous injection of KRAS siRNA encapsulated in iRGD-exosomes showed potent tumor growth inhibition in a mouse model [72]. Transient receptor potential polycystic 2 (TRPP2) enhances the metastasis and invasion of human laryngeal squamous cell carcinoma by regulating EMT. TRPP2 small interfering RNA (siRNA) was encapsulated in HEK293T cell-derived exosomes and delivered to FaDu cells (Pharynx Squamous Cell Carcinoma). TRPP2 small interfering RNA (siRNA) inhibits EMT in FaDu cells Also, EMT marker E-Cadherin expression level increased, and the level of vimentin and N-Cadherin decreased [73]. Thus, compared to other available conventional delivery systems, exosomes are an ideal drug delivery system for cancer therapeutics.

## GREAT BEGINNING OF THE CRISPR/CAS SYSTEM IN HUMAN TRIALS

The plethora of roles for CRISPR/Cas9 as a powerful remedy against critical diseases has been employed in clinical trials to examine its efficiency in humans. In the current year 2021, CRISPR/Cas9 has made a big opening for therapeutics applied to translational medicine. The therapies inclined on chronic urinary tract infections, cancers of the lung and blood, Leber congenital amaurosis eye disease, blood disorders such as sickle cell disease and beta-thalassemia and protein-folding disorders titled Hereditary transthyretin amyloidosis.

In the area of precise gene knockout technology for cancer treatment, CRISPR has been used as a competent tool for transforming T cells by introducing plasmid-enclosing guide RNA targeting programmed cell death protein 1 and Cas9 for lung cancer development. Programmed cell death protein 1 (PD-1) is a surface protein integrated into immune cells that restrain the usual functioning of the immune system by evading the inflammatory response and recognition of other foreign substances, thereby escaping normal cell death. Its Ligand (PD-L1) association is triggered by various molecular players and processes in the WNT, JAK/STAT, MAPK, and Hedgehog pathways involved in metastasis [75]. Transformed T cells are segregated from non-transformed cells, undergo multiplication, and are injected into non-small cell lung cancer patients in order to silence the PD-1 gene and succeed in the apoptosis of tumor cells [76]. The foremost attempt of CRISPR on human marker fixing of impaired tumor obstructing multiple genes (TCR α chain, TCR β chain, and PDCD1) related to refractory cancer. The affirmative results were obtained without any cytokine release ailment and nearly half of the abdominal size reduction, considering that CRISPR gene editing is a revolutionary process against several cancer models [77]. Therefore, the CRISPR/Cas system can be a crucial inhibitor of the metastatic cascade.

## DIFFERENT DELIVERY SYSTEMS FOR CRISPR/CAS

Achieving efficient delivery of the CRISPR/Cas9 system to its target is an essential step in gene editing. Therefore, the development of a novel delivery system with high efficiency, low immunogenicity, and cytotoxicity is critical for therapeutic applications. The off-target effects of the CRISPR System can lead to unwanted changes in the genome. The system must be properly entered into the target cell, and it can only perform more accurately and efficiently. For *in vivo* application of the CRISPR/Cas system, the elements of the CRISPR/Cas9 system should remain stable before reaching its target site and must be successfully taken up by the recipient cells and protected from endolysosomal degradation; subsequently, the CRISPR system must enter the nucleus to initiate gene editing. CRISPR/Cas9-based plasmids must travel through the cytosol to the nucleus for transcription. Therefore, using a proper delivery system is important to prevent unwanted side effects and improve safety at both the extracellular and intracellular levels [78].

CRISPR systems are delivered in three different forms: mRNA for Cas9 translation alongside a separate guide RNA, DNA plasmid encoding both the Cas9 protein and the guide RNA, and Cas9 protein with guide RNA (ribonucleoprotein complex). The delivery system must be chosen based on the volume of accommodation and the *in vivo*, *in vitro*, and *ex vivo* applications.

CRISPR/Cas9 delivery systems can be classified into non-viral vector systems and viral vectors (Table **3**). Viral vectors include adeno-associated viruses (AAVs), adenoviral vectors (AdV), lentiviral vectors (LV), and bacteriophages [79]. AVV are the most commonly used viral vectors because of their high titers, low immunogenicity, and low genomic integration rate. They are used in gene augmentation therapy for small genes in human clinical trials and gene editing in cells and animal models. The packaging capacity of the virus is 4.7 kb, so more than one vector is needed for delivery. In a dual virus, one AAV expresses Cas9, while the other expresses sgRNA and donor template DNA. In some cases, the gene will exceed 9 kb to solve this problem, and have developed a triple AAV approach [79, 80]. Adenoviruses are non-enveloped, double-stranded viruses with a genome range of 34–43 kb and two flanked ITR sequences. It transduces both dividing and nondividing cells. The genome remains extrachromosomal and does not integrate into the host genome. The latest generation of AdVs is an ideal delivery system for CRISPR/Cas9. The absence of the viral gene in the genome increases packaging capacity by up to 35 kb. This limits the potential off-target effects of the CRISPR/Cas9 system. They have a high transduction efficiency and low human symptoms. However, the viral capsid may still elicit acute-phase immune responses. AdV delivery using CRISPR/Cas9 has been used to establish disease models, develop tools for drug discovery, and treat existing diseases [79, 81].

**Table 3. List of delivery systems for CRISPR/Cas.**

| Sl. No | Strategies | Advantage | Limitation | References |
|---|---|---|---|---|
| 1 | AVV | low genomic integration rate. Low immunogenicity | limited packaging capacity | [79, 80] |
| 2 | AdV | High efficiency delivery | viral capsid might induce acute phase immune responses | [79, 81] |
| 3 | LV | Persistent gene transfer | Unwanted off-target effect | [79, 82] |
| 4 | Microinjection | Guaranteed delivery to the cells, reproducible, less toxic to the cell | Time consuming, need a skilled person, mainly used for *in vitro* | [78, 86] |
| 5 | Electroporation | Transfection efficiency is high | Nonspecific transfection, in some cell induce cell death | [78, 87] |
| 6 | Hydrodynamic delivery | Virus-free; low cost; ease | Traumatic to tissue | [78, 88] |
| 7 | Lipid nanoparticle | Low cost Virus free | Endosomal degradation of cargo | [78, 89] |
| 8 | Gold nanoparticle | Virus free | Nonspecific inflammatory response | [78, 90] |
| 9 | CCPs | Virus-free can deliver intact RNP | Variable penetrating capacity, Extensive optimization is required | [78, 91] |
| 10 | Itop | High efficiency, Virus free | Not preferable for *in vivo* | [83,97] |

The lentivirus (LV) is a single-stranded spherical RNA virus. They transduce both dividing and nondividing cells. They had a packaging capacity of 8 kb. They cause unwanted off-target effects when combined with CRISPR/Cas9. These are then integrated into the host genome. Because most labs cannot generate non-integrating LVs, LV vectors are used less often than AAVs and AdVs, and LVs are most commonly used to create disease models [79, 82]. LV vectors are deleted from all viral genes and do not activate the immune system. Insertional mutagenesis, carcinogenesis, and immunogenicity are the main concerns of viral delivery systems. In addition, the difficulty in large-scale production and the limited insertion size limit their further application. Viral vector-mediated delivery will remain in the system for 4-6 years and create many off-target effects. Cas9 is a bacterial (foreign) protein that induces an MHC-1-mediated immune response. Humans already have immunity against viruses and limit viral-mediated CRISPR delivery *in vivo* [83].

Non-viral delivery methods are on the rise because of the limitations of viral-based CRISPR delivery. A non-viral system does not persist in the host system for long. Compared to viral delivery systems, non-viral systems are less toxic and more efficient [84]. Non-viral delivery approaches can be further classified into physical and chemical-mediated delivery. Non-viral delivery systems face many obstacles. The first obstacle is the effective encapsulation of the editing tools into delivery vectors because of the large size and different charge properties of Cas9 protein, mRNA, and donor DNA. The second obstacle is the stability of this complex under physiological conditions. The third obstacle is the host immune response triggered by the elements of the CRISPR/Cas9 system, which is derived from bacteria, and the fourth obstacle is the insufficient accumulation of non-viral vector-mediated CRISPR/Cas9 systems in the targeted tissues. Cellular uptake is the next obstacle owing to the selective transmission of the hydrophobic and negatively charged plasma membrane. Endosomal and lysosomal degradation are also critical for efficient CRISPR/Cas9 delivery because of the acidic environment (pH 5.0–6.2) and hydrolases [85].

As previously mentioned, non-viral delivery can be classified into chemical and physical methods. The physical methods include microinjection, electroporation, and hydrodynamic delivery. In the microinjection method, nucleases and donor templates are directly delivered into cells by penetrating the cell membrane using glass microcapillaries with fine tips. This method requires a high level of sophistication and manual skills. This is a low-throughput process, but it is suitable for all types of CRISPR/Cas9 systems. This method is highly specific, reproducible, and less toxic to cells; however, it induces cell damage, limits their application, and is primarily used for *in vitro* and *ex vivo* applications and is not preferred for *in vivo* applications [78, 86].

Electroporation is an extensively used method for the delivery of nucleic acids and proteins to cell lines. During electroporation, membrane permeability increased. All types of CRISPR/Cas9 systems can be delivered by this method, and transfection efficiency is very high; however, it induces cell death and causes non-specific transfection. They are mostly used in *in vitro* and *ex vivo* applications and are not preferred for *in vivo* [78, 87]. Hydrodynamic delivery involves rapidly pushing a large-volume (8–10% body weight) solution containing the gene-editing cargo into an animal's bloodstream, preferably through the tail vein in mice. The hydrodynamic pressure created by the injection temporarily enhances the permeability of the endothelial and parenchymal cells, allowing the intake of the CRISPR/Cas9 system [78, 88].

Lipid nanoparticle-mediated, gold nanoparticle (AuNP)-mediated, cell-penetrating peptide-mediated, and iTOP-mediated delivery are examples of chemical delivery systems. The gold particle delivery system contains four components: a core gold nanoparticle, short DNA oligo donor, endosomal disrupter polymer, and CRISPR system. Short DNA Oligo's donor, which is conjugated to the core gold nanoparticle this DNA further complexed with the Cas9 RNP. The resulting complex was coated with the endosomal disrupter polymer PAsp (DET). Endosomal disrupter polymers promote endocytosis and disrupt endosomes. AuNPs are inert and do not trigger an immune response against the nanoparticles themselves. It has been used for *in vitro*, *in vivo,* and *ex vivo* applications. The entire Cas9: sgRNA RNP complex was delivered using this method [78, 89].

Lipid nanoparticles/liposomes were used to deliver both Cas9 and sgRNA genetic material (either plasmid DNA or mRNA) and Cas9: sgRNA RNP complexes. The method is suitable for *in vivo, ex vivo,* and *in vitro* studies, allowing extensive testing on various scales of cell populations. The absence of viral particles reduces immunogenicity and renders the delivery system safer for applications. Once the lipid nanoparticles cross the cell membrane, they are encased within the endosome and are more prone to degradation by lysosomal components. If it escapes degradation, it must translocate to the nuclease to perform gene editing; however, this method is less efficient [78, 90]. iTOP is a novel method for delivering native proteins and other compounds to cells. A hyperosmolar buffer containing sodium chloride and propanbetaine (a transduction compound) stimulates macropinocytosis, leading to the cellular uptake of cargo. This method was effective for Cas9 and sgRNA. They have Lower efficiency in primary cells than electroporation and microinjection, and are not suitable for *in vivo* applications [78, 91].

Cell-penetrating peptides (CPPs) are short stretches of amino acids that are polycationic, amphipathic, or non-polar. Different types of CCP are needed for the uptake of different types of proteins, and based on the CCP type, the efficiency of intake will vary. Extensive optimization of each cargo is required, so it is mainly used for *in vitro* and *ex vivo* delivery. They are less efficient, and once within the cell, the Cas9-sgRNA complex must translocate to the nuclease [78, 92]. Each delivery system has its advantages and disadvantages. The delivery system should be chosen based on its accommodation capacity and *in vivo*, *ex vivo*, and *in vitro* applications. Exosomes can be used as a delivery system for CRISPR/Cas, but they have not been explored extensively.

## EXOSOMAL-BASED DELIVERY FOR CRISPR

$NAD^+$ ADP-ribosyltransferase 1 (PARP-1) is a nuclear enzyme involved in cellular division and genomic maintenance. Poly (ADP-ribose) polymerase-1 performs bilateral responsibility for chromatin reorganization, telomeric preservation, and genome repair at one extreme. It also acts as an agent of redness, swelling, joint stiffness, pain, and itchiness with deleterious effects on immune cells in its incurable pattern. Stirring up of PARP-1 was observed as a warning indication of DNA impairment and reactive oxygen species stress; however, infection with Helicobacter pylori and Epstein–Barr virus causes genetic alteration in PARP-1, affecting the base excision repair mechanism, resulting in its upregulation in gastric histology sections and shortening the life span of patients [93]. PARP-1 regulates p53 at its C-terminal domain, allowing increased hypoxia-inducible factor α 1 to be involved in cancerous growth [94]. Enhanced PARP-1 expression was observed in triple-negative breast cancer based on microarray evaluation influenced by BRCA gene transformation in the majority of patients compared with healthy samples [95].

The superior therapeutic approach focuses on the subjugation of PARP-1 by CRISPR sgRNA-Cas9 encapsulated conveyance by exosomes inhibiting ovarian cancer. In xenograft BALB/ C nude mice implanted with SKOV3 ovarian adenocarcinoma cells, exosomes were electroporated with Cas9 and sgRNA, prohibiting a peculiar PARP-1 gene sequence, and were intravenously infused to enable frameshift alteration. The coalition of PARP-1 interrupted by CRISPR/Cas9-charged exosomes and platinum cisplatin resulted in an improved strategy for impeding an approximately 57% rapid increase in cancer cells and nearly 27.56% of cell death [96]. Hence, exosomes can be considered powerful vehicles carrying CRISPR elements to energize the apoptotic mechanism and eliminate neoplasms (Fig. **2**).

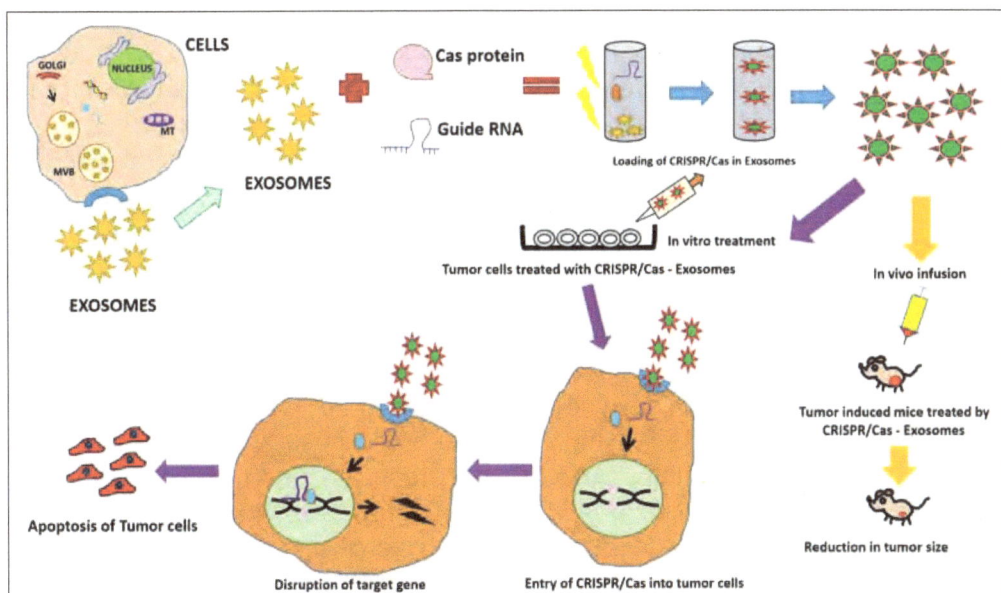

**Fig. (2).** Novel scheme for CRISPR/Cas9 delivery by means of Exosomes.

## CONCLUSION

Cancer is a dreadful disease, and constant therapeutic modalities are necessary to improve its treatment options. Exosomes are nano-vesicles of the measurement nearly 30-150 nm liberated by all kinds of living cells under natural as well as pathological conditions. We discuss the pros and cons of delivering CRISPR/Cas9 through the exosome system and their mechanism of action. It is evident that exosomal delivery of CRISPR/CAS9 assembly is key for treating cancer.

## FUTURE PERSPECTIVE

Cancer is a leading cause of mortality worldwide. Undesired mutations in human DNA cause uncontrolled cell proliferation, leading to cancer. Efficient therapeutic options for metastatic cancer are limited because they are detected at later stages. Metastasis is a complex process involving crosstalk between many molecules. Understanding the precise molecular mechanism occurring inside tumor cells, in other words, monitoring the expression of each oncogene and tumor suppressor biomolecule that undergoes genetic alteration and its resolution at the right interval in accordance with the stage of cancer, is extremely important.

Victory against cancer will be achieved by early detection of raised oncogenic biomarker expression in body fluids rather than a person waiting for the extreme symptoms to show up and attain his worst health condition. Many studies have demonstrated the treatment of cancer, but their survival rates remain low. For this reason, there is a necessity for splendid technology that strongly targets cancer cells to eliminate and prevent relapse. CRISPR-based therapy is a discussion theme that exercises Cas9 and guides RNA for the breakdown of target gene sequences in order to revive the immune system and promote cancer cell death. Thereafter, in order to obtain positive laboratory experimental results on CRISPR, the technology looks forward to more human trials focusing on efficient targeting of a particular gene without affecting other neighboring gene sequences (*i.e.*, with no side effects). The exosome dynamics confirmed its biocompatibility and weak immunogenicity for drug delivery, which can directly interact with target cells for effortless conveyance. The motive behind employing exosomes loaded with CRISPR/Cas9 is to help maintain their stability and allow their rapid incorporation into the host cell. The current paradigm of CRISPR/Cas9 delivered by exosomes targeting PARP-1 turned out to be promising in expediting tumor cell death and inhibiting malignancy. Hence, there is hope for the treatment of metastatic cancers by broadening the sphere of CRISPR/Cas9 technology in conjunction with exosomes to safeguard the lives of patients.

## REFERENCES

[1]   Sung H, Ferlay J, Siegel RL, *et al.* Global cancer statistics 2020: Globocan estimates of incidence and mortality worldwide for 36 cancers in 185 countries. CA Cancer J Clin 2021; 71(3): 209-49.
[http://dx.doi.org/10.3322/caac.21660] [PMID: 33538338]

[2]   Sanner T, Grimsrud TK. Nicotine: Carcinogenicity and effects on response to cancer treatment - a review. Front Oncol 2015; 5(Aug): 196.
[http://dx.doi.org/10.3389/fonc.2015.00196] [PMID: 26380225]

[3]   Gilbert ES. Ionising radiation and cancer risks: what have we learned from epidemiology? Int J Radiat Biol 2009; 85(6): 467-82.
[http://dx.doi.org/10.1080/09553000902883836] [PMID: 19401906]

[4]   Schiller JT, Lowy DR. Virus infection and human cancer: an overview. Recent Results Cancer Res 2014; 193: 1-10.
[http://dx.doi.org/10.1007/978-3-642-38965-8_1] [PMID: 24008290]

[5]   Blackadar CB. Historical review of the causes of cancer. World J Clin Oncol 2016; 7(1): 54-86.
[http://dx.doi.org/10.5306/wjco.v7.i1.54] [PMID: 26862491]

[6]   Garber JE, Offit K. Hereditary cancer predisposition syndromes. J Clin Oncol 2005; 23(2): 276-92.
[http://dx.doi.org/10.1200/JCO.2005.10.042] [PMID: 15637391]

[7]   Seyfried TN, Huysentruyt LC. On the origin of cancer metastasis. Crit Rev Oncog 2013; 18(1-2): 43-73.
[http://dx.doi.org/10.1615/CritRevOncog.v18.i1-2.40] [PMID: 23237552]

[8]   Scheel BI, Holtedahl K. Symptoms, signs, and tests: The general practitioner's comprehensive approach towards a cancer diagnosis. Scand J Prim Health Care 2015; 33(3): 170-7.
[http://dx.doi.org/10.3109/02813432.2015.1067512] [PMID: 26375323]

[9]   Harding C, Stahl P. Pages 650-658. Biochem Biophys Res Commun 1983; 113(2): 650-8.
[http://dx.doi.org/10.1016/0006-291X(83)91776-X] [PMID: 6870878]

[10]  Johnstone RM, Adam M, Hammond JR, Orr L, Turbide C. Vesicle formation during reticulocyte maturation. Association of plasma membrane activities with released vesicles (exosomes). J Biol Chem 1987; 262(19): 9412-20.

[http://dx.doi.org/10.1016/S0021-9258(18)48095-7] [PMID: 3597417]

[11]   Hu Q, Su H, Li J, *et al.* Clinical applications of exosome membrane proteins. Precis Clin Med 2020; 3 (1): 54-66.
[http://dx.doi.org/10.1093/pcmedi/pbaa007] [PMID: 32257533]

[12]   Bu H, He D, He X, Wang K. Exosomes: Isolation, analysis, and applications in cancer detection and therapy. ChemBioChem 2019; 20(4): 451-61.
[http://dx.doi.org/10.1002/cbic.201800470] [PMID: 30371016]

[13]   Wang W, Zhu N, Yan T, *et al.* The crosstalk: exosomes and lipid metabolism. Cell Commun Signal 2020; 18(1): 119.
[http://dx.doi.org/10.1186/s12964-020-00581-2] [PMID: 32746850]

[14]   Munagala R, Aqil F, Jeyabalan J, Gupta RC. Bovine milk-derived exosomes for drug delivery. Cancer Lett 2016; 371(1): 48-61.
[http://dx.doi.org/10.1016/j.canlet.2015.10.020] [PMID: 26604130]

[15]   Behzadi E, Hosseini HM, Halabian R, Fooladi AAI. Macrophage cell-derived exosomes/staphylococcal enterotoxin B against fibrosarcoma tumor. Microb Pathog 2017; 111: 132-8.
[http://dx.doi.org/10.1016/j.micpath.2017.08.027] [PMID: 28843722]

[16]   Xiao-Jie L, Hui-Ying X, Zun-Ping K, Jin-Lian C, Li-Juan J. CRISPR-Cas9: a new and promising player in gene therapy. J Med Genet 2015; 52(5): 289-96.
[http://dx.doi.org/10.1136/jmedgenet-2014-102968] [PMID: 25713109]

[17]   Lundgren M, Charpentier E, Fineran PC. CRISPR: Methods and protocols. Cris Methods Protoc 2015; 1311: 1-366.

[18]   Hille F, Charpentier E. CRISPR-Cas: biology, mechanisms and relevance. Philos Trans R Soc Lond B Biol Sci 2016; 371(1707): 371.
[PMID: 27672148]

[19]   Torres-Ruiz R, Rodriguez-Perales S. CRISPR-Cas9 technology: applications and human disease modelling. Brief Funct Genomics 2017; 16(1): 4-12.
[http://dx.doi.org/10.1093/bfgp/elw025] [PMID: 27345434]

[20]   Uddin F, Rudin CM, Sen T. CRISPR gene therapy: Applications, limitations, and implications for the future. Front Oncol 2020; 10(August): 1387.
[http://dx.doi.org/10.3389/fonc.2020.01387] [PMID: 32850447]

[21]   Ahmed AA, Etemadmoghadam D, Temple J, *et al.* Driver mutations in *TP53* are ubiquitous in high grade serous carcinoma of the ovary. J Pathol 2010; 221(1): 49-56.
[http://dx.doi.org/10.1002/path.2696] [PMID: 20229506]

[22]   McCann AH, Kirley A, Carney DN, *et al.* Amplification of the MDM2 gene in human breast cancer and its association with MDM2 and p53 protein status. Br J Cancer 1995; 71(5): 981-5.
[http://dx.doi.org/10.1038/bjc.1995.189] [PMID: 7734324]

[23]   Bonapace L, Coissieux MM, Wyckoff J, *et al.* Cessation of CCL2 inhibition accelerates breast cancer metastasis by promoting angiogenesis. Nature 2014; 515(7525): 130-3.
[http://dx.doi.org/10.1038/nature13862] [PMID: 25337873]

[24]   Huang F, Chen J, Wang Z, Lan R, Fu L, Zhang L. δ-Catenin promotes tumorigenesis and metastasis of lung adenocarcinoma. Oncol Rep 2018; 39(2): 809-17.
[PMID: 29251319]

[25]   Aboubakar Nana F, Vanderputten M, Ocak S. Role of focal adhesion kinase in small-cell lung cancer and its potential as a therapeutic target. Cancers (Basel) 2019; 11(11): 1683.
[PMID: 31671774]

[26]   Ji HF, Pang D, Fu SB, *et al.* Overexpression of focal adhesion kinase correlates with increased lymph node metastasis and poor prognosis in non-small-cell lung cancer. J Cancer Res Clin Oncol 2013;

139(3): 429-35.
[http://dx.doi.org/10.1007/s00432-012-1342-8] [PMID: 23143646]

[27]    Sossey-Alaoui K, Su G, Malaj E, Roe B, Cowell JK. WAVE3, an actin-polymerization gene, is truncated and inactivated as a result of a constitutional t(1;13)(q21;q12) chromosome translocation in a patient with ganglioneuroblastoma. Oncogene 2002; 21(38): 5967-74.
[http://dx.doi.org/10.1038/sj.onc.1205734] [PMID: 12185600]

[28]    Sossey-Alaoui K, Safina A, Li X, *et al.* Down-regulation of WAVE3, a metastasis promoter gene, inhibits invasion and metastasis of breast cancer cells. Am J Pathol 2007; 170(6): 2112-21.
[http://dx.doi.org/10.2353/ajpath.2007.060975] [PMID: 17525277]

[29]    Fernando HS, Sanders AJ, Kynaston HG, Jiang WG. WAVE3 is associated with invasiveness in prostate cancer cells. Urol Oncol 2010; 28(3): 320-7.
[http://dx.doi.org/10.1016/j.urolonc.2008.12.022] [PMID: 19395286]

[30]    Cai Y, Yousef A, Grandis JR, Johnson DE. NSAID therapy for PIK3CA-Altered colorectal, breast, and head and neck cancer. Adv Biol Regul 2020; 75(September): 100653.
[http://dx.doi.org/10.1016/j.jbior.2019.100653] [PMID: 31594701]

[31]    Finetti F, Terzuoli E, Giachetti A, *et al.* mPGES-1 in prostate cancer controls stemness and amplifies epidermal growth factor receptor-driven oncogenicity. Endocr Relat Cancer 2015; 22(4): 665-78.
[http://dx.doi.org/10.1530/ERC-15-0277] [PMID: 26113609]

[32]    Panza E, De Cicco P, Ercolano G, *et al.* Differential expression of cyclooxygenase-2 in metastatic melanoma affects progression free survival. Oncotarget 2016; 7(35): 57077-85.
[http://dx.doi.org/10.18632/oncotarget.10976] [PMID: 27494851]

[33]    Wang D, Xia D, Dubois RN. The crosstalk of PTGS2 and EGF signaling pathways in colorectal cancer. Cancers (Basel) 2011; 3(4): 3894-908.
[http://dx.doi.org/10.3390/cancers3043894] [PMID: 24213116]

[34]    Jana D, Sarkar DK, Ganguly S, *et al.* Role of Cyclooxygenase 2 (COX-2) in Prognosis of Breast Cancer. Indian J Surg Oncol 2014; 5(1): 59-65.
[http://dx.doi.org/10.1007/s13193-014-0290-y] [PMID: 24669166]

[35]    Zeppernick F, Ahmadi R, Campos B, *et al.* Stem cell marker CD133 affects clinical outcome in glioma patients. Clin Cancer Res 2008; 14(1): 123-9.
[http://dx.doi.org/10.1158/1078-0432.CCR-07-0932] [PMID: 18172261]

[36]    Liou GY. CD133 as a regulator of cancer metastasis through the cancer stem cells. Int J Biochem Cell Biol 2019; 106: 1-7.
[http://dx.doi.org/10.1016/j.biocel.2018.10.013] [PMID: 30399449]

[37]    Saadatmand S, Vos JR, Hooning MJ, *et al.* This article has been accepted for publication and undergone full peer review but has not been through the copyediting, typesetting, pagination and proofreading process which may lead to differences between this version and the Version of Record. Please c. Laryngoscope 2014; (2): 2-31.

[38]    Huang H. Matrix metalloproteinase-9 (MMP-9) as a cancer biomarker and MMP-9 biosensors: Recent advances. Sensors (Basel) 2018; 18(10): 3249.
[http://dx.doi.org/10.3390/s18103249] [PMID: 30262739]

[39]    Zeng Y, Abdallah A, Lu JP, *et al.* δ-Catenin promotes prostate cancer cell growth and progression by altering cell cycle and survival gene profiles. Mol Cancer 2009; 8(1): 19.
[http://dx.doi.org/10.1186/1476-4598-8-19] [PMID: 19284555]

[40]    Li W, Cho MY, Lee S, Jang M, Park J, Park R. CRISPR-Cas9 mediated CD133 knockout inhibits colon cancer invasion through reduced epithelial-mesenchymal transition. PLoS One 2019; 14(8): e0220860.
[http://dx.doi.org/10.1371/journal.pone.0220860] [PMID: 31393941]

[41]    Constanzo JD, Tang KJ, Rindhe S, *et al.* PIAS1-FAK Interaction promotes the survival and

progression of non-small cell lung cancer. Neoplasia 2016; 18(5): 282-93.
[http://dx.doi.org/10.1016/j.neo.2016.03.003] [PMID: 27237320]

[42]   Zhu G, Pan C, Bei JX, *et al.* Mutant p53 in cancer progression and targeted therapies. Front Oncol 2020; 10: 595187.
[http://dx.doi.org/10.3389/fonc.2020.595187] [PMID: 33240819]

[43]   Ercolano G, De Cicco P, Rubino V, *et al.* Knockdown of PTGS2 by CRISPR/CAS9 system designates a new potential gene target for melanoma treatment. Front Pharmacol 2019; 10(December): 1456.
[http://dx.doi.org/10.3389/fphar.2019.01456] [PMID: 31920649]

[44]   Bledzka K, Schiemann B, Schiemann WP, Fox P, Plow EF, Sossey-Alaoui K. The WAVE3-YB1 interaction regulates cancer stem cells activity in breast cancer. Oncotarget 2017; 8(61): 104072-89.
[http://dx.doi.org/10.18632/oncotarget.22009] [PMID: 29262622]

[45]   Sossey-Alaoui K, Safina A, Li X, *et al.* Down-regulation of WAVE3, a metastasis promoter gene, inhibits invasion and metastasis of breast cancer cells. Am J Pathol 2007; 170(6): 2112-21.
[http://dx.doi.org/10.2353/ajpath.2007.060975] [PMID: 17525277]

[46]   Huleihel L, Hussey GS, Naranjo JD, *et al.* Matrix-bound nanovesicles within ECM bioscaffolds. Sci Adv 2016; 2(6): e1600502.
[http://dx.doi.org/10.1126/sciadv.1600502] [PMID: 27386584]

[47]   Jeppesen DK, Fenix AM, Franklin JL, *et al.* Reassessment of Exosome Composition. Cell 2019; 177(2): 428-445.e18.
[http://dx.doi.org/10.1016/j.cell.2019.02.029] [PMID: 30951670]

[48]   Tian T, Zhu YL, Hu FH, Wang YY, Huang NP, Xiao ZD. Dynamics of exosome internalization and trafficking. J Cell Physiol 2013; 228(7): 1487-95.
[http://dx.doi.org/10.1002/jcp.24304] [PMID: 23254476]

[49]   Zhang L, Yu D. Exosomes in cancer development, metastasis, and immunity. Biochim Biophys Acta Rev Cancer 2019; 1871(2): 455-68.
[http://dx.doi.org/10.1016/j.bbcan.2019.04.004] [PMID: 31047959]

[50]   Li P, Kaslan M, Lee SH, Yao J, Gao Z. Progress in exosome isolation techniques. Theranostics 2017; 7(3): 789-804.
[http://dx.doi.org/10.7150/thno.18133] [PMID: 28255367]

[51]   Bachurski D, Schuldner M, Nguyen PH, *et al.* Extracellular vesicle measurements with nanoparticle tracking analysis - An accuracy and repeatability comparison between NanoSight NS300 and ZetaView. J Extracell Vesicles 2019; 8(1): 1596016.
[http://dx.doi.org/10.1080/20013078.2019.1596016] [PMID: 30988894]

[52]   Deng F, Miller J. A review on protein markers of exosome from different bio-resources and the antibodies used for characterization. J Histotechnol 2019; 42(4): 226-39.
[http://dx.doi.org/10.1080/01478885.2019.1646984] [PMID: 31432761]

[53]   Yang C, Merlin D. Nanoparticle-mediated drug delivery systems for the treatment of IBD: Current perspectives. Int J Nanomedicine 2019; 14: 8875-89.
[http://dx.doi.org/10.2147/IJN.S210315] [PMID: 32009785]

[54]   Yang B, Chen Y, Shi J. Exosome biochemistry and advanced nanotechnology for next-generation theranostic platforms. Adv Mater 2019; 31(2): e1802896.
[http://dx.doi.org/10.1002/adma.201802896] [PMID: 30126052]

[55]   Sun D, Zhuang X, Xiang X, *et al.* A novel nanoparticle drug delivery system: the anti-inflammatory activity of curcumin is enhanced when encapsulated in exosomes. Mol Ther 2010; 18(9): 1606-14.
[http://dx.doi.org/10.1038/mt.2010.105] [PMID: 20571541]

[56]   Bagheri E, Abnous K, Farzad SA, Taghdisi SM, Ramezani M, Alibolandi M. Targeted doxorubicin-loaded mesenchymal stem cells-derived exosomes as a versatile platform for fighting against colorectal cancer. Life Sci 2020; 261(July): 118369.

[http://dx.doi.org/10.1016/j.lfs.2020.118369] [PMID: 32882265]

[57]   Yu M, Gai C, Li Z, *et al.* Targeted exosome-encapsulated erastin induced ferroptosis in triple negative breast cancer cells. Cancer Sci 2019; 110(10): 3173-82.
[http://dx.doi.org/10.1111/cas.14181] [PMID: 31464035]

[58]   Tian Y, Li S, Song J, *et al.* A doxorubicin delivery platform using engineered natural membrane vesicle exosomes for targeted tumor therapy. Biomaterials 2014; 35(7): 2383-90.
[http://dx.doi.org/10.1016/j.biomaterials.2013.11.083] [PMID: 24345736]

[59]   Nie H, Xie X, Zhang D, *et al.* Use of lung-specific exosomes for miRNA-126 delivery in non-small cell lung cancer. Nanoscale 2020; 12(2): 877-87.
[http://dx.doi.org/10.1039/C9NR09011H] [PMID: 31833519]

[60]   Liang G, Zhu Y, Ali DJ, Tian T, Xu H, Si K, *et al.* Engineered exosomes for targeted co-delivery of miR-21 inhibitor and chemotherapeutics to reverse drug resistance in colon cancer. J Nanobiotechnology 2020; 18(1): 1-15.
[http://dx.doi.org/10.1186/s12951-019-0560-5] [PMID: 31898555]

[61]   Dad HA, Gu TW, Zhu AQ, Huang LQ, Peng LH. Plant exosome-like nanovesicles: emerging therapeutics and drug delivery nanoplatforms. Mol Ther 2021; 29(1): 13-31.
[http://dx.doi.org/10.1016/j.ymthe.2020.11.030] [PMID: 33278566]

[62]   Alvarez-Erviti L, Seow Y, Yin H, Betts C, Lakhal S, Wood MJA. Delivery of siRNA to the mouse brain by systemic injection of targeted exosomes. Nat Biotechnol 2011; 29(4): 341-5.
[http://dx.doi.org/10.1038/nbt.1807] [PMID: 21423189]

[63]   Atay S, Gercel-Taylor C, Taylor DD. Human trophoblast-derived exosomal fibronectin induces pro-inflammatory IL-1β production by macrophages. Am J Reprod Immunol 2011; 66(4): 259-69.
[http://dx.doi.org/10.1111/j.1600-0897.2011.00995.x] [PMID: 21410811]

[64]   Lin D, Zhang H, Liu R, *et al.* iRGD-modified exosomes effectively deliver *CPT1A* siRNA to colon cancer cells, reversing oxaliplatin resistance by regulating fatty acid oxidation. Mol Oncol 2021; 15(12): 3430-46.
[http://dx.doi.org/10.1002/1878-0261.13052] [PMID: 34213835]

[65]   Faruqu FN, Xu L, Al-Jamal KT. Preparation of exosomes for siRNA delivery to cancer cells. J Vis Exp 2018; 2018(142)
[http://dx.doi.org/10.3791/58814-v] [PMID: 30582600]

[66]   Pascucci L, Coccè V, Bonomi A, *et al.* Paclitaxel is incorporated by mesenchymal stromal cells and released in exosomes that inhibit *in vitro* tumor growth: a new approach for drug delivery. J Control Release 2014; 192: 262-70.
[http://dx.doi.org/10.1016/j.jconrel.2014.07.042] [PMID: 25084218]

[67]   Fuhrmann G, Serio A, Mazo M, Nair R, Stevens MM. Active loading into extracellular vesicles significantly improves the cellular uptake and photodynamic effect of porphyrins. J Control Release 2015; 205: 35-44.
[http://dx.doi.org/10.1016/j.jconrel.2014.11.029] [PMID: 25483424]

[68]   Wahlgren J, De L Karlson T, Brisslert M, *et al.* Plasma exosomes can deliver exogenous short interfering RNA to monocytes and lymphocytes. Nucleic Acids Res 2012; 40(17): e130.
[http://dx.doi.org/10.1093/nar/gks463] [PMID: 22618874]

[69]   Sato YT, Umezaki K, Sawada S, *et al.* Engineering hybrid exosomes by membrane fusion with liposomes. Sci Rep 2016; 6(1): 21933.
[http://dx.doi.org/10.1038/srep21933] [PMID: 26911358]

[70]   Dominique C. Hinshaw1, Lalita A. Shevde1,2. HHS Public Access. Physiol Behav 2016; 176(1): 139-48.

[71]   Hood JL. Post isolation modification of exosomes for nanomedicine applications. Nanomedicine (Lond) 2016; 11(13): 1745-56.

[http://dx.doi.org/10.2217/nnm-2016-0102] [PMID: 27348448]

[72]    Kamerkar S, LeBleu VS, Sugimoto H, *et al.* Exosomes facilitate therapeutic targeting of oncogenic KRAS in pancreatic cancer. Nature 2017; 546(7659): 498-503.
[http://dx.doi.org/10.1038/nature22341] [PMID: 28607485]

[73]    Wang C, Chen L, Huang Y, *et al.* Exosome-delivered TRPP2 siRNA inhibits the epithelial-mesenchymal transition of FaDu cells. Oncol Lett 2019; 17(2): 1953-61.
[PMID: 30675260]

[74]    Kim MS, Haney MJ, Zhao Y, *et al.* Development of exosome-encapsulated paclitaxel to overcome MDR in cancer cells. Nanomedicine 2016; 12(3): 655-64.
[http://dx.doi.org/10.1016/j.nano.2015.10.012] [PMID: 26586551]

[75]    Han Y, Liu D, Li L. PD-1/PD-L1 pathway: current researches in cancer. Am J Cancer Res 2020; 10(3): 727-42. Available from: http://www.ncbi.nlm.nih.gov/pubmed/32266087
[PMID: 32266087]

[76]    Lacey SF, Fraietta JA. First Trial of CRISPR-Edited T cells in Lung Cancer. Trends Mol Med. 2020; 26(8): 713–5.
[http://dx.doi.org/10.1016/j.molmed.2020.06.001]

[77]    Stadtmauer EA, Fraietta JA, Davis MM, *et al.* CRISPR-engineered T cells in patients with refractory cancer. Science (80-). 2020; 367(6481): 1–20.
[http://dx.doi.org/1126/science.aba7365]

[78]    Lino CA, Harper JC, Carney JP, Timlin JA. Delivering CRISPR: a review of the challenges and approaches. Drug Deliv 2018; 25(1): 1234-57.
[http://dx.doi.org/10.1080/10717544.2018.1474964] [PMID: 29801422]

[79]    Xu CL, Ruan MZC, Mahajan VB, Tsang SH. Viral delivery systems for crispr. Viruses 2019; 11(1): 28.
[http://dx.doi.org/10.3390/v11010028] [PMID: 30621179]

[80]    Samulski RJ, Muzyczka N. AAV-mediated gene therapy for research and therapeutic purposes. Annu Rev Virol 2014; 1(1): 427-51.
[http://dx.doi.org/10.1146/annurev-virology-031413-085355] [PMID: 26958729]

[81]    Voets O, Tielen F, Elstak E, *et al.* Highly efficient gene inactivation by adenoviral CRISPR/Cas9 in human primary cells. PLoS One 2017; 12(8): e0182974.
[http://dx.doi.org/10.1371/journal.pone.0182974] [PMID: 28800587]

[82]    Naldini L, Blömer U, Gallay P, Ory D, Mulligan R, Gage FH, *et al.In vivo* gene delivery and stable transduction of nondividing cells by a lentiviral vector. Science (80-). 1996; 272(5259): 263–7.
[http://dx.doi.org/10.1126/science.272.5259.263]

[83]    van Montfoort N, van der Aa E, Woltman AM. Understanding MHC class I presentation of viral antigens by human dendritic cells as a basis for rational design of therapeutic vaccines. Front Immunol 2014; 5(APR): 182.
[http://dx.doi.org/10.3389/fimmu.2014.00182] [PMID: 24795724]

[84]    Nayerossadat N, Maedeh T, Ali PA. Viral and nonviral delivery systems for gene delivery. Adv Biomed Res 2012; 1(1): 27.
[http://dx.doi.org/10.4103/2277-9175.98152] [PMID: 23210086]

[85]    Li L, Hu S, Chen X. Non-viral delivery systems for CRISPR/Cas9-based genome editing: Challenges and opportunities. Biomaterials 2018; 171: 207-18.
[http://dx.doi.org/10.1016/j.biomaterials.2018.04.031] [PMID: 29704747]

[86]    Horii T, Arai Y, Yamazaki M, *et al.* Validation of microinjection methods for generating knockout mice by CRISPR/Cas-mediated genome engineering. Sci Rep 2014; 4(1): 4513.
[http://dx.doi.org/10.1038/srep04513] [PMID: 24675426]

[87]    Hashimoto M, Takemoto T. Electroporation enables the efficient mRNA delivery into the mouse zygotes and facilitates CRISPR/Cas9-based genome editing. Sci Rep 2015; 5(1): 11315.
[http://dx.doi.org/10.1038/srep11315] [PMID: 26066060]

[88]    Yin H, Xue W, Chen S, *et al.* Genome editing with Cas9 in adult mice corrects a disease mutation and phenotype. Nat Biotechnol 2014; 32(6): 551-3.
[http://dx.doi.org/10.1038/nbt.2884] [PMID: 24681508]

[89]    Mout R, Ray M, Yesilbag Tonga G, *et al.* Direct cytosolic delivery of crispr/cas9-ribonucleoprotein for efficient gene editing. ACS Nano 2017; 11(3): 2452-8.
[http://dx.doi.org/10.1021/acsnano.6b07600] [PMID: 28129503]

[90]    Wang M, Zuris JA, Meng F, *et al.* Efficient delivery of genome-editing proteins using bioreducible lipid nanoparticles. Proc Natl Acad Sci USA 2016; 113(11): 2868-73.
[http://dx.doi.org/10.1073/pnas.1520244113] [PMID: 26929348]

[91]    D'Astolfo DS, Pagliero RJ, Pras A, *et al.* Efficient intracellular delivery of native proteins. Cell 2015; 161(3): 674-90.
[http://dx.doi.org/10.1016/j.cell.2015.03.028] [PMID: 25910214]

[92]    Ramakrishna S, Kwaku Dad AB, Beloor J, Gopalappa R, Lee SK, Kim H. Gene disruption by cell-penetrating peptide-mediated delivery of Cas9 protein and guide RNA. Genome Res 2014; 24(6): 1020-7.
[http://dx.doi.org/10.1101/gr.171264.113] [PMID: 24696462]

[93]    Afzal H, Yousaf S, Rahman F, *et al.* PARP1: A potential biomarker for gastric cancer. Pathol Res Pract 2019; 215(8): 152472.
[http://dx.doi.org/10.1016/j.prp.2019.152472] [PMID: 31174925]

[94]    Schiewer MJ, Knudsen KE. Transcriptional roles of PARP1 in cancer. Mol Cancer Res 2014; 12(8): 1069-80.
[http://dx.doi.org/10.1158/1541-7786.MCR-13-0672] [PMID: 24916104]

[95]    Ossovskaya V, Koo IC, Kaldjian EP, Alvares C, Sherman BM. Upregulation of poly (ADP-Ribose) polymerase-1 (PARP1) in triple-negative breast cancer and other primary human tumor types. Genes Cancer 2010; 1(8): 812-21.
[http://dx.doi.org/10.1177/1947601910383418] [PMID: 21779467]

[96]    Kim SM, Yang Y, Oh SJ, Hong Y, Seo M, Jang M. Cancer-derived exosomes as a delivery platform of CRISPR/Cas9 confer cancer cell tropism-dependent targeting. J Control Release 2017; 266: 8-16.
[http://dx.doi.org/10.1016/j.jconrel.2017.09.013] [PMID: 28916446]

# CHAPTER 2

# Cancer Stem Cells and Their Role in Chemo-Resistance

**Vaishali Ji[1], Chandra Kishore[2,\*]** and **Krishna Prakash[3]**

[1] *Department of Botany, Patna Science College, Patna, Bihar, India*

[2] *Department of Pulmonary, Critical Care and Sleep Medicine, Icahn School of Medicine at Mount Sinai, New York, USA*

[3] *ICAR-Indian Agricultural Research Institute (IARI), Hazaribagh, Jharkhand, India*

**Abstract:** Cancer stem cells (CSCs) are found to be responsible for chemoresistance and disease relapse because of their ability to self-renew and capacity to differentiate into heterogeneous lineages of cancer cells. The in-depth knowledge of molecular mechanisms and their characteristics that ultimately lead to treatment failure might help in finding novel targets and make the drugs effective for a longer time. In this chapter, we will try to understand the key features and characteristic mechanisms that regulate CSC function at the molecular level in drug resistance as well as recent developments in therapeutic approaches for targeting CSCs. The novel insights into the role of CSCs in chemo-resistance will provide better therapeutic rationales for treating cancer. This chapter will also discuss the basics of conventional chemotherapies, different theories of CSC, molecular and cellular mechanisms of CSC self-defense, and how all these factors are ultimately involved in chemoresistance.

**Keywords:** Cancer, Cancer therapy, Drug-resistant, Stem cells, Transporter proteins.

## INTRODUCTION

Since the identification of cancer stem cells (CSCs) in the tumor, the understanding of carcinogenesis and chemotherapy approaches has changed a lot. Research has focused a lot on the involvement of cancer stem cells in carcinogenesis, drug resistance, and metastasis. Bone marrow stem cells are required for continuous replenishment of blood cells and they consist of long-term renewing stem cells, short-term renewing stem cells, and nonrenewable multipotent progenitors that can only differentiate into various types of blood cells in the bone marrow. There needs to be a proper balance in cell renewal and cell

---
\* **Corresponding author Chandra Kishore:** Department of Pulmonary, Critical Care and Sleep Medicine, Icahn School of Medicine at Mount Sinai, New York, USA; E-mails: ckcanres@gmail.com, chandra.kishore@mssm.edu

**Ashok Kumar Pandurangan (Ed.)**

division and any aberrant changes can lead to blood cancer development. Pluripotent stem cells are present in the organs that have the ability of self-renewal and differentiate into organ-specific cells and aberrant proliferation of these cells is involved in or aggravates the solid cancer development and growth. In the mammary gland tissues, three types of cells have been identified-myoepithelial cells, ductal epithelial cells, and milk-producing alveolar cells- but the clonal population can develop into all the functional types of mammary gland cells. Human mammary epithelial cells can be developed into spheroids that consist of the three main types of mammary cells. One of the important characteristics of normal stem cells which remain quiescent and stay most of the time in the SubGo phase is self-renewal and pluripotency. Stem cells can repair DNA and also accumulate carcinogen-induced mutations with time. But whether cancer stem cells arise from pre-existing normal stem cells after the accumulation of mutation or cancer stem cells and normal stem cells are independent is still a topic of contention. Stem cells are relatively more resistant to toxins and radiation and this might be a possible cause of the development of resistance in cancer stem cells in a longer course of treatment. A better understanding of normal/cancer stem cell biology can give a better idea to deal with cancer development and resistance to the treatments.

## Normal Stem Cells and Cancer Stem Cells Linked to Carcinogenesis

Cancer stem cells are present in the tumors and play an important role in different types of blood cancers and solid cancers. These stem cells might be the source of the development and reemergence of cancer after chemotherapy. Cancer stem cells, which are a very small fraction of the tumor have the potential to grow into tumors when transplanted at new sites but the rest of the tumor cells lack this regenerative power. It is a general perception that leukemia originates from the stem cell population that gets transformed and produces a large colony of cells that have lost the potential of self-renewal and differentiation. Teratocarcinoma is an important example of the presence of pluripotent cells in tumors [1]. Stem cells present in the tumor have been shown to express organ-specific biomarkers (Table 2). The pluripotent stem cells present in the tumor might arise from the normal stem cells that had accumulated mutations or from the differentiated cells that had acquired the capacity of self-renewal and stem cell properties [2]. Cancer stem cells have many properties similar to normal stem cells and hence sometimes it becomes very tough to distinguish between them. Normal stem cells might provide the properties of drug resistance, a longer resting phase, active DNA repair capacity, and anti-apoptotic potential, and also similar characteristics are present in cancer stem cells [3]. The study of the detailed mechanism of development of drug resistance in normal or cancer stem cells of the tumor might prove new drug targets and a better strategy to manage the cancer disease.

## Transporter Proteins in Stem Cells and Cancer

Stem cells have the properties of self-renewal and differentiation as well as quiescence for a longer time interval. They also require a special microenvironment consisting of unique cells, stroma, and growth factors for their survival and maintenance. Stem cells are shown to express very high levels of ABC drug transporter proteins [4]. Hematopoietic stem cells express very high levels of ABCG2 [5] proteins, and two of the most extensively studied ABC transporter genes are ABCB1 and ABCG2 [6]. ABCC1 gene has also been shown to be overexpressed in multidrug-resistant cancer cells [7]. The ABC transporter superfamily plays an important role in normal physiology and helps in transporting the drugs across the placenta and intestine. They have also an important role in the blood-testis barrier [8] and blood-brain barrier [9]. These transporters efflux the toxic chemicals from the cells utilizing the energy of ATP hydrolysis and protect the cells from harmful effects. The drug-transporting property of stem cells is also utilized for their isolation and analysis in blood cancers. Hoechst 33342 and rhodamine 123 dyes are accumulated inside the cells but the stem cells expressing ABCG2 and ABCB1 throw out these dyes outside the cell [10]. These low fluorescent stem cell populations because of efflux are called dull cells or side population (SP) cells [11]. The side population of stem cells can be isolated from many organs and they might represent lineage-specific stem cells.

## Chemotherapy Resistance in Cancer and Cancer Stem Cells

There are multiple ways by which a cancer cell can acquire resistance to chemotherapeutic drugs such as drug efflux, mutation and/or overexpression of drug targets, metabolizing or inactivating the drugs [12]. Typically, cancer cells that re-emerge at primary or secondary sites after the chemotherapy cycles are multiple drug-resistant, and because of the selective advantage, they overtake the tumor population. Cancer stem cells have the natural tendency to resist chemotherapy because of the expression of ABC transporters, quiescence nature, and DNA repair capabilities, and these characteristics allow tumor cells to survive chemotherapy and help tumor cells regrow by releasing various factors. According to the acquired resistance model, cancer stem cells or their close progeny acquires resistance to the drugs [13]. Based on the recent experience with imatinib (Glivec) in leukemia, it was found that ABC-mediated efflux is not the only responsible factor behind drug resistance in cancer stem cells. In the case of leukemia, mutation in ABL is the stronger reason behind imatinib resistance as compared to the drug efflux [14]. DNA repair capacity and overexpression of antiapoptotic pathways also play an important role in drug resistance [15]. Since stem cells are quiescent and non-dividing cells hence, they are generally refractory to the drugs targeting the cell cycle or cell division [16]. Since quiescence is an important aspect of stem cells, we need to develop drugs that can attack nondividing cells including stem cells.

## Controlling Drug-Resistant Cancer Cells

In the early phases, ABCB1 inhibitor drugs such as verapamil and cyclosporin A were used along with other chemotherapy drugs assuming that these drug transporter inhibitors might control the chemotherapy-resistant cancer cells but the results were not so promising [17]. The second generation of drug transporter inhibitors such as PSC833 and VX-710 underwent clinical trials but the results were largely negative as ABCB1 inhibitors were shown to interact with the chemotherapy regimens. The reason for the failure of these drugs can also be attributed to the expression of additional drug transporters such as ABCC1 and ABCG2, which were not targeted by the ABCB1 inhibitors. ABC transporter inhibitors along with chemotherapy drugs might be a better strategy to overcome drug resistance and in many studies, these transporter inhibitors have been explained as cancer stem cell sensitizing agents [18]. It has also been suggested that drug transporter inhibitors work better when combined with stem cell targeting agents. Most of the clinical trials have focused on ABCB1 but the targeting of ABCG2 that is overexpressed on stem cells also needs to be extensively studied [19]. The compound fumitremorgin C (FTC) has been shown to target ABCG2 but the toxicity of the drug has limited its further study [20]. FTC derivative Ko143 [21] has been shown to have lower toxicity and higher specificity for ABCG2 in mice and ABCB1 inhibitor GF120918 [22] inhibits ABCG2 in *in vitro* and *in vivo* models. We need to develop and identify a potent, non-toxic, and specific transporter inhibitor against ABCB1, ABCG2, and ABCC1 to see a better effect on drug efflux inhibition. To find a drug that selectively kills cancer stem cells and not the normal stem cells or to find a therapeutic window to selectively kill cancer stem cells without disturbing the normal stem cells will be a challenging task more specifically in bone marrow as normal stem cells are required for normal functioning of the body [23]. Important ABC transporters involved in drug efflux are mentioned in Table **1**.

Table 1. ABC drug efflux transporters and drug or their substrate.

| Gene/Protein | Effluxed Drugs/Substrates |
|---|---|
| *ABCA2*/ABCA2 | Estramustine [25] |
| *ABCB1*/PGP or MDR1 | Colchicine, doxorubicin, etoposide, vinblastine, paclitaxel, Digoxin, saquinivir [26], |
| *ABCC1*/MRP1 | Doxorubicin, daunorubicin, vincristine, etoposide, colchicine, camptothecins, methotrexate, Rhodamine [27] |

*(Table 1) cont.....*

| Gene/Protein | Effluxed Drugs/Substrates |
|---|---|
| *ABCC2*/MRP2 | Vinblastine, cisplatin, doxorubicin, methotrexate, Sulfinpyrazone [28] |
| *ABCC3*/MRP3 | Methotrexate, etoposide [29] |
| *ABCC4*/MRP4 | 6-mercaptopurine, methotrexate, 6-thioguanine and metabolites, PMEA, cAMP, cGMP [30] |
| *ABCC5*/MRP5 | 6-mercaptopurine, 6-thioguanine, and metabolites, PMEA, cAMP, cGMP [31] |
| *ABCC6*/MRP6 | Etoposide [32] |
| *ABCC11*/MRP8 | 5-fluorouracil, PMEA, cAMP, cGMP [33] |
| *ABCG2*/MXR or BCRP | Mitoxantrone, topotecan, doxorubicin, daunorubicin, irinotecan, imatinib, methotrexate, Pheophorbide A, Hoechst, 33342, rhodamine [34] |

**Table 2. Markers expressed on cancer stem cells of different classes of cancer.**

| Classes of Cancer | CSC Markers Expressed on Cells |
|---|---|
| Head and neck cancer | CD133$^+$, CD44$^+$, SSEA-1$^+$ [37] |
| Lung cancer | CD133$^+$, CD44$^+$, ABCG2, ALDH, CD87$^+$, SP, CD90$^+$ [38] |
| Melanoma | CD20$^+$, ABCB5$^+$, CD271$^+$, CD133$^+$, ALDH$^+$ [39] |
| Colon cancer | CD133$^+$, CD44$^+$, EpCAM$^+$, ESA, ALDH, CD24$^+$, CD166$^+$ [40] |
| Pancreatic cancer | CD44$^+$, CD24$^+$, CD133$^+$, ESA, ABCG2, ALDH, EpCAM$^+$ [41] |
| Prostate cancer | ABCG2, ALDH, $\alpha2\beta1$, CD133$^+$, CD44$^+$ [42] |
| Breast cancer | ALDH-1, CD24$^-$, CD133$^+$, CD44$^+$, EpCAM$^+$ [43] |
| Leukemia (AML) | CD123$^+$, CD34$^+$, CD38$^-$ [44] |
| Gastric cancer | CD24$^+$, CD133$^+$, CD44$^+$ [45] |
| Brain cancer | CD44$^+$, CD36$^+$, CD90$^+$, CD133$^+$, EGFR$^+$, L1CAM$^+$ [46] |
| Bladder cancer | CD44+, CD44v6$^+$, ALDH+ [47] |
| Ovarian | CD24+, ALDH+, CD44+, CD133+, EpCAM [48] |
| Acute myeloid leukemia | CD34+, CD38−, CD90+, CD71+, CD19+, CD20+, CD44+, CD10+, CD45RA+, CD123 [49] |
| Cervical cancer | ABCG2+, CD133+, CD49f+, ALDH+ [50] |
| Laryngeal cancer | ALDH+, CD44+, CD133+ [51] |
| Nasopharyngeal cancer | CD44+, CD133+, ALDH+, CD24+ [52] |
| Esophageal cancer | ITGA7+, CD44+, ALDH+, CD133+, CD90+ [53] |
| Oral squamous cell carcinoma | CD44+/CD24-, ITGA7+ [54] |
| Cutaneous squamous cell carcinoma | CD44+, CD133+ [55] |
| Multiple myeloma | CD138−, CD19+, CD27+ [56] |
| Malignant mesothelioma | CD9+, CD24+, CD26+ [57] |

*(Table 2) cont.....*

| Classes of Cancer | CSC Markers Expressed on Cells |
|---|---|
| Renal cell carcinoma | CD133+, ALDH+, CXCR4+, CD44+, CD105+ [58] |
| Gallbladder cancer | CD44+/CD133+ [59] |

The concept of quiescent stem cells armed with multiple drug transporter and their inhibition is more exciting for its application in those tumors in which anticancer drugs kill most of the cancer cells and few cancer stem cells survive but in those cancer models such as kidney, pancreas, and colon cancer models where most cancer cells survive and few cancer cells die in response to chemotherapy, this model doesn't have much potential [24].

Cancer stem cells (CSCs) or tumor-initiating cells (TICs) have been widely studied for their origin and the ways to target them effectively. First cancer stem cells were shown as a CD34$^+$/CD38$^-$ subpopulation of leukemia cells by Bonnet and Dick in 1997, which had the potential to form tumors in NOD/SCID mice [35]. The first report for the presence of cancer stem cells in solid cancers was given by the presence of CD44$^+$/CD24$^-$/ $^{low}$ Lineage− cells in human breast cancer cells [36]. Later on, cancer stem cells were reported in several cancers such as the cancers of skin, brain, lung, liver, pancreas, colon, breast, *etc.* The origin and source of cancer stem cells are not very clear and some of the potential sources of origin might be adult stem cells and adult progenitor cells that have accumulated mutations or differentiated cells or cancer cells that have obtained the properties of stem cells by dedifferentiation. CSCs play an important role in chemoresistance, radioresistance, disease relapse, and cell quiescence. Since most of the chemotherapeutic drugs target dividing cells, CSCs can easily escape the drugs because of the lesser frequency of cell division.

**Cell Signaling in Cancer Stem Cells Cancer Therapy**

Cancer stem cells have the nature of self-renewal and differentiation, which helps in maintaining the number of copies as well as forming the newer types of cells. Cancer stem cells are now known to be involved in the regulation of several aspects of malignancy such as tumor recurrence, metastasis of the cancer cells, heterogeneity in the tumor population, resistance to chemotherapeutic drugs, and radio-resistance. CSCs are maintained by multiple cell-signaling pathways such as Wnt signaling, NF-κB, Notch, Hedgehog, JAK-STAT, PI3K/AKT/mTOR, TGF/SMAD, and several extracellular factors such as vascular niches, hypoxia, cancer-associated macrophages, mesenchymal stem cells, and fibroblasts, extracellular matrix, and exosomes. Several molecules, vaccines, antibodies, and CAR-T cells have been designed to specifically target the CSCs. But cancer stem cells find some other ways to evade these pathways. Oct4, Sox2, Nanog, KLF4, and MYC are some of the transcription factors known to maintain the stem cell state of the cell. Oct4 has been shown to act as a master regulator that controls the self-renewal, pluripotency, and maintenance of stem cells. Oct4 is known to be highly expressed in cancer stem cells. The overexpression of Oct4 is related to glioma grades and promotes hepatocellular carcinoma stem cells. Some of the chemotherapeutic drugs such as cisplatin, etoposide, Adriamycin, paclitaxel, and gamma radiation have been shown to induce the expression of Oct4 in lung tumors and CD133+ cells are more resistant to the drugs. Oct4 expression is associated with poor outcomes in breast cancer and knockdown of Oct4 suppresses the stemness of germ cell tumors. Sox 2 is involved in the development and maintenance of embryonic stem cells and it is one of the transcription factors that are involved in the maintenance of cancer stem cells. A higher expression of Sox2 induces xenograft glioma and the suppression of Sox2 controls the glioblastoma cell proliferation and tumor formation. Sox2 is known to maintain tumor-initiating cells in osteosarcoma and its downregulation controls the tumorigenicity. Osteosarcoma cells having lost the expression of Sox2 can't form osteosphere and differentiate into osteoblast. Sox2 is overexpressed in cutaneous squamous cell carcinoma and promotes cancer metastasis. Nanog is involved in self-renewal and multiple transcriptional regulatory functions. Abnormal expression of Nanog has been found in many human cancers such as breast cancer, lung cancer, head and neck cancer, brain cancer, cervical cancer, and gastric cancer. Higher expression of Nanog protein is linked with lymph node positivity in colorectal cancer. Higher expression of Nanog in colorectal cancer is associated with enhanced colony formation and tumorigenicity *in vivo*. Gastric cancer patients having a higher expression of Nanog have a lower survival rate.

KLF4 plays an important role in multiple physiological processes. KLF4 can activate or inhibit the transcription in a context-dependent manner and it has oncogenic or tumor suppressor roles depending on the type of cancer. KLF4 acts as an anticancer factor in intestinal and gastric cancers and it is downregulated in colorectal and gastric cancer stem cells. Downregulation of KLF4 is also observed in liver cancer, bladder cancer, non-small-cell lung carcinoma, anaplastic meningioma, and esophageal cancer. Overexpression of KLF4 in breast cancer stem cells is correlated with an aggressive phenotype in canine mammary tumors. Hence, KLF4 can act as an oncogene as well as a tumor suppressor depending on the context. MYC acts as an oncogene and regulates a large number of protein-coding and noncoding genes that are involved in cell metabolism and self-renewal, growth, and differentiation of cancer stem cells. MYC gene is one of the most commonly activated oncogenes in different types of cancer but the overexpression of MYC alone is not sufficient to induce cancer.

Aberrant Wnt signaling is found in multiple cancers such as colon cancer, breast cancer, thyroid cancer, and esophageal cancer. Wnt signaling plays an important role in the regulation of cancer stem cells, apoptosis, and dedifferentiation. The notch pathway regulates leukemia, breast cancer, lung cancer, and glioblastoma. Notch acts as an oncogene as well as a tumor suppressor gene. Notch is downregulated in breast cancer, skin cancer, liver cancer, prostate cancer, and non-small cell lung cancer. Activation of the notch pathway leads to cell survival, self-renewal, metastasis, and anti-apoptotic in cancer stem cells. An abnormal Hedgehog signaling pathway is observed in bladder cancer, breast cancer, lung cancer, gastric cancer, pancreatic cancer, and medulloblastoma. Hedgehog signaling is involved in tumorigenesis, tumor growth, and regulation of residual cancer cells after therapy. Aberrant Hedgehog signaling plays an important role in cancer stem cell development and maintenance. Hh signaling is involved in the self-renewal, maintenance, proliferation, and tumorigenicity of cancer stem cells in lung adenocarcinoma. NF-κB is involved in immune and inflammatory responses and induces cell survival, proliferation, and differentiation. Overexpression of NF-κB is reported in gastrointestinal, genitourinary, gynecological, head and neck, and breast cancers as well as multiple myelomas and blood cancers. NF-κB is involved in cell survival, proliferation, metastasis, and tumorigenesis. NF-κB induces angiogenesis and adhesion and helps cancer to progress. NF-κB is involved in inflammation, self-renewal, maintenance, and metastasis of the cancer stem cells. JAK/STAT pathway is involved in cell proliferation, apoptosis, differentiation, and immune regulation. JAK/STAT pathway is involved in hematopoiesis, survival, self-renewal, and neurogenesis of embryonic stem cells. Overexpression of STAT3 promotes cell survival and maintains stemness in breast cancer stem cells. TGF/SMAD signaling is involved in cell proliferation, differentiation, apoptosis, and homeostasis in cancer and cancer stem cells. Upregulation of TGF-β1 enhances the smad4, CD133 in liver cancer stem cells. TGF-β/SMAD pathway acts as a tumor suppressor in the early stages of cancer but acts as an inducer of cancer in the later advanced stages of cancer. PI3K/AKT/mTOR signaling pathway is known to be involved in glioblastoma multiforme. Suppression of PTEN in neural stem cells causes the development of cancerous phenotypes and induces growth, antiapoptotic characteristics, and increased cell migration and invasion. Peroxisome proliferator-activated receptors (PPARs) signaling pathways are linked to carcinogenesis and they are involved in prostate cancer, breast cancer, pancreatic cancer, leukemia, glioblastoma, neuroblastoma, and glioblastoma. The involvement of PPARs in CSCs is not well understood but there are some reports about PPARγ involvement in CSCs development and maintenance. These signaling pathways are not linear but crosstalk to each other to regulate cancer stem cells. Wnt signaling and NF-κB pathway work together to promote cell survival and proliferation of CSCs. Suppression of Notch1 induces NF-kB activity and promotes the CD133-positive cells in melanoma CSCs. NF-kB and

JAK/STAT pathways act in collaboration to promote self-renewal of cancer stem cells in hepatocellular carcinoma. PI3K/mTOR signaling induces the expression of STAT3, which helps in the survival and proliferation of breast CSCs. Some of the drugs in different stages of clinical trials are summarised in Table **3**.

**Table 3. Drugs acting on cell signaling pathways in different stages of clinical trials.**

| Cell Signaling Components | Drugs |
|---|---|
| Hedgehog signaling-Smoothened | Vismodegib, Sonidegib, Glasdegib, Taladegib, Patidegib [60], |
| Notch inhibitors -γSecretase | MK-0752, RO4929097, Nirogacestat [61], |
| Pan -Notch | Crenigacestat, AL101, CB-103, BMS-906024, |
| DLL4 | Demcizumab, Brontictuzumab, Enoticumab, MEDI0639, |
| Wnt inhibitor | Ipafricept, Vantictumab, PRI-724, CWP232291, LGK974, ETC-1922159 [62, 63] |
| TGFB | Galunisertib, LY3200882, AVID200, Trabedersen, Fresolimumab, Vactosertib, NIS793 [64] |
| JAK | Ruxolitinib, AZD4205, SAR302503, SB1518 [65] |
| PI3K | Alpelisib, Buparlisib, BYL719, SF1126, SAR245409 [66], |

Overactivation of cancer stem cell signaling pathways or prolonged use of chemotherapeutic drugs cause resistance in cancer stem cells and hence the cancer tumors that respond to the treatment initially stop responding to the treatment. These resistant CSCs are responsible for chemo and radiotherapy resistance of the tumor. Hence eliminating these cancer stem cells should be the primary strategy in the treatment of cancer.

## CONCLUSION

Cancer stem cells are one of the major factors in the development of chemo and radiotherapy resistance in cancer treatment and they apply various strategies to evade chemotherapeutic drugs. We need to find ways to efficiently target these cancer stem cells to manage cancer properly and inhibit cancer reemergence and resistance.

## REFERENCES

[1]     Mintz B, Cronmiller C, Custer RP. Somatic cell origin of teratocarcinomas. Proc Natl Acad Sci USA 1978; 75(6): 2834-8.
[http://dx.doi.org/10.1073/pnas.75.6.2834] [PMID: 275854]

[2]     Reya T, Morrison SJ, Clarke MF, Weissman IL. Stem cells, cancer, and cancer stem cells. Nature 2001; 414(6859): 105-11.
[http://dx.doi.org/10.1038/35102167] [PMID: 11689955]

[3]     Dean M, Fojo T, Bates S. Tumour stem cells and drug resistance. Nat Rev Cancer 2005; 5(4): 275-84.
        [http://dx.doi.org/10.1038/nrc1590] [PMID: 15803154]

[4]     Dean M. ABC transporters, drug resistance, and cancer stem cells. J Mammary Gland Biol Neoplasia
        2009; 14(1): 3-9.
        [http://dx.doi.org/10.1007/s10911-009-9109-9] [PMID: 19224345]

[5]     Raaijmakers MHGP. ATP-binding-cassette transporters in hematopoietic stem cells and their utility as
        therapeutical targets in acute and chronic myeloid leukemia. Leukemia 2007; 21(10): 2094-102.
        [http://dx.doi.org/10.1038/sj.leu.2404859] [PMID: 17657220]

[6]     Rees DC, Johnson E, Lewinson O. ABC transporters: the power to change. Nat Rev Mol Cell Biol
        2009; 10(3): 218-27.
        [http://dx.doi.org/10.1038/nrm2646] [PMID: 19234479]

[7]     Cole SPC. Multidrug resistance protein 1 (MRP1, ABCC1), a "multitasking" ATP-binding cassette
        (ABC) transporter. J Biol Chem 2014; 289(45): 30880-8.
        [http://dx.doi.org/10.1074/jbc.R114.609248] [PMID: 25281745]

[8]     Mruk DD, Su L, Cheng CY. Emerging role for drug transporters at the blood–testis barrier. Trends
        Pharmacol Sci 2011; 32(2): 99-106.
        [http://dx.doi.org/10.1016/j.tips.2010.11.007] [PMID: 21168226]

[9]     de Boer AG, van der Sandt ICJ, Gaillard PJ. The role of drug transporters at the blood-brain barrier.
        Annu Rev Pharmacol Toxicol 2003; 43(1): 629-56.
        [http://dx.doi.org/10.1146/annurev.pharmtox.43.100901.140204] [PMID: 12415123]

[10]    Bertoncello I, Williams B. Hematopoietic stem cell characterization by Hoechst 33342 and rhodamine
        123 staining. Methods Mol Biol 2004; 263: 181-200.
        [http://dx.doi.org/10.1385/1-59259-773-4:181] [PMID: 14976367]

[11]    Wu C, Alman BA. Side population cells in human cancers. Cancer Lett 2008; 268(1): 1-9.
        [http://dx.doi.org/10.1016/j.canlet.2008.03.048] [PMID: 18487012]

[12]    Alfarouk KO, Stock CM, Taylor S, *et al.* Resistance to cancer chemotherapy: failure in drug response
        from ADME to P-gp. Cancer Cell Int 2015; 15(1): 71.
        [http://dx.doi.org/10.1186/s12935-015-0221-1] [PMID: 26180516]

[13]    Rosa R, Monteleone F, Zambrano N, Bianco R. *In vitro* and *in vivo* models for analysis of resistance to
        anticancer molecular therapies. Curr Med Chem 2014; 21(14): 1595-606.
        [http://dx.doi.org/10.2174/09298673113209990226] [PMID: 23992330]

[14]    Milojkovic D, Apperley J. Mechanisms of resistance to imatinib and second-generation tyrosine
        inhibitors in chronic myeloid leukemia. Clin Cancer Res 2009; 15(24): 7519-27.
        [http://dx.doi.org/10.1158/1078-0432.CCR-09-1068] [PMID: 20008852]

[15]    Brown JM, Wilson G. Apoptosis genes and resistance to cancer therapy: what does the experimental
        and clinical data tell us? Cancer Biol Ther 2003; 2(5): 477-90.
        [http://dx.doi.org/10.4161/cbt.2.5.450] [PMID: 14614312]

[16]    Yano S, Takehara K, Tazawa H, *et al.* Cell-cycle-dependent drug-resistant quiescent cancer cells
        induce tumor angiogenesis after chemotherapy as visualized by real-time FUCCI imaging. Cell Cycle
        2017; 16(5): 406-14.
        [http://dx.doi.org/10.1080/15384101.2016.1220461] [PMID: 27715464]

[17]    Ansbro MR, Shukla S, Ambudkar SV, Yuspa SH, Li L. Screening compounds with a novel high-
        throughput ABCB1-mediated efflux assay identifies drugs with known therapeutic targets at risk for
        multidrug resistance interference. PLoS One 2013; 8(4): e60334.
        [http://dx.doi.org/10.1371/journal.pone.0060334] [PMID: 23593196]

[18]    Shukla S, Ohnuma S, Ambudkar SV. Improving cancer chemotherapy with modulators of ABC drug
        transporters. Curr Drug Targets 2011; 12(5): 621-30.

[http://dx.doi.org/10.2174/138945011795378540] [PMID: 21039338]

[19]   Toyoda Y, Takada T, Suzuki H. Inhibitors of human ABCG2: From technical background to recent updates with clinical implications. Front Pharmacol 2019; 10: 208.
[http://dx.doi.org/10.3389/fphar.2019.00208] [PMID: 30890942]

[20]   Allen JD, van Loevezijn A, Lakhai JM, *et al.* Potent and specific inhibition of the breast cancer resistance protein multidrug transporter *in vitro* and in mouse intestine by a novel analogue of fumitremorgin C. Mol Cancer Ther 2002; 1(6): 417-25.
[PMID: 12477054]

[21]   Weidner LD, Zoghbi SS, Lu S, *et al.* The Inhibitor Ko143 Is Not Specific for ABCG2. J Pharmacol Exp Ther 2015; 354(3): 384-93.
[http://dx.doi.org/10.1124/jpet.115.225482] [PMID: 26148857]

[22]   de Bruin M, Miyake K, Litman T, Robey R, Bates SE. Reversal of resistance by GF120918 in cell lines expressing the ABC half-transporter, MXR. Cancer Lett 1999; 146(2): 117-26.
[http://dx.doi.org/10.1016/S0304-3835(99)00182-2] [PMID: 10656616]

[23]   Li L, Neaves WB. Normal stem cells and cancer stem cells: the niche matters. Cancer Res 2006; 66(9): 4553-7.
[http://dx.doi.org/10.1158/0008-5472.CAN-05-3986] [PMID: 16651403]

[24]   Chen W, Dong J, Haiech J, Kilhoffer MC, Zeniou M. Cancer stem cell quiescence and plasticity as major challenges in cancer therapy. Stem Cells Int 2016; 2016(1): 1740936.
[http://dx.doi.org/10.1155/2016/1740936] [PMID: 27418931]

[25]   Davis W Jr, Tew KD. ATP-binding cassette transporter-2 (ABCA2) as a therapeutic target. Biochem Pharmacol 2018; 151: 188-200.
[http://dx.doi.org/10.1016/j.bcp.2017.11.018] [PMID: 29223352]

[26]   Leschziner GD, Andrew T, Pirmohamed M, Johnson MR. ABCB1 genotype and PGP expression, function and therapeutic drug response: a critical review and recommendations for future research. Pharmacogenomics J 2007; 7(3): 154-79.
[http://dx.doi.org/10.1038/sj.tpj.6500413] [PMID: 16969364]

[27]   Peterson BG, Tan KW, Osa-Andrews B, Iram SH. High-content screening of clinically tested anticancer drugs identifies novel inhibitors of human MRP1 (ABCC1). Pharmacol Res 2017; 119: 313-26.
[http://dx.doi.org/10.1016/j.phrs.2017.02.024] [PMID: 28258008]

[28]   Le MT, Phan TV, Tran-Nguyen VK, Tran TD, Thai KM. Prediction model of human ABCC2/MRP2 efflux pump inhibitors: a QSAR study. Mol Divers 2021; 25(2): 741-51.
[http://dx.doi.org/10.1007/s11030-020-10047-9] [PMID: 32048150]

[29]   Ali I, Welch MA, Lu Y, Swaan PW, Brouwer KLR. Identification of novel MRP3 inhibitors based on computational models and validation using an *in vitro* membrane vesicle assay. Eur J Pharm Sci 2017; 103: 52-9.
[http://dx.doi.org/10.1016/j.ejps.2017.02.011] [PMID: 28238947]

[30]   Chen Y, Yuan X, Xiao Z, Jin H, Zhang L, Liu Z. Discovery of novel multidrug resistance protein 4 (MRP4) inhibitors as active agents reducing resistance to anticancer drug 6-Mercaptopurine (6-MP) by structure and ligand-based virtual screening. PLoS One 2018; 13(10): e0205175.
[http://dx.doi.org/10.1371/journal.pone.0205175] [PMID: 30321196]

[31]   Borst P, de Wolf C, van de Wetering K. Multidrug resistance-associated proteins 3, 4, and 5. Pflugers Arch 2007; 453(5): 661-73.
[http://dx.doi.org/10.1007/s00424-006-0054-9] [PMID: 16586096]

[32]   Eadie LN, Dang P, Goyne JM, Hughes TP, White DL. ABCC6 plays a significant role in the transport of nilotinib and dasatinib, and contributes to TKI resistance *in vitro*, in both cell lines and primary patient mononuclear cells. PLoS One 2018; 13(1): e0192180.

[http://dx.doi.org/10.1371/journal.pone.0192180] [PMID: 29385210]

[33]   Toyoda Y, Ishikawa T. Pharmacogenomics of human ABC transporter ABCC11 (MRP8): potential risk of breast cancer and chemotherapy failure. Anticancer Agents Med Chem 2010; 10(8): 617-24.
[http://dx.doi.org/10.2174/187152010794473975] [PMID: 21182469]

[34]   Henrich CJ, Robey RW, Bokesch HR, *et al.* New inhibitors of ABCG2 identified by high-throughput screening. Mol Cancer Ther 2007; 6(12): 3271-8.
[http://dx.doi.org/10.1158/1535-7163.MCT-07-0352] [PMID: 18089721]

[35]   Bonnet D, Dick JE. Human acute myeloid leukemia is organized as a hierarchy that originates from a primitive hematopoietic cell. Nat Med 1997; 3(7): 730-7.
[http://dx.doi.org/10.1038/nm0797-730] [PMID: 9212098]

[36]   Hwang-Verslues WW, Kuo WH, Chang PH, *et al.* Multiple lineages of human breast cancer stem/progenitor cells identified by profiling with stem cell markers. PLoS One 2009; 4(12): e8377.
[http://dx.doi.org/10.1371/journal.pone.0008377] [PMID: 20027313]

[37]   Major AG, Pitty LP, Farah CS. Cancer stem cell markers in head and neck squamous cell carcinoma. Stem Cells Int 2013; 2013: 1-13.
[http://dx.doi.org/10.1155/2013/319489] [PMID: 23533441]

[38]   Masciale V, Grisendi G, Banchelli F, *et al.* Isolation and identification of cancer stem-like cells in adenocarcinoma and squamous cell carcinoma of the lung: A pilot study. Front Oncol 2019; 9: 1394.
[http://dx.doi.org/10.3389/fonc.2019.01394] [PMID: 31921651]

[39]   Parmiani G. Melanoma cancer stem cells: Markers and functions. Cancers (Basel) 2016; 8(3): 34.
[http://dx.doi.org/10.3390/cancers8030034] [PMID: 26978405]

[40]   Munro MJ, Wickremesekera SK, Peng L, Tan ST, Itinteang T. Cancer stem cells in colorectal cancer: a review. J Clin Pathol 2018; 71(2): 110-6.
[http://dx.doi.org/10.1136/jclinpath-2017-204739] [PMID: 28942428]

[41]   Gzil A, Zarębska I, Bursiewicz W, Antosik P, Grzanka D, Szylberg Ł. Markers of pancreatic cancer stem cells and their clinical and therapeutic implications. Mol Biol Rep 2019; 46(6): 6629-45.
[http://dx.doi.org/10.1007/s11033-019-05058-1] [PMID: 31486978]

[42]   Moltzahn F, Thalmann GN. Cancer stem cells in prostate cancer. Transl Androl Urol 2013; 2(3): 242-53.
[PMID: 26816738]

[43]   Ricardo S, Vieira AF, Gerhard R, *et al.* Breast cancer stem cell markers CD44, CD24 and ALDH1: expression distribution within intrinsic molecular subtype. J Clin Pathol 2011; 64(11): 937-46.
[http://dx.doi.org/10.1136/jcp.2011.090456] [PMID: 21680574]

[44]   Ding Y, Gao H, Zhang Q. The biomarkers of leukemia stem cells in acute myeloid leukemia. Stem Cell Investig 2017; 4(3): 19.
[http://dx.doi.org/10.21037/sci.2017.02.10] [PMID: 28447034]

[45]   Takaishi S, Okumura T, Wang TC. Gastric cancer stem cells. J Clin Oncol 2008; 26(17): 2876-82.
[http://dx.doi.org/10.1200/JCO.2007.15.2603] [PMID: 18539967]

[46]   Abou-Antoun TJ, Hale JS, Lathia JD, Dombrowski SM. Brain cancer stem cells in adults and children: cell biology and therapeutic implications. Neurotherapeutics 2017; 14(2): 372-84.
[http://dx.doi.org/10.1007/s13311-017-0524-0] [PMID: 28374184]

[47]   Tran MN, Goodwin Jinesh G, McConkey DJ, Kamat AM. Bladder cancer stem cells. Curr Stem Cell Res Ther 2010; 5(4): 387-95.
[http://dx.doi.org/10.2174/157488810793351640] [PMID: 20955163]

[48]   Burgos-Ojeda D, Rueda BR, Buckanovich RJ. Ovarian cancer stem cell markers: Prognostic and therapeutic implications. Cancer Lett 2012; 322(1): 1-7.
[http://dx.doi.org/10.1016/j.canlet.2012.02.002] [PMID: 22334034]

[49]    Horton SJ, Huntly BJP. Recent advances in acute myeloid leukemia stem cell biology. Haematologica 2012; 97(7): 966-74.
        [http://dx.doi.org/10.3324/haematol.2011.054734] [PMID: 22511496]

[50]    Organista-Nava J, Gómez-Gómez Y, Garibay-Cerdenares OL, Leyva-Vázquez MA, Illades-Aguiar B. Cervical cancer stem cell-associated genes: Prognostic implications in cervical cancer. Oncol Lett 2019; 18(1): 7-14.
        [http://dx.doi.org/10.3892/ol.2019.10307] [PMID: 31289465]

[51]    Greco A, Rizzo MI, De Virgilio A, *et al.* Cancer stem cells in laryngeal cancer: what we know. Eur Arch Otorhinolaryngol 2016; 273(11): 3487-95.
        [http://dx.doi.org/10.1007/s00405-015-3837-9] [PMID: 26585332]

[52]    Wei P, Niu M, Pan S, *et al.* Cancer stem-like cell: a novel target for nasopharyngeal carcinoma therapy. Stem Cell Res Ther 2014; 5(2): 44.
        [http://dx.doi.org/10.1186/scrt433] [PMID: 25158069]

[53]    Harada K, Pool Pizzi M, Baba H, Shanbhag ND, Song S, Ajani JA. Cancer stem cells in esophageal cancer and response to therapy. Cancer 2018; 124(20): 3962-4.
        [http://dx.doi.org/10.1002/cncr.31697] [PMID: 30368777]

[54]    Baillie R, Tan ST, Itinteang T. Cancer stem cells in oral cavity squamous cell carcinoma: A review. Front Oncol 2017; 7: 112.
        [http://dx.doi.org/10.3389/fonc.2017.00112] [PMID: 28626726]

[55]    Chen D, Wang CY. Targeting cancer stem cells in squamous cell carcinoma. Precis Clin Med 2019; 2(3): 152-65.
        [http://dx.doi.org/10.1093/pcmedi/pbz016] [PMID: 31598386]

[56]    Gao M, Kong Y, Yang G, Gao L, Shi J. Multiple myeloma cancer stem cells. Oncotarget 2016; 7(23): 35466-77.
        [http://dx.doi.org/10.18632/oncotarget.8154] [PMID: 27007154]

[57]    Ghani FI, Yamazaki H, Iwata S, *et al.* Identification of cancer stem cell markers in human malignant mesothelioma cells. Biochem Biophys Res Commun 2011; 404(2): 735-42.
        [http://dx.doi.org/10.1016/j.bbrc.2010.12.054] [PMID: 21163253]

[58]    Corrò C, Moch H. Biomarker discovery for renal cancer stem cells. J Pathol Clin Res 2018; 4(1): 3-18.
        [http://dx.doi.org/10.1002/cjp2.91] [PMID: 29416873]

[59]    Manohar R, Li Y, Fohrer H, *et al.* Identification of a candidate stem cell in human gallbladder. Stem Cell Res (Amst) 2015; 14(3): 258-69.
        [http://dx.doi.org/10.1016/j.scr.2014.12.003] [PMID: 25765520]

[60]    Sheikh A, Alvi AA, Aslam HM, Haseeb A. Hedgehog pathway inhibitors – current status and future prospects. Infect Agent Cancer 2012; 7(1): 29.
        [http://dx.doi.org/10.1186/1750-9378-7-29] [PMID: 23116301]

[61]    Espinoza I, Miele L. Notch inhibitors for cancer treatment. Pharmacol Ther 2013; 139(2): 95-110.
        [http://dx.doi.org/10.1016/j.pharmthera.2013.02.003] [PMID: 23458608]

[62]    Zhang Y, Wang X. Targeting the Wnt/β-catenin signaling pathway in cancer. J Hematol Oncol 2020; 13(1): 165.
        [http://dx.doi.org/10.1186/s13045-020-00990-3] [PMID: 33276800]

[63]    Kishore C, Sundaram S, Karunagaran D. Vitamin K3 (menadione) suppresses epithelial-mesenchymal-transition and Wnt signaling pathway in human colorectal cancer cells. Chem Biol Interact 2019; 309: 108725.
        [http://dx.doi.org/10.1016/j.cbi.2019.108725] [PMID: 31238027]

[64]    Huang CY, Chung CL, Hu TH, Chen JJ, Liu PF, Chen CL. Recent progress in TGF-β inhibitors for cancer therapy. Biomed Pharmacother 2021; 134: 111046.

[http://dx.doi.org/10.1016/j.biopha.2020.111046] [PMID: 33341049]

[65]   Quintás-Cardama A, Verstovsek S. Molecular pathways: Jak/STAT pathway: mutations, inhibitors, and resistance. Clin Cancer Res 2013; 19(8): 1933-40.
[http://dx.doi.org/10.1158/1078-0432.CCR-12-0284] [PMID: 23406773]

[66]   Mishra R, Patel H, Alanazi S, Kilroy MK, Garrett JT. PI3K Inhibitors in Cancer: Clinical Implications and Adverse Effects. Int J Mol Sci 2021; 22(7): 3464.
[http://dx.doi.org/10.3390/ijms22073464] [PMID: 33801659]

**CHAPTER 3**

# Importance of Natural Compounds Targeting the Mitophagic Process in Breast Cancer Treatment

Prathibha Sivaprakasam[1], Karthikeyan Chandrabose[2], Sureshkumar Anandasadagopan[3], Hariprasth Lakshmanan[4] and Ashok Kumar Pandurangan[1,*]

[1] *School of Life Sciences, B.S. Abdur Rahman Crescent Institute of Science and Technology, Seethakathi Estate, GST road, Vandalur-600048, Chennai, Tamil Nadu, India*

[2] *Department of Pharmacy, Indira Gandhi National Tribal University, Amarkantak, Madhya Pradesh, India*

[3] *Department of Biochemistry and Biotechnology Lab, CSIR-Central Leather Research Institute (CLRI), Adyar, Chennai, India*

[4] *Department of Biochemistry, School of Life Sciences - Ooty Campus, JSS Academy of Higher Education and Research, Mysuru, Karnataka, India*

**Abstract:** Breast cancer is a serious concern among women and the second most common cancer worldwide with an estimated 2.3 million new cases reported in the year 2020 alone. Most breast cancers are *carcinomas*, which can be further classified into invasive and *in-situ* carcinomas depending on their infiltrating ability. Also, another classification of breast cancers exists based on the presence or absence of hormone receptors on the cell surface namely Triple-negative breast cancer (TNBC), Basal-like BC, Claudin low, HER2+, Luminal A and Luminal B. The diagnosis and treatment for the above-mentioned subtypes prove to be quite challenging. A special form of autophagy in which the damaged or defective mitochondria are detected by the autophagy machinery and are finally digested by the lysosomes is known as mitophagy. Recent investigations have reported that the mechanisms governing mitochondrial activities are critical for cancer therapy. Since most of the chemically synthesised drugs in recent times have not been shown to increase the overall survival rates in BC patients and on the contrary have resulted in many side effects, new strategies, and innovative chemo-preventive agents are required to augment the efficacy of existing cancer regimens. Phytochemicals, naturally occurring plant compounds, are important sources for new medications in cancer therapies which may thus prove to be better than their existing chemotherapeutic counterparts. Hence, the incorporation of such phytochemicals favouring mitophagic dysregulations alongside existing treatment regimes (endocrine therapy, chemotherapy, surgical exclusions) may prove to be effective in minimizing the side effects associated with these treatments.

\* **Corresponding author Ashok Kumar Pandurangan:** School of Life Sciences, B.S. Abdur Rahman Crescent Institute of Science and Technology, Seethakathi Estate, GST road, Vandalur-600048, Chennai, Tamil Nadu, India; E-mail: panduashokkumar@gmail.com

**Ashok Kumar Pandurangan (Ed.)**

**Keywords:** Breast cancer, Chemo-preventive agents, Mitophagy, Natural compounds, Triple negative breast cancer.

## INTRODUCTION

Cancer is a unique disease that can occur in different parts of the human body. Breast Cancer (BC) is very common in women and is better defined as the unchecked growth of malignant cells in the mammary epithelial tissues. This disease affects both genders, however, it is more predominant among females and its incidence rises dramatically with age [1]. Various studies have shown that lung cancer in the male population is seconded by breast cancer in women proving to be the main source of cancer-related mortality across the globe, with almost 1.7 million new cases and 521,900 deaths in 2012 alone, when contrasted with 1.38 million new cases and 458,000 deaths during 2008 [2, 3]. This records around 25% of all new disease cases and 15% of all cancer-related deaths among women [2, 4, 5]. An expected 231,840 (29%) new instances of the invasive form of breast cancer were analysed among females in the US during 2015, in contrast to 105,590 (13%) instances of lung cancers in a similar populace [6].

BC is a diverse condition with promising prospects with many biochemical modifications that occur throughout the disease's course. Similar to developments in other cancer types, current advances in tumour sequencing technology have led to the discovery of molecular targets and pathways that are engaged in the carcinogenesis development of BC and the advancement of the tumor [7, 8].

Mitophagy is an adaptive response that is reported to be induced by various stress factors thereby eventually aiding in the removal of damaged mitochondria [9]. When it pertains to carcinogenesis, autophagy, and mitochondrial clearance seem to function as a process that is recruited on demand by growing cancer cells in order to alter significant malignant characteristics throughout cancer onset and progression [10]. In recent years, there has been increasing evidence that mitophagy pathways are important regulators of cancer cell mitochondrial mass and dynamics, redox homeostasis, bioenergetics, oncogene-driven metabolic transformation, and cell death signals. This is associated with the fact that mitochondrial biology and metabolic adaptability are critical in the progression of cancer as well as in response to anticancer treatments. There is a growing consensus that mitophagy is a highly adaptable system that assists cancer cells in their metabolic transformations and survival inside the hostile tumour microenvironment [9].

Chemotherapeutic drugs harbour their advantages and drawbacks. Therefore, the National Comprehensive Cancer Network (NCCN) recommends combination therapy of anti-cancer drugs. Chemotherapy, however, has negative effects on both malignant and normal cells. Recent findings have proven that chemotherapy for breast cancer might induce cardiotoxicity [11].

Flavonoids, alkaloids, polysaccharides, essential oils, quinonoids, terpenoids, coumarins, and saponins are endogenous chemical components of plant extracts. Numerous researchworks have shown that natural plant compounds have anti-inflammatory, antiviral, antioxidant, neuroprotective, and cardioprotective characteristics [12]. Many *in vitro* and *in vivo* research, as well as clinical trials, have shown that natural products possess anticarcinogenic and chemo-preventive benefits on malignant cells involving DNA repair, cell proliferation, differentiation, apoptosis, carcinogen metabolism, angiogenesis, and progression. Hence, the synergistic effects of natural products and chemotherapeutic medicines eventually reduce toxicity and drug resistance [11]. This review thus highlights the treatment strategies for breast cancer, their negative impacts, the role of mitophagy in breast cancer, and the use of various natural compounds as effective drugs against mitophagy to hinder tumor progression.

## Breast Cancer Statistics

As per a precise examination of BC cases in 187 nations worldwide, the frequency of breast malignancy expanded from 641,000 cases in 1980 to 1,643,000 cases in 2010, suggesting a yearly increment of 3.1% [13]. It served as an important reason for malignancy-related mortality in ladies in the less developed regions (324,000 deaths accounting for 14.3% of the aggregate) and is presently considered the second most incessant reason for cancer-related deaths in females in developing countries too (198,000 deaths accounting to 15.4%) [2]. However, the rate of incidence greatly differed across nations like Northern America, Australia, and New Zealand having a higher occurrence in contrast with Africa and Asia having a lower incidence [3]. Though Europe reported the maximum BC cases with individual nations like Belgium and Denmark (119.9 and 105.0 per 100,000 separately) exceeding the incidence table (IARC 2014), North American and West European countries reported the maximum cases in region-wise distribution. The last occurrence was seen in Eastern Asia and Central America. Despite the fact that frequency rates stayed most elevated in the developed countries, mortality was generally a lot higher in the less developed regions [4]. According to recent reports, although the well-developed nations account for around 2.3 million new BC cases, approximately only 6,85,000 cases have been reported as mortality [2, 5].

Various surveys state that patterns in occurrence are influenced by ethnicity and age in various populations. For instance, in developing nations it had been accounted that females of reproductive age were twice as liable to develop BC than females aged 50 and above, accounting for nearly 66% of cases worldwide [13]. In the USA, the BC incidence rate diminished nearly 7% among the white populace from 2002 to 2003 and stayed stable from 2007 to 2011. However, it had a 0.3% upsurge (annual rate) among the black populace during 2007 and 2011 [6]. Various studies conducted in Sweden [14] and Iraq [15] reported that age and ethnicity play a pivotal role in BC diagnosis.

An ongoing statistical study (2019) being conducted in the United States reports that nearly 268,600 new instances of the invasive form of BC and 48,100 instances of Ductal Carcinoma *In Situ* (DCIS) may be diagnosed and also that 41,760 mortality may occur from this. Another important study states that nearly 82% of women aged greater than fifty years of age, develop BC and approximately 90% of BC-related mortality occurs in this age group [16].

As indicated by Globocan in the year 2012, India, the United States, and China together record approximately 33% of the BC burden worldwide. India accounted for an 11.54% increment and 13.82% mortality in the BC cases during 2008-2012 [2, 3]. This upsurge in the mortality rate is attributed to the dearth of BC screening, diagnosis only in the advanced stage, and insufficiency in proper medical facilities.

## Breast Cancer and Indian Scenario

As per the survey conducted by the Indian Council of Medical Research (ICMR) in metropolitan cities from 1982 to 2005, the incidence of BC has nearly doubled [17], and also the BC incidence seen in Indian females is a decade younger (premenopausal age) than the Western population [12 - 15].

The Population Based Cancer Registries (PBCRs) in India have accounted for various factors such as industrialization, fast urbanization, aging, and an increase in population to influence the incidence and death of BC cases. Also, BMI, obesity, waist-to-hip proportion, low parity, breastfeeding, negligence in physical activity and diet, liquor and tobacco consumption, smoking, marital status, locality (urban/rural), lack of awareness, illiteracy, lack of early diagnostic aids, monetary constraints and certain environmental factors were believed to pose as significant factors contributing to the increase in BC incidence [18]. However, the development of BC in women of younger age is yet unidentified. Another important factor is that a larger part of patients here are diagnosed only at a progressed and metastatic stage of BC. Hence a multidisciplinary strategy is the need of the hour to treat BC to reduce both its incidence and mortality among the Indian population, which may include conducting improved awareness programs, up taking preventive measures, organizing screening programs for early diagnosis and accessibility of treatment facilities [19].

## Mitophagy

Latest trend in research focuses on mitochondria and its role in cancer genesis and progression. Contradicting the Warburg hypothesis where mitochondria are portrayed as a silent organelle, they seem to be hyperactive in promoting tumor cell survival *via* malignant reprograming of various tumor-related genes thereby supplying the tumorigenic environment with surplus energy for tumorigenesis, regulation of redox homeostasis and effectively suppressing necrosis and apoptosis [20].

Intrinsic features of mitochondrial activity in cancer cells cause tumorigenic cells to be selectively modified, including variations in the mitochondrial membrane potential ($\Delta\psi$m), which provides a putative target for anti-cancer treatment. Mitochondrial redox conjugated to triphenylphosphonium (TPP) molecules leverage these variations and accumulate as a selective therapeutic strategy within the mitochondria.

Mitophagy is believed to be context-dependent in a tumorigenic environment as it is mainly influenced by the metabolic needs and the cancer stage. In normal cells, before undergoing neoplastic transformations, mitophagy is anti-tumorigenic in nature as it is involved in selective degradation of mitochondria that are dysfunctional and prevent Reactive Oxygen Species (ROS) accumulation that possibly triggers cancers. However, in cancer cells, mitophagy becomes a pro-survival strategy when the mitochondria are specifically targeted with compounds that are prone to induce apoptosis and necrosis [21].

The therapeutic efficiency of chemotherapy (CT) may be improved by controlling mitophagy through pharmacological approaches by using drugs that are non-toxic inducers of mitophagy like Urolithin A [22] and the p62-mediated mitophagy inducer (PMI) [23]. However surprisingly, anti-mitophagic molecules like the mitochondrial translocator protein (TSPO) are overexpressed only in aggressive cancer forms implying that molecular mitophagy control is embedded in the disease's pathophysiology.

Drug resistance limits the efficacy of CT despite the fact that it is the most widely used BC treatment strategy owing to factors like drug target alterations, pro-survival pathway inductions, and dysfunctional cell death inductions [24, 25]. Hence, anti-cancer drug sensitivity enhancement through new specific targets in order to suppress drug resistance has been effectively under study for the past few decades [26].

Mitophagy is a selective autophagic process that promotes tumorigenesis and cell survival in various tumors by eliminating dysfunctional mitochondria [21].

Oxidative stress and faulty mitochondria are the main reasons contributing to the toxicity of various chemotherapeutic drugs [22, 23], and the drug resistance in cancer cells is believed to be owing to the mitophagic removal of such damaged mitochondria [26]. However, excessive mitochondrial depletion in cells may instigate cell metabolic disorders and even cell death [27]. Hence, mitophagy likely assumes a dual role in resistance to cancer drugs mainly relying upon cell types and various other conditions.

## Mitophagy and Cancer

Expanding proof from different investigations has proven that mitophagic dysregulation in tumorigenesis is an etiological factor. Mutations in the Parkin gene lead to mitochondrial damage resulting from elevated levels of ROS and also hinder mitophagy progression [28]. Various cancer types have been reported for the PARK2 gene (Parkin) mutations, which are located in the FRA6E, 6q26 region of chromosome 6. Recent research-oriented experiments have proven that mitophagic inhibition promotes tumorigenesis whereas functional mitophagy facilitates the progression of tumors [29].

### *Mutations in PARK2 (Parkin)*

Dysfunctional mitochondria are polyubiquitinated with the aid of Parkin, an E3 ubiquitin ligase. Juvenile autosomal-recessive Parkinsonism is associated with homozygous mutations in the PARK2 or PARK6 genes [30]. The PARK2 gene is situated at the most vulnerable site of chromosome 6 (FRA6E, 6q26) eventually making it susceptible to all kinds of genetic mutations [31]. To emphasize the above statement, studies on various cell lines displayed enhanced tumorigenesis, and the knockout mice model (Parkin knockout) is more susceptible to cancers of the liver [32, 33]. Many cancer types including colon, gliomas, lung, and melanoma harbour PARK2 aberrations [30, 31, 34 - 37], suggesting that the PARK2 gene is tumor suppressive in nature [38]. A recent study was performed on the PARK2 gene of the XTC.UC1 cells and Hürthle tumor cells revealed the presence of a homozygous point mutation where valine was substituted with leucine (V380 L) resulting in auto-ubiquitination malfunctioning and Parkin's suppressed E3 ligase functioning [39]. However, when a wild-type Parkin gene was introduced into the XTC.UC1 cells, it eventually sensitized the cells to cell death *via* membrane depolarization thereby emphasizing the fact that an increase in tumorigenesis is observed when the PARK2 gene undergoes mutations.

## Mitophagy Mediated by HIF1α - BNIP3, NIX, and FUNDC1

### *HIF1α and the Tumor Microenvironment*

In general, the tumor microenvironment of solid tumors is profoundly hypoxic leading to the upregulation of an ACE transcriptional controller of hypoxic reactions namely - HIF1α. The potential of metastasis and the progression of cancerous cells, along with the sustenance of Cancer Stem Cells (CSCs) are greatly enhanced owing to the favourable hypoxic tumor microenvironment [40, 41]. PARK2 mutations inhibit mitophagy in tumorigenesis, whereas, aberrations in BCL2 Interacting Protein 3 (BNIP3) facilitate functionally active mitophagy during metastasis and tumor progression, which is better explained by the fact that the diminished agility of the cancer cells is solely because of the mitochondrial damages incurred by the cells during the start of tumorigenesis [42]. On the contrary, in the sense of tumour progression, NIX and FUNDC1 have not been thoroughly analysed, and need further study. Hence, enhanced mitophagy during cancer progression might be an adaptive response by cancerous cells to strengthen their survival rates [41, 42].

### *BNIP3 and NIX in Cancer Mitophagy*

Reports state that an LC3 Interacting Region (LIR) present in the BNIP3 and NIX genes is associated with Atg8 in hypoxic conditions and induces mitophagy *via* HIF1α [43], however, the part played by BNIP3 in cancer progression and tumorigenesis is still ambiguous. ShRNA lentiviral knockdown of the BNIP3 gene decreased cell proliferation and vascular mimicry in a melanoma cell line by restructuring the cytoskeletal actin thereby depicting its pro-tumorigenic role [44]. In a similar manner, the upregulation of BNIP3 in hepatocellular tumor cells was induced by ERK/HIF1α while the mTOR/S6K1 pathway was suppressed to activate autophagy and increase anoikis resistance [45]. In addition, hypoxia-induced over-expression of BNIP3 was reported in the adenoid cystic tumor cells, whereas autophagic inhibition led to suppressed invasion of tumours [46].

Various other studies conducted on BNIP3 portray it as a prominent cancer suppressor gene possessing many anti-cancer features, which was confirmed in mice models, where faulty BNIP3 expressions lead to mitophagic irregularities, eventually leading to increased metastasis of mammary tumorigenesis [47]. It is also reported that an increased level of aggressiveness was seen in pancreatic cell lines, in which BNIP3 was epigenetically silenced [48], which was confirmed through immunohistochemical results of samples obtained from the pancreas of cancer patients [46]. Research findings also stated that the survival rates were very low in nearly 59% of patients who exhibited undetectable/trace levels of BNIP3 expressions and the only rational answer stated is that BNIP3 can be spliced alternatively by exon 3 removal, ultimately yielding a short splice version with PKM2-dependent survival properties [46, 47]. Hence, it is proved that BNIP3 likely acts as a suppressor gene with its erratic transcriptional regulation *via* Sp3 and alternative splicing activities imposing it with pro-tumorigenic properties [48, 49], yet, unlike BNIP3, NIX's position in cancer progression remains largely unclear, and further analysis is needed.

## *FUNDC1 in Cancer Mitophagy*

FUNDC1's significance in cancer-related mitophagy is not as clear as its role in hypoxia-associated mitophagy, as it was only recently discovered in 2012. Nevertheless, extensive research on its function in the future can possibly highlight new cancer mitophagy study targets. A recent study states that being a special receptor of the mitochondrial membrane (outer), FUNDC1 binds to LC3 with the aid of its LIR motif triggering mitophagy (hypoxia-induced) [50]. Mitochondrial uncouplers and hypoxic condition favour the upregulation and translocation of ULK1 - a crucial mitophagy regulator, into dysfunctional mitochondria where phosphorylation of FUNDC1 occurs (ULK1 aided) at serine 17 permitting LC3- FUNDC1 binding. Extensive study in this regard also enlightened the finding that mitophagy, which is hypoxia-mediated is effectively regulated by the BCL2L1-PGAM5-FUNDC1 axis [51]. Similar findings reveal that FUNDC1's mitophagic property is greatly influenced by the status of phosphorylation of Tyr18 in the LIR region, which assumes the role of a 'Molecular Switch' [52]. FUNDC1's molecular pathways have only recently started to unravel and it remains to be seen if FUNDC1 can still play a major role in the mitophagy of cancer.

## KRAS Mutations and Cancer Mitophagy

A proto-oncogene of immense significance is KRAS, which generally undergoes single nucleotide aberrations leading to its hyperactivation [53], induction of the PI3K proliferative pathway, and GLUT1 stimulation, which acts as a metabolic switch in aerobic glycolysis [54, 55]. Generally, pancreatic, colorectal, and lung tumors express mutations in the KRAS gene [56, 57]. Numerous research findings emphasise that an increase in autophagy-mediated tumor progression is seen in cancer forms with KRAS mutations. One such study conducted on the Rat2 cells with oncogenic KRASV12 mutations proved the restoration of normal mitochondrial respiratory functions through autophagic hindrance and these findings were further validated with correlative data displaying increased LC3-II levels in hepatocellular tumor cells with diminished glucose levels and KRAS[V12] mutations [58, 59]. Further studies conducted on mice models harbouring non-small lung cancer cells reported that the carcinoma and adenoma form of cells changed to a more benign but rare condition of oncocytoma cells, owing to the loss of Atg7 as a result of KRAS$^{G12D}$ gene upregulation. However, an increase in the number of damaged mitochondria was observed in the above-stated case [60]. In a similar manner, lung tumor progression was found to be impaired in Atg5 mutant mice exhibiting KRAS$^{G12D}$ aberrations [61]. Therefore, it is evident that increased mitophagy-mediated cancer progression is observed in tumors with KRAS mutations, which is unlike the case in normal tumor environments where mitophagy hinders progression during tumorigenesis.

## Biological Role of Mitophagy

Cells have developed complex mechanisms to sustain cellular homeostasis and one among the many ways is mitophagy, a catabolic pathway that selectively degrades excessive or damaged mitochondria, proteins, and other organelles within lysosomes [62] by autophagy in response to different stresses [63, 64]. Unlike canonical autophagy, only those mitochondria expressing mitophagic receptors on its surface are targeted *via* mitophagy. The best examples for this include the lipid-mediated system (ceramide), the microtubule-related proteins 1 light chain 3 (LC3)-interacting region (LIR)-linked receptor system [*e.g.*, B-cell lymphoma 2 (BCL2) protein-interacting protein 3 (BNIP3) and BNIP3-like (BNIP3L)] and the Parkin/PTEN-induced putative kinase 1 (PINK1) receptor system [65]. The process of mitophagy signaling in mammalian cells is represented in Fig. (**1**).

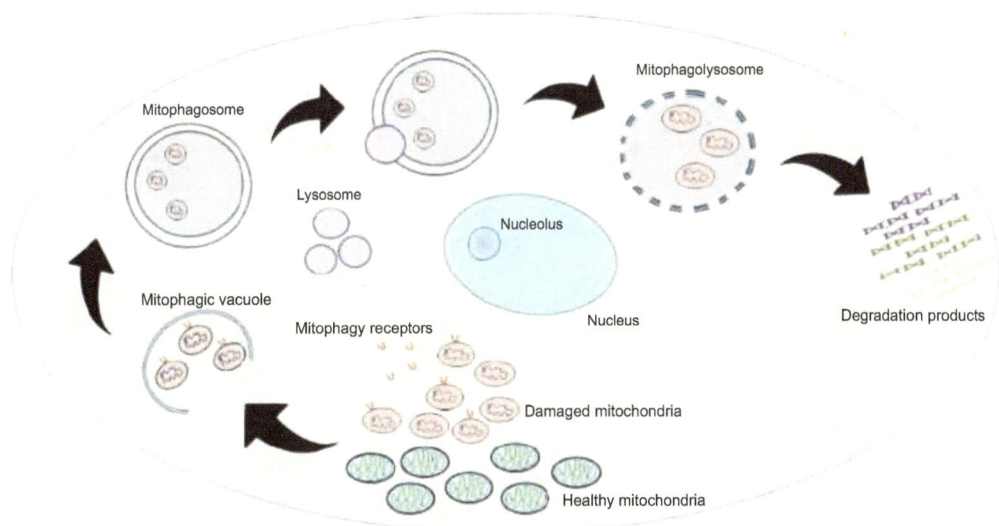

**Fig. (1).** The process of mitophagy in mammalian cells.

In response to different stress conditions, autophagy may serve as a survival mechanism for cancer cells but the role of canonical autophagy in cancer is still unexplained clearly [66, 67]. Mitophagy can be associated with numerous physiological mechanisms and disorders and a few of the best examples owing to a deficient mitophagic pathway include cardiac ailments, the onset of Parkinson's disease, and an impaired natural killer cell's memory [68, 69]. Additionally, recent research proves that mitophagic dysfunction also induces tumorigenesis and neoplastic upregulation [70] and the induction of mitophagy in macrophages has also been reported to prevent the progression of colitis-associated cancer [71]. It has also been reported that the ROS from the mitochondria plays an important role in metastasis and tumorigenesis [72] and that the loss of BNIP3 and the consequent mitophagic dysfunction contribute to ROS increment and metastasis of the mammary neoplastic progression [70, 71].

## Manipulating Mitophagy as a Potential Target for Cancer Therapy

The realm of anti-cancer therapy has now included studying various autophagic regulators like hydro chloroquine and chloroquine, which are presently in their clinical phases [71]. Though a little vague, various studies on cancer therapy improvement involving mitophagic pathway manipulations are also underway [70, 71]. The clinical outcome of apoptosis/necrosis induced *via* mitophagy or cancer-therapy-dependent cell survival is based on the various clinical therapies used and also on the type of cells. Fig. (2) shows the role of mitophagy signaling in cancer and resistance to chemotherapeutic drugs.

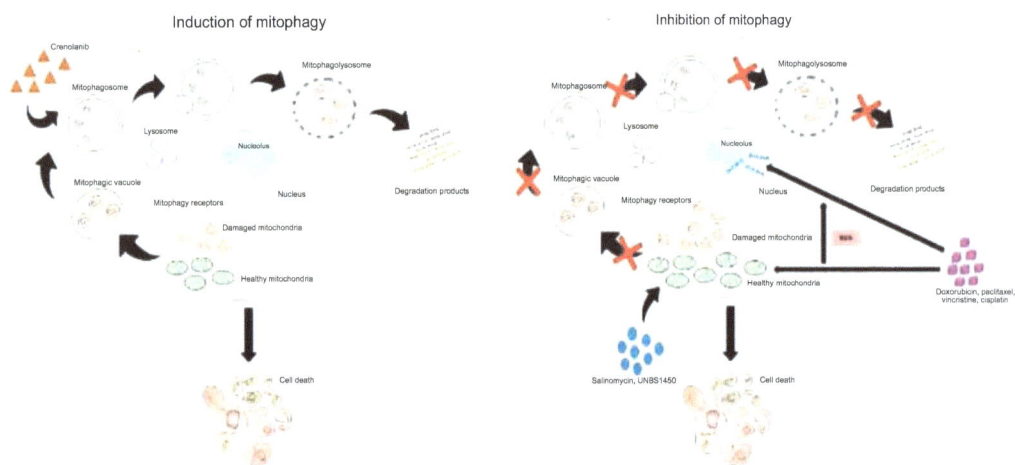

**Fig. (2).** The controversial role of mitophagy in cancer drug resistance.

## Induction of Mitophagy Increases Cancer Cell Death and Chemotherapy Sensitivity

One of the significant molecules that are involved in the effective regulation of mitophagy is Ceramide, which is also an important candidate for sphingolipid metabolism [72]. Recent findings have elaborated that CerS1/C18-ceramide specifically mediates lethal mitophagy, which is B-cell lymphoma 2-related X (BAX)/BCL2 antagonist/killer 1 (BAK1)- and is also caspase-independent. Ceramide enables lipidated LC3 formation, which, with the aid of Dynamin-Related Protein 1 (DRP1)-mediated mitochondrial fission, binds to ceramide on the mitochondrial membrane, effectively targeting autophagolysosomes to mitochondria and eventually inducing lethal mitophagy in tumor cells [73, 74]. Cell death and other related metabolic disorders in a tumorigenic environment are induced when extensive mitochondrial depletion without proper mitochondrial biogenesis or metabolic plasticity takes place [75]. The myocytes present in the cardiac tissue initiate a protective response by triggering DRP1-mediated fission induced by BNIP3, which is also an essential step for mitophagy [76]. However, elucidation of the fundamental mechanism of multiple effects of DRP1 between cancer cells and myocytes of the cardiovascular tissues will aid in better development of anticancer drugs.

Immature hematopoietic cells express a membrane-bound receptor tyrosine kinase - FMS-like tyrosine kinase 3 (FLT3) and mutations in this FLT3 region, in patients (nearly 30%) with Acute Myelogenous Leukaemia (AML), have been reported recently emphasizing the fact that an Internal Tandem Duplication (ITD) is the most common form of FLT3 mutation in the juxtamembrane region (FLT3-ITD) [77, 78]. Crenolanib, sorafenib, and quizartinib (AC220) are prominent FLT3-ITD inhibitors that demonstrated efficient results against treatment in preclinical models of AML, however not in clinical phase trials as they had gained drug resistance by then [79, 80]. But interestingly, a ceramide analogue drug, which is also mitochondria-targeted (LCL-461) has successfully proven to minimize crenolanib resistance by instigating deadly mitophagy in FLT3-ITD+ AML in both *in vitro* and *in vivo* scenarios [81, 82]. Considering this mode of induction of the lethal mitophagy by ceramide and ceramide-like drugs, the FLT3-ITD+ AML is likely to become a potential target for other cancer types as well and extensive research in this field is warranted.

### Inhibition of Mitophagy Enhances Drug Sensitivity

A large number of studies have shown that genetic and pharmacological targeting of various stages of the autophagic/mitophagic mechanism can effectively downregulate mitophagy. The best examples in this regard include: silencing

BNIP3, BNIP3L, Parkin, PINK1 and autophagy-related 5 (ATG5) mitophagic/autophagic genes [72, 73], administration of LY294002 and 3-methyladenine which are excellent inhibitors of phosphoinositide-3-kinase (PI3K) that prevent autophagosomes formation [83, 84] and making use of drugs like bafilomycin A1, liensinine, chloroquine and leupeptin, which possess the efficacy in autophagolysosome degradation and prevention of lysosome-autophagosomes fusion [85 - 87].

## Classical Inhibitors of Mitophagy

An efficient DNA-damaging agent and the most common drug of choice for cancer treatment is Doxorubicin, which induces toxicity in cancer cells *via* upregulation of mitochondrial dysfunction and excessive superoxide formation [80, 88]. Studies have shown that post doxorubicin treatment in colorectal tumor stem cells, the levels of the mitophagic regulator BNIP3L were increased but on the contrary, the sensitivity of colorectal tumor stem cells towards doxorubicin was enhanced when mitophagy was inhibited *via* silencing the BNIP3L gene [89].

Apart from being a prominent coccidiostat ionophore and antibacterial drug of choice, Salinomycin is known to possess anti-cancer activity *via* mitochondrial hyperpolarization. Activation of mitochondrial dynamic fusion and fission processes in salinomycin-treated cells contributes to changes in mitochondrial mass and the preservation of mitochondrial function, respectively. Hence, the damaged mitochondria are eliminated from the salinomycin-treated cells *via* mitophagy, which acts as the pro-survival mechanism of action owing to the reason that the damaged mitochondria devour excess ATP and liberate toxic ROS in abundance thereby stalling cellular homeostasis. Moreover, the sensitivity of both tumors and cancer stem cells towards salinomycin increased greatly when mitophagic inhibition was combined with ATG5 knockout [90].

There are actually a number of new medicines being investigated for anticancer therapies and in conjunction with such possible anticancer products are the mitophagic inhibitors, which effectively aid in improving the cytotoxicity. One such drug is the UNBS1450, which is a sodium channel antagonist and also a potent anti-cancer candidate. Apoptosis is stalled in the stromal neuroblastoma SH-N-AS cell line through mitophagy resulting in enhanced UNBS1450 resistance. Therefore, effective autophagic inhibition *via*, autophagy-related 7 (ATG7), Beclin-1and small inhibitory RNAs targeting ATG5 ultimately sensitizes the SK-N-AS cells by reactivating the apoptotic mode of cell death in them [91].

## Novel Inhibitors of Mitophagy

The seed embryo of *Nelumbo nucifera* is known as a rich source of an isoquinoline alkaloid - Liensinine, which efficiently sensitizes BC cells to various classical chemotherapeutic medications like paclitaxel, cisplatin, doxorubicin, and vincristine by inhibiting mitophagy. Liensinine was found to inhibit the fusion of lysosomes and autophagosomes thereby facilitating the accumulation of mitophagosomes. It was believed that liensinine shares the same mode of action as that of hydroxychloroquine, bafilomycin A1, and chloroquine, but differs in the mechanism of blockade of fusion of lysosome with autophagosome by altering (alkalinizing) the pH of the lysosomes and also significantly alters the activity of lysosomal hydrolases. Later studies however confirmed that the change in the lysosomal pH was independent of liensinine treatment and also that it is not essential for inhibition of autophagosome-lysosome fusion and cathepsin progression directed by liensinine [92]. A research study portrays the important role held by a small GTP-binding protein ras-related protein 7A (RAB7A) in the biogenesis of lysosomes, the final maturation of late autophagic vacuoles and also a crucial part in the late endocytic pathway [93]. But, the employment of RAB7A to lysosomes was hindered by liensinine thereby subsequently stalling the cathepsin transportation (endocytic pathway-dependent) into the lysosomes and also disrupting the fusion between the lysosomes and the autophagosomes [92], thereby proving the only possible mechanism of sensitizing cancerous cells to doxorubicin-initiated apoptosis as liensinine effectively halts mitophagy/ autophagy.

## Role of Natural Compounds in Mitophagy

Mitophagy is a major process needed for the proper maintenance of various cellular functions. Induction of mitophagy and the elimination of faulty mitochondria through mitophagy takes place in two steps: triggering of autophagy and autophagic recognition by damaged mitochondria removal [94, 95]. Researchers in the past few decades have developed an interest in studying the effects of different natural compounds (animal and vegetable origin) found in dietary sources [94]. In recent times, many of these natural compounds have been extensively examined for their capacity to control mitochondrial homeostasis. Recent findings from various experimental studies concerning the effects of different natural compounds on mitophagy are listed below:

### *Withaferin*

Withaferin A (WA) is extracted from *Withania somnifera* and is considered to be a prominent steroidal lactone. It displays an array of features including anti-cancer, Reactive Oxygen Species (ROS) modulation, and immune-modulatio-

-like primordial properties [96]. WA treatment in breast cancer cells effectively suppresses the assembling of Complex III and Poly-Ethylene-Glycol induced mitochondrial fusion. It was also found to reduce Optic Atrophy Protein 1 (OPA1), Mitofusin1 (Mfn1), and Mitofusin2 (Mfn2) expression levels, which are also found to be involved in the mitochondrial fusion process [97]. ROS-mediated paraptosis characterized by inflation of both mitochondria and endoplasmic reticulum, large vacuole formation, and inadequate apoptotic or autophagic morphology was observed in MCF-7 and MDA-MB-231 cells upon WA treatment, thereby proving its ability as a potential candidate in breast cancer treatment [98].

### Curcumin

Curcumin is a potent polyphenolic agent derived from *Curcuma longa* or turmeric, as it is known locally. It has been found to harbour umpteen anticancer effects on the onset and/or the development of various cancers. Many studies on curcumin report that it effectively enhances apoptosis and inhibits the proliferation of cancerous cells found in the colon, lungs, and breasts, and even in the prostate region. It also plays a pivotal role in various signalling pathways – HER2, ER, p53, NF-$\kappa$B, MAPK, Akt, Notch-1, Wnt/$\beta$-catenin, AP-1, JAK/STAT, AMPK/COX-2, Sonic Hedgehog and various other apoptotic signaling cascades [99].

Curcumin when administered alone or in combination with either radiation or chemotherapy alters the expression of many genes that are associated with apoptosis. In specific, it hinders the expression of Bcl-2 (anti-apoptotic gene) and enhances the caspase cascade, PUMA, and Bax expression levels (pro-apoptotic genes). An elaborate study on breast cancer stem cells reveals that curcumin enhances the sensitivity of mitomycin C leading to apoptosis *via* Bcl-2 [100]. Another finding emphasized that curcumin attenuates apoptosis receptor expression on the surface of cancer cells by interacting with ROS [99]. Upon curcumin treatment, TNBC cells (MDA-MB-231) displayed elevated levels of caspase 9 activity, Apaf-1, and also the liberation of cytochrome c, confirming that curcumin facilitates mitochondria-dependent mode of cell death [101].

### Gingerol

Gingerol is a therapeutically remarkable bioactive ingredient obtained from ginger, well known to have anti-diabetic, antioxidant, and anti-cancer-like properties. A detailed study on the effects of gingerol on cancer cells reveals that it triggers various morphological alterations such as DNA fragmentation and a substantial increase in TUNEL-positive cells. It also effectively led to the mitochondrial membrane potential depolarization and enhanced expression levels of PARP and caspase 3 [102].

## Thymoquinone

The active component obtained from the *Nigella sativa* seeds is Thymoquinone, which has been documented to exhibit anti-cancer, antioxidant, anti-inflammatory, and antimicrobial-like properties used to treat various ailments. Thymoquinone triggers apoptosis and prevents cell proliferation in numerous types of cancerous cells. Pre-treatment with thymoquinone and betulinic acid in conjunction with gemcitabine confers a synergistic role in suppressing the expression of PKM2 leading to cell proliferation hindrance [103, 104].

## Artepillin C

The Brazilian green propolis is known to harbour a predominant bioactive ingredient, namely Artepillin C, which exhibits significant antiproliferative, proapoptotic, antimetastatic, and cytotoxic traits [105]. Artepillin C was found to cause apoptosis in TRAIL-resistant LNCaP cells *via* both extrinsic (receptor-mediated) and intrinsic (mitochondrial) pathways. It upregulated TRAIL-R2 expression, downregulated NF-κB activity, activated caspases 3 & 8, and obstructed the mitochondrial membrane potential significantly [106]. Another similar study demonstrates that Artepillin C possesses antileukemic effects partly by obstructing the membrane potential of mitochondria and increasing the Fas antigen expression [105].

## Cucurbitacin B

Cucurbitacin B is a natural bioactive ingredient found copiously in cucumbers and in the traditional Chinese herbal medication - Pedicellus Melo, displays an anti-inflammatory effect and also suppresses tumor development in many cancers as a small molecule of STAT3 inhibitor [107]. It effectively hinders the phosphorylation of ACLY (ATP citrate lyase) and leads to apoptosis *via* the upregulation of the mitochondrial apoptotic pathway [108, 109].

## Triptolide

A potent diterpenoid triperoxide component – Triptolide, is found in the plant species *Tripterygium wilfordii Hook f.* which exhibits a wide range of anti-cancer traits. It has been reported that Triptolide influences the SIRT3-GSK-3β cascade thereby facilitating the translocation of Bax into the mitochondria, ultimately diminishing the membrane potential of mitochondria [110]. Recent findings state that by altering the NF-κB pathway (signaling), triptolide depolarizes the mitochondrial membrane and also achieves G2/M phase arrest in the cell cycle [111]. Similarly, acetylation of complexes I and II leading to their loss of enzyme activity and hindered mitochondrial translocation of SIRT3 from the cytosol is achieved in triptolide-treated p53-deficient tumor cells [112]. Another such study revealed that cancer cells upon triptolide administration lead to ROS production and Ca2+ release thereby triggering the G0/G1 phase cell cycle arrest that ends in apoptosis and autophagy of the cells [113].

## Allicin

Among the many functionally active ingredients obtained from freshly crushed garlic is allicin [114], which triggered the p-53-associated mode of cell death in tumor cells. Another finding confirmed that mitochondrial degradation was observed in allicin-treated cancer cells as it potentially hindered the PI3K/mTOR signaling pathway, suppressed the levels of p53 and Bcl-2 in the cytoplasm and upregulated Beclin-1 and AMPK pathways [115]. It was also reported that allicin effectively released cytochrome c, translocated Bax to the mitochondria, and led to the phosphorylation of the JNK-activated Bcl-2 family and ultimately to the upregulation of mitophagic pathways in treated tumor cells [116].

## Jolkinolide B

The roots of Euphorbia fischeriana Steud, harbour a potentially significant therapeutic compound - Jolkinolide B (JB), that hinders cancer progression *via* several pathways and mechanisms [117]. Studies conducted on various cancer cell lines prove that JB efficiently suppressed the membrane potential of mitochondria while enhancing the levels of $Ca^{2+}$ (both mitochondrial and intracellular) leading to apoptosis [118]. It was also found that JB suppressed the lactic acid production in tumor cells and also reduced the expression levels of Glut1, Glut3, Glut4, Ldh-a, Hk2, caspases 3& 9, Bcl-2 genes while enhancing the production of ROS and Bax expressions [117].

## Chalocomoracin

A unique phenomenon is observed in the mulberry leaves, which have been infected by a specific fungus, where, in order to curb further fungal germination, a significant bioactive compound (secondary metabolite) is produced-Chalocomoracin (CMR) [119]. Various studies conducted on CMR emphasise that it has a range of biological functions against a variety of pathogens, including MRSA (Methicillin-Resistant *Staphylococcus Aureus*), Rhinovirus, and even on human tumors [120].

Increased oxidative stress, calpain activity, and release of $Ca^{2+}$ in excess within the cells are observed when CMR is administered to MDA-MB-231 (TNBC) cells resulting in altered mitochondrial membrane potential. This in turn leads to the upregulation of PINK1 and activation of Parkin leading to ubiquitination of cells. Since the rate of division is greater in the tumor cells, excess ubiquitination occurs ultimately resulting in the accumulation of ubiquitinated proteins causing excessive damage in comparison to normal cells [119]. CMR-assisted vesicular vacuolation had also been witnessed which was associated with ER stress as a consequence of mitophagy triggered *via* ROS. Therefore, mitophagy from CMR treatment could be an innovative approach to cancer therapeutics [121].

## CONCLUSION

Conclusively, the above-listed research exploration brings into focus the mitochondrial life-cycle regulation as a key effector in cancer cell divergence and uncovers various therapeutic implications for the pharmacological calibration of mitophagy ultimately leading ways to conquer chemotherapeutic resistance. Extensive research shows that dietary bioactive compounds derived from natural sources are important in both preventing and curing cancers and many other ailments. They are believed to be substantially rich and vital sources for drug screening and also pivotal representatives in determining the actual molecular mechanisms in tumorous conditions. The regulatory properties of such naturally occurring products on mitophagy are exerted over multiple mechanisms and on several molecular targets, which indicates the potential usage of these compounds as therapeutic agents in several diseased conditions in relation to dysfunctional mitochondria resulting in mitophagy. Hence, detailed studies on the basic mechanisms may aid in designing and developing specified therapeutic agents and drastically diminish the side effects of these mediators.

## AUTHOR'S CONTRIBUTION

All the authors have contributed equally to the data collection, analysis, interpretation, writing and finalization of this review article.

## REFERENCES

[1]    Lukong KE. Understanding breast cancer – The long and winding road. BBA Clin 2017; 7: 64-77.
       [http://dx.doi.org/10.1016/j.bbacli.2017.01.001] [PMID: 28194329]

[2]    Ferlay J, Soerjomataram I, Dikshit R, *et al.* Cancer incidence and mortality worldwide: Sources, methods and major patterns in GLOBOCAN 2012. Int J Cancer 2015; 136(5): E359-86.
       [http://dx.doi.org/10.1002/ijc.29210] [PMID: 25220842]

[3]    Ferlay J, Shin HR, Bray F, Forman D, Mathers C, Parkin DM. Estimates of worldwide burden of cancer in 2008: GLOBOCAN 2008. Int J Cancer 2010; 127(12): 2893-917.
       [http://dx.doi.org/10.1002/ijc.25516] [PMID: 21351269]

[4]     International Agency for Research on Cancer. "World cancer factsheet." Cancer Research UK, 2014. Available from: http://www. cruk. org/cancerstats

[5]     Torre LA, Bray F, Siegel RL, Ferlay J, Lortet-Tieulent J, Jemal A. Global cancer statistics, 2012. CA Cancer J Clin 2015; 65(2): 87-108.
        [http://dx.doi.org/10.3322/caac.21262] [PMID: 25651787]

[6]     Cancer facts & figures 2015. American Cancer Society 2015.

[7]     Casasent AK, Edgerton M, Navin NE. Genome evolution in ductal carcinoma *in situ* : invasion of the clones. J Pathol 2017; 241(2): 208-18.
        [http://dx.doi.org/10.1002/path.4840] [PMID: 27861897]

[8]     Feng Y, Spezia M, Huang S, *et al.* Breast cancer development and progression: Risk factors, cancer stem cells, signaling pathways, genomics, and molecular pathogenesis. Genes Dis 2018; 5(2): 77-106.
        [http://dx.doi.org/10.1016/j.gendis.2018.05.001] [PMID: 30258937]

[9]     Vara-Perez M, Felipe-Abrio B, Agostinis P. Mitophagy in cancer: a tale of adaptation. Cells 2019; 8(5): 493.
        [http://dx.doi.org/10.3390/cells8050493] [PMID: 31121959]

[10]    Twig G, Shirihai OS. The interplay between mitochondrial dynamics and mitophagy. Antioxid Redox Signal 2011; 14(10): 1939-51.
        [http://dx.doi.org/10.1089/ars.2010.3779] [PMID: 21128700]

[11]    Zhang Y, Li H, Zhang J, *et al.* The combinatory effects of natural products and chemotherapy drugs and their mechanisms in breast cancer treatment. Phytochem Rev 2020; 19(5): 1179-97.
        [http://dx.doi.org/10.1007/s11101-019-09628-w]

[12]    Mohan A, Narayanan S, Sethuraman S, Maheswari Krishnan U. Combinations of plant polyphenols & anti-cancer molecules: a novel treatment strategy for cancer chemotherapy. Anticancer Agents Med Chem 2013; 13(2): 281-95.
        [http://dx.doi.org/10.2174/1871520611313020015] [PMID: 22721388]

[13]    Forouzanfar MH, Foreman KJ, Delossantos AM, *et al.* Breast and cervical cancer in 187 countries between 1980 and 2010: a systematic analysis. Lancet 2011; 378(9801): 1461-84.
        [http://dx.doi.org/10.1016/S0140-6736(11)61351-2] [PMID: 21924486]

[14]    Hemminki K, Mousavi SM, Sundquist J, Brandt A. Does the breast cancer age at diagnosis differ by ethnicity? A study on immigrants to Sweden. Oncologist 2011; 16(2): 146-54.
        [http://dx.doi.org/10.1634/theoncologist.2010-0104] [PMID: 21266400]

[15]    Majid RA, Mohammed HA, Hassan HA, Abdulmahdi WA, Rashid RM, Hughson MD. A population-based study of Kurdish breast cancer in northern Iraq: Hormone receptor and HER2 status. A comparison with Arabic women and United States SEER data. BMC Womens Health 2012; 12(1): 16.
        [http://dx.doi.org/10.1186/1472-6874-12-16] [PMID: 22727195]

[16]    Siegel RL, Miller KD, Jemal A. Cancer statistics, 2019. CA Cancer J Clin 2019; 69(1): 7-34.
        [http://dx.doi.org/10.3322/caac.21551] [PMID: 30620402]

[17]    Ali I, Wani WA, Saleem K. Cancer scenario in India with future perspectives. Cancer Ther. 2011; 8, 56–70.

[18]    Malvia S, Bagadi SA, Dubey US, Saxena S. Epidemiology of breast cancer in Indian women. Asia Pac J Clin Oncol 2017; 13(4): 289-95.
        [http://dx.doi.org/10.1111/ajco.12661] [PMID: 28181405]

[19]    Ju YS, Alexandrov LB, Gerstung M, Martincorena I, Nik-Zainal S, Ramakrishna M, *et al.* Origins and functional consequences of somatic mitochondrial DNA mutations in human cancer. Elife. 2014;3: 1–28.
        [http://dx.doi.org/10.7554/eLife.02935]

[20]    Chourasia AH, Boland ML, Macleod KF. Mitophagy and cancer. Cancer Metab 2015; 3(1): 4.

[http://dx.doi.org/10.1186/s40170-015-0130-8] [PMID: 25810907]

[21]   Ryu D, Mouchiroud L, Andreux PA, *et al.* Urolithin A induces mitophagy and prolongs lifespan in C. elegans and increases muscle function in rodents. Nat Med 2016; 22(8): 879-88.
       [http://dx.doi.org/10.1038/nm.4132] [PMID: 27400265]

[22]   East DA, Fagiani F, Crosby J, *et al.* PMI: a ΔΨm independent pharmacological regulator of mitophagy. Chem Biol 2014; 21(11): 1585-96.
       [http://dx.doi.org/10.1016/j.chembiol.2014.09.019] [PMID: 25455860]

[23]   Holohan C, Van Schaeybroeck S, Longley DB, Johnston PG. Cancer drug resistance: an evolving paradigm. Nat Rev Cancer 2013; 13(10): 714-26.
       [http://dx.doi.org/10.1038/nrc3599] [PMID: 24060863]

[24]   Fojo T, Bates S. Strategies for reversing drug resistance. Oncogene. 2003; 22(6): 7512–23.
       [http://dx.doi.org/10.1038/sj.onc.1206951]

[25]   Scatena R, Bottoni P, Botta G, Martorana GE, Giardina B. The role of mitochondria in pharmacotoxicology: a reevaluation of an old, newly emerging topic. Am J Physiol Cell Physiol 2007; 293(1): C12-21.
       [http://dx.doi.org/10.1152/ajpcell.00314.2006] [PMID: 17475665]

[26]   Fulda S, Galluzzi L, Kroemer G. Targeting mitochondria for cancer therapy. Nat Rev Drug Discov 2010; 9(6): 447-64.
       [http://dx.doi.org/10.1038/nrd3137] [PMID: 20467424]

[27]   Yan C, Luo L, Guo CY, *et al.* Doxorubicin-induced mitophagy contributes to drug resistance in cancer stem cells from HCT8 human colorectal cancer cells. Cancer Lett 2017; 388(December): 34-42.
       [http://dx.doi.org/10.1016/j.canlet.2016.11.018] [PMID: 27913197]

[28]   Kubli DA, Gustafsson ÅB. Mitochondria and Mitophagy. Circ Res 2012; 111(9): 1208-21.
       [http://dx.doi.org/10.1161/CIRCRESAHA.112.265819] [PMID: 23065344]

[29]   Bernardini JP, Lazarou M, Dewson G. Parkin and mitophagy in cancer. Oncogene 2017; 36(10): 1315-27.
       [http://dx.doi.org/10.1038/onc.2016.302] [PMID: 27593930]

[30]   Chang JY, Yi HS, Kim HW, Shong M. Dysregulation of mitophagy in carcinogenesis and tumor progression. Biochim Biophys Acta Bioenerg 2017; 1858(8): 633-40.
       [http://dx.doi.org/10.1016/j.bbabio.2016.12.008] [PMID: 28017650]

[31]   Shimura H, Hattori N, Kubo S, *et al.* Familial Parkinson disease gene product, parkin, is a ubiquitin-protein ligase. Nat Genet 2000; 25(3): 302-5.
       [http://dx.doi.org/10.1038/77060] [PMID: 10888878]

[32]   Matsuda S, Nakanishi A, Minami A, Wada Y, Kitagishi Y. Functions and characteristics of PINK1 and Parkin in cancer. Front Biosci (Landmark Ed) 2015; 20(3): 491-501.
       [http://dx.doi.org/10.2741/4321]

[33]   Tay SP, Yeo CWS, Chai C, *et al.* Parkin enhances the expression of cyclin-dependent kinase 6 and negatively regulates the proliferation of breast cancer cells. J Biol Chem 2010; 285(38): 29231-8.
       [http://dx.doi.org/10.1074/jbc.M110.108241] [PMID: 20630868]

[34]   Veeriah S, Taylor BS, Meng S, *et al.* Somatic mutations of the Parkinson's disease–associated gene PARK2 in glioblastoma and other human malignancies. Nat Genet 2010; 42(1): 77-82.
       [http://dx.doi.org/10.1038/ng.491] [PMID: 19946270]

[35]   D'Amico AG, Maugeri G, Magro G, Salvatorelli L, Drago F, D'Agata V. Expression pattern of parkin isoforms in lung adenocarcinomas. Tumour Biol 2015; 36(7): 5133-41.
       [http://dx.doi.org/10.1007/s13277-015-3166-z] [PMID: 25656612]

[36]   Maugeri G, Grazia D'Amico A, Maria Rasà D, *et al.* Expression profile of Wilms Tumor 1 (WT1) isoforms in undifferentiated and all-trans retinoic acid differentiated neuroblastoma cells. Genes

Cancer 2016; 7(1-2): 47-58.
[http://dx.doi.org/10.18632/genesandcancer.94] [PMID: 27014421]

[37]  Lee S, She J, Deng B, *et al.* Multiple-level validation identifies *PARK2* in the development of lung cancer and chronic obstructive pulmonary disease. Oncotarget 2016; 7(28): 44211-23.
[http://dx.doi.org/10.18632/oncotarget.9954] [PMID: 27329585]

[38]  Hu HH, Kannengiesser C, Lesage S, *et al.* PARKIN Inactivation Links Parkinson's Disease to Melanoma. J Natl Cancer Inst 2015; 108(3): 1-8.
[PMID: 26683220]

[39]  Poulogiannis G, McIntyre RE, Dimitriadi M, *et al. PARK2* deletions occur frequently in sporadic colorectal cancer and accelerate adenoma development in *Apc* mutant mice. Proc Natl Acad Sci USA 2010; 107(34): 15145-50.
[http://dx.doi.org/10.1073/pnas.1009941107] [PMID: 20696900]

[40]  Lee WJ, Chien MH, Chow JM, *et al.* Nonautophagic cytoplasmic vacuolation death induction in human PC-3M prostate cancer by curcumin through reactive oxygen species -mediated endoplasmic reticulum stress. Sci Rep 2015; 5(1): 10420.
[http://dx.doi.org/10.1038/srep10420] [PMID: 26013662]

[41]  Hill RP, Subarsky P. The hypoxic tumor microenvironment and metastatic progression. Clin Exp Metastasis 2015; 20: 237-50.
[http://dx.doi.org/10.1023/a:1022939318102]

[42]  Semenza GL. The hypoxic tumor microenvironment: A driving force for breast cancer progression. Biochim Biophys Acta Mol Cell Res 2016; 1863(3): 382-91.
[http://dx.doi.org/10.1016/j.bbamcr.2015.05.036] [PMID: 26079100]

[43]  Ray R, Chen G, Vande Velde C, *et al.* BNIP3 heterodimerizes with Bcl-2/Bcl-X(L) and induces cell death independent of a Bcl-2 homology 3 (BH3) domain at both mitochondrial and nonmitochondrial sites. J Biol Chem 2000; 275(2): 1439-48.
[http://dx.doi.org/10.1074/jbc.275.2.1439] [PMID: 10625696]

[44]  Maes H, Van Eygen S, Krysko DV, *et al.* BNIP3 supports melanoma cell migration and vasculogenic mimicry by orchestrating the actin cytoskeleton. Cell Death Dis 2014; 5(3): e1127.
[http://dx.doi.org/10.1038/cddis.2014.94] [PMID: 24625986]

[45]  Sun L, Li T, Wei Q, *et al.* Upregulation of BNIP3 mediated by ERK/HIF-1α pathway induces autophagy and contributes to anoikis resistance of hepatocellular carcinoma cells. Future Oncol 2014; 10(8): 1387-98.
[http://dx.doi.org/10.2217/fon.14.70] [PMID: 25052749]

[46]  Wu H, Huang S, Chen Z, Liu W, Zhou X, Zhang D. Hypoxia-induced autophagy contributes to the invasion of salivary adenoid cystic carcinoma through the HIF-1α/BNIP3 signaling pathway. Mol Med Rep 2015; 12(5): 6467-74.
[http://dx.doi.org/10.3892/mmr.2015.4255] [PMID: 26323347]

[47]  Okami J, Simeone DM, Logsdon CD. Silencing of the hypoxia-inducible cell death protein BNIP3 in pancreatic cancer. Cancer Res 2004; 64(15): 5338-46.
[http://dx.doi.org/10.1158/0008-5472.CAN-04-0089] [PMID: 15289340]

[48]  Erkan M, Kleeff J, Esposito I, *et al.* Loss of BNIP3 expression is a late event in pancreatic cancer contributing to chemoresistance and worsened prognosis. Oncogene 2005; 24(27): 4421-32.
[http://dx.doi.org/10.1038/sj.onc.1208642] [PMID: 15856026]

[49]  Gang H, Dhingra R, Lin J, *et al.* PDK2-mediated alternative splicing switches Bnip3 from cell death to cell survival. J Cell Biol 2015; 210(7): 1101-15.
[http://dx.doi.org/10.1083/jcb.201504047] [PMID: 26416963]

[50]  Huang Y, Shen P, Chen X, *et al.* Transcriptional regulation of BNIP3 by Sp3 in prostate cancer. Prostate 2015; 75(14): 1556-67.

[http://dx.doi.org/10.1002/pros.23029] [PMID: 26012884]

[51]   Liu L, Feng D, Chen G, *et al.* Mitochondrial outer-membrane protein FUNDC1 mediates hypoxia-induced mitophagy in mammalian cells. Nat Cell Biol 2012; 14(2): 177-85.
[http://dx.doi.org/10.1038/ncb2422] [PMID: 22267086]

[52]   Wu H, Xue D, Chen G, *et al.* The BCL2L1 and PGAM5 axis defines hypoxia-induced receptor-mediated mitophagy. Autophagy 2014; 10(10): 1712-25.
[http://dx.doi.org/10.4161/auto.29568] [PMID: 25126723]

[53]   Kuang Y, Ma K, Zhou C, *et al.* Structural basis for the phosphorylation of FUNDC1 LIR as a molecular switch of mitophagy. Autophagy 2016; 12(12): 2363-73.
[http://dx.doi.org/10.1080/15548627.2016.1238552] [PMID: 27653272]

[54]   Flemming A. Double-pronged approach to combat mutant KRAS. Nat Rev Drug Discov 2013; 12(3): 188-9.
[http://dx.doi.org/10.1038/nrd3969] [PMID: 23449300]

[55]   Weinberg F, Hamanaka R, Wheaton WW, *et al.* Mitochondrial metabolism and ROS generation are essential for Kras-mediated tumorigenicity. Proc Natl Acad Sci USA 2010; 107(19): 8788-93.
[http://dx.doi.org/10.1073/pnas.1003428107] [PMID: 20421486]

[56]   Ying H, Kimmelman AC, Lyssiotis CA, *et al.* Oncogenic Kras maintains pancreatic tumors through regulation of anabolic glucose metabolism. Cell 2012; 149(3): 656-70.
[http://dx.doi.org/10.1016/j.cell.2012.01.058] [PMID: 22541435]

[57]   Kerr EM, Gaude E, Turrell FK, Frezza C, Martins CP. Mutant Kras copy number defines metabolic reprogramming and therapeutic susceptibilities. Nature 2016; 531(7592): 110-3.
[http://dx.doi.org/10.1038/nature16967] [PMID: 26909577]

[58]   Karachaliou N, Mayo C, Costa C, *et al.* KRAS mutations in lung cancer. Clin Lung Cancer 2013; 14(3): 205-14.
[http://dx.doi.org/10.1016/j.cllc.2012.09.007] [PMID: 23122493]

[59]   Smit VTHBM, Boot AJM, Smits AMM, Fleuren GJ, Cornelisse CJ, Bos JL. KRAS codon 12 mutations occur very frequently in pancreatic adenocarcinomas. Nucleic Acids Res 1988; 16(16): 7773-82.
[http://dx.doi.org/10.1093/nar/16.16.7773] [PMID: 3047672]

[60]   Chan TL, Zhao W, Leung SY, Yuen ST. BRAF and KRAS mutations in colorectal hyperplastic polyps and serrated adenomas. Cancer Res 2003; 63(16): 4878-81.
[PMID: 12941809]

[61]   Kim JH, Kim HY, Lee YK, *et al.* Involvement of mitophagy in oncogenic K-Ras-induced transformation. Autophagy 2011; 7(10): 1187-98.
[http://dx.doi.org/10.4161/auto.7.10.16643] [PMID: 21738012]

[62]   Guo JY, Karsli-Uzunbas G, Mathew R, *et al.* Autophagy suppresses progression of K-ras-induced lung tumors to oncocytomas and maintains lipid homeostasis. Genes Dev 2013; 27(13): 1447-61.
[http://dx.doi.org/10.1101/gad.219642.113] [PMID: 23824538]

[63]   Rao S, Tortola L, Perlot T, *et al.* A dual role for autophagy in a murine model of lung cancer. Nat Commun 2014; 5(1): 3056.
[http://dx.doi.org/10.1038/ncomms4056] [PMID: 24445999]

[64]   Galluzzi L, Pietrocola F, Bravo-San Pedro JM, *et al.* Autophagy in malignant transformation and cancer progression. EMBO J 2015; 34(7): 856-80.
[http://dx.doi.org/10.15252/embj.201490784] [PMID: 25712477]

[65]   Youle RJ, Narendra DP. Mechanisms of mitophagy. Nat Rev Mol Cell Biol 2011; 12(1): 9-14.
[http://dx.doi.org/10.1038/nrm3028] [PMID: 21179058]

[66]   Zhu J, Wang KZQ, Chu CT. After the banquet. Autophagy 2013; 9(11): 1663-76.

[http://dx.doi.org/10.4161/auto.24135] [PMID: 23787782]

[67]   Hamacher-Brady A, Brady NR. Mitophagy programs: mechanisms and physiological implications of mitochondrial targeting by autophagy. Cell Mol Life Sci 2016; 73(4): 775-95.
[http://dx.doi.org/10.1007/s00018-015-2087-8] [PMID: 26611876]

[68]   Apel A, Herr I, Schwarz H, Rodemann HP, Mayer A. Blocked autophagy sensitizes resistant carcinoma cells to radiation therapy. Cancer Res 2008; 68(5): 1485-94.
[http://dx.doi.org/10.1158/0008-5472.CAN-07-0562] [PMID: 18316613]

[69]   Jarauta V, Jaime P, Gonzalo O, *et al.* Inhibition of autophagy with chloroquine potentiates carfilzomib-induced apoptosis in myeloma cells *in vitro* and *in vivo*. Cancer Lett 2016; 382(1): 1-10.
[http://dx.doi.org/10.1016/j.canlet.2016.08.019] [PMID: 27565383]

[70]   Liang DH, Choi DS, Ensor JE, Kaipparettu BA, Bass BL, Chang JC. The autophagy inhibitor chloroquine targets cancer stem cells in triple negative breast cancer by inducing mitochondrial damage and impairing DNA break repair. Cancer Lett 2016; 376(2): 249-58.
[http://dx.doi.org/10.1016/j.canlet.2016.04.002] [PMID: 27060208]

[71]   Yan C, Li TS. Dual role of mitophagy in cancer drug resistance. Anticancer Res 2018; 38(2): 617-21.
[PMID: 29374684]

[72]   Gewirtz DA. The four faces of autophagy: implications for cancer therapy. Cancer Res 2014; 74(3): 647-51.
[http://dx.doi.org/10.1158/0008-5472.CAN-13-2966] [PMID: 24459182]

[73]   Yan C, Luo L, Goto S, *et al.* Enhanced autophagy in colorectal cancer stem cells does not contribute to radio-resistance. Oncotarget 2016; 7(29): 45112-21.
[http://dx.doi.org/10.18632/oncotarget.8972] [PMID: 27129175]

[74]   Pickrell AM, Youle RJ. The roles of PINK1, parkin, and mitochondrial fidelity in Parkinson's disease. Neuron 2015; 85(2): 257-73.
[http://dx.doi.org/10.1016/j.neuron.2014.12.007] [PMID: 25611507]

[75]   Redmann M, Dodson M, Boyer-Guittaut M, Darley-Usmar V, Zhang J. Mitophagy mechanisms and role in human diseases. Int J Biochem Cell Biol 2014; 53: 127-33.
[http://dx.doi.org/10.1016/j.biocel.2014.05.010] [PMID: 24842106]

[76]   Chourasia AH, Tracy K, Frankenberger C, *et al.* Mitophagy defects arising from BNip3 loss promote mammary tumor progression to metastasis. EMBO Rep 2015; 16(9): 1145-63.
[http://dx.doi.org/10.15252/embr.201540759] [PMID: 26232272]

[77]   Guo W, Sun Y, Liu W, *et al.* Small molecule-driven mitophagy-mediated NLRP3 inflammasome inhibition is responsible for the prevention of colitis-associated cancer. Autophagy 2014; 10(6): 972-85.
[http://dx.doi.org/10.4161/auto.28374] [PMID: 24879148]

[78]   Prasad S, Gupta SC, Tyagi AK. Reactive oxygen species (ROS) and cancer: Role of antioxidative nutraceuticals. Cancer Lett 2017; 387: 95-105.
[http://dx.doi.org/10.1016/j.canlet.2016.03.042] [PMID: 27037062]

[79]   Sentelle RD, Senkal CE, Jiang W, *et al.* Ceramide targets autophagosomes to mitochondria and induces lethal mitophagy. Nat Chem Biol 2012; 8(10): 831-8.
[http://dx.doi.org/10.1038/nchembio.1059] [PMID: 22922758]

[80]   Zhou J, Li G, Zheng Y, *et al.* A novel autophagy/mitophagy inhibitor liensinine sensitizes breast cancer cells to chemotherapy through DNM1L-mediated mitochondrial fission. Autophagy 2015; 11(8): 1259-79.
[http://dx.doi.org/10.1080/15548627.2015.1056970] [PMID: 26114658]

[81]   Dany M, Ogretmen B. Ceramide induced mitophagy and tumor suppression. Biochim Biophys Acta Mol Cell Res 2015; 1853(10): 2834-45.
[http://dx.doi.org/10.1016/j.bbamcr.2014.12.039] [PMID: 25634657]

[82]    Dany M, Gencer S, Nganga R, *et al.* Targeting FLT3-ITD signaling mediates ceramide-dependent mitophagy and attenuates drug resistance in AML. Blood 2016; 128(15): 1944-58.
[http://dx.doi.org/10.1182/blood-2016-04-708750] [PMID: 27540013]

[83]    Lee Y, Lee HY, Hanna RA, Gustafsson AB. Mitochondrial autophagy by bnip3 involves drp1-mediated mitochondrial fission and recruitment of parkin in cardiac myocytes. Am J Physiol - Hear Circ Physiol. 2011; 301(5): 1924–31.
[http://dx.doi.org/10.1152/ajpheart.00368.2011]

[84]    Kindler T, Lipka DB, Fischer T. FLT3 as a therapeutic target in AML: still challenging after all these years. Blood 2010; 116(24): 5089-102.
[http://dx.doi.org/10.1182/blood-2010-04-261867] [PMID: 20705759]

[85]    Stein EM, Tallman MS. Emerging therapeutic drugs for AML. Blood 2016; 127(1): 71-8.
[http://dx.doi.org/10.1182/blood-2015-07-604538] [PMID: 26660428]

[86]    Mauro-Lizcano M, Esteban-Martínez L, Seco E, *et al.* New method to assess mitophagy flux by flow cytometry. Autophagy 2015; 11(5): 833-43.
[http://dx.doi.org/10.1080/15548627.2015.1034403] [PMID: 25945953]

[87]    Radogna F, Cerella C, Gaigneaux A, Christov C, Dicato M, Diederich M. Cell type-dependent ROS and mitophagy response leads to apoptosis or necroptosis in neuroblastoma. Oncogene 2016; 35(29): 3839-53.
[http://dx.doi.org/10.1038/onc.2015.455] [PMID: 26640148]

[88]    Luanpitpong S, Chanvorachote P, Nimmannit U, *et al.* Mitochondrial superoxide mediates doxorubicin-induced keratinocyte apoptosis through oxidative modification of ERK and Bcl-2 ubiquitination. Biochem Pharmacol 2012; 83(12): 1643-54.
[http://dx.doi.org/10.1016/j.bcp.2012.03.010] [PMID: 22469513]

[89]    Zhang S, Liu X, Bawa-Khalfe T, *et al.* Identification of the molecular basis of doxorubicin-induced cardiotoxicity. Nat Med 2012; 18(11): 1639-42.
[http://dx.doi.org/10.1038/nm.2919] [PMID: 23104132]

[90]    Jangamreddy JR, Ghavami S, Grabarek J, *et al.* Salinomycin induces activation of autophagy, mitophagy and affects mitochondrial polarity: Differences between primary and cancer cells. Biochim Biophys Acta Mol Cell Res 2013; 1833(9): 2057-69.
[http://dx.doi.org/10.1016/j.bbamcr.2013.04.011] [PMID: 23639289]

[91]    Hyttinen JMT, Niittykoski M, Salminen A, Kaarniranta K. Maturation of autophagosomes and endosomes: A key role for Rab7. Biochim Biophys Acta Mol Cell Res 2013; 1833(3): 503-10.
[http://dx.doi.org/10.1016/j.bbamcr.2012.11.018] [PMID: 23220125]

[92]    Wang K, Klionsky DJ. Mitochondria removal by autophagy. Autophagy 2011; 7(3): 297-300.
[http://dx.doi.org/10.4161/auto.7.3.14502] [PMID: 21252623]

[93]    Liu Y, Zhou J, Wang L, *et al.* A cyanine dye to probe mitophagy: simultaneous detection of mitochondria and autolysosomes in live cells. J Am Chem Soc 2016; 138(38): 12368-74.
[http://dx.doi.org/10.1021/jacs.6b04048] [PMID: 27574920]

[94]    Gibellini L, Bianchini E, De Biasi S, Nasi M, Cossarizza A, Pinti M. Natural compounds modulating mitochondrial functions. Evidence-based Complement Altern Med 2015; p. 527209.
[http://dx.doi.org/10.1155/2015/527209]

[95]    Tao F, Zhang Y, Zhang Z. The role of herbal bioactive components in mitochondria function and cancer therapy. Evidence-based Complement Altern Med 2019; p. 3868354.
[http://dx.doi.org/10.1155/2019/3868354]

[96]    Chang HW, Li RN, Wang HR, *et al.* Withaferin a induces oxidative stress-mediated apoptosis and dna damage in oral cancer cells. Front Physiol 2017; 8(SEP): 634.
[http://dx.doi.org/10.3389/fphys.2017.00634] [PMID: 28936177]

[97]     Sehrawat A, Samanta SK, Hahm ER, St Croix C, Watkins S, Singh SV. Withaferin A-mediated apoptosis in breast cancer cells is associated with alterations in mitochondrial dynamics. Mitochondrion 2019; 47: 282-93.
[http://dx.doi.org/10.1016/j.mito.2019.01.003] [PMID: 30685490]

[98]     Ghosh K, De S, Das S, Mukherjee S, Sengupta Bandyopadhyay S. Withaferin A induces ROS-mediated paraptosis in human breast cancer cell-lines MCF-7 and MDA-MB-231. PLoS One 2016; 11(12): e0168488.
[http://dx.doi.org/10.1371/journal.pone.0168488] [PMID: 28033383]

[99]     Zhou QM, Sun Y, Lu YY, Zhang H, Chen QL, Su SB. Curcumin reduces mitomycin C resistance in breast cancer stem cells by regulating Bcl-2 family-mediated apoptosis. Cancer Cell Int 2017; 17(1): 84.
[http://dx.doi.org/10.1186/s12935-017-0453-3] [PMID: 28959140]

[100]    Zhou GZ, Li AF, Sun YH, Sun GC. A novel synthetic curcumin derivative MHMM-41 induces ROS-mediated apoptosis and migration blocking of human lung cancer cells A549. Biomed Pharmacother 2018; 103(April): 391-8.
[http://dx.doi.org/10.1016/j.biopha.2018.04.086] [PMID: 29674274]

[101]    Gogada R, Amadori M, Zhang H, *et al.* Curcumin induces Apaf-1-dependent, p21-mediated caspase activation and apoptosis. Cell Cycle 2011; 10(23): 4128-37.
[http://dx.doi.org/10.4161/cc.10.23.18292] [PMID: 22101335]

[102]    Chakraborty D, Bishayee K, Ghosh S, Biswas R, Kumar Mandal S, Rahman Khuda-Bukhsh A. [6]-Gingerol induces caspase 3 dependent apoptosis and autophagy in cancer cells: Drug–DNA interaction and expression of certain signal genes in HeLa cells. Eur J Pharmacol 2012; 694(1-3): 20-9.
[http://dx.doi.org/10.1016/j.ejphar.2012.08.001] [PMID: 22939973]

[103]    Pandita A, Kumar B, Manvati S, Vaishnavi S, Singh SK, Bamezai RNK. Synergistic combination of gemcitabine and dietary molecule induces apoptosis in pancreatic cancer cells and down regulates PKM2 expression. PLoS One 2014; 9(9): e107154.
[http://dx.doi.org/10.1371/journal.pone.0107154] [PMID: 25197966]

[104]    Chan GCF, Cheung KW, Sze DMY. The immunomodulatory and anticancer properties of propolis. Clin Rev Allergy Immunol 2013; 44(3): 262-73.
[http://dx.doi.org/10.1007/s12016-012-8322-2] [PMID: 22707327]

[105]    Szliszka E, Zydowicz G, Mizgala E, Krol W. Artepillin C (3,5-diprenyl-4-hydroxycinnamic acid) sensitizes LNCaP prostate cancer cells to TRAIL-induced apoptosis. Int J Oncol 2012; 41(3): 818-28.
[http://dx.doi.org/10.3892/ijo.2012.1527] [PMID: 22735465]

[106]    Kimoto T, Aga M, Hino K, *et al.* Apoptosis of human leukemia cells induced by Artepillin C, an active ingredient of Brazilian propolis. Anticancer Res 2001; 21(1A): 221-8.https://pubmed.ncbi.nlm.nih.gov/11299738/ [Internet].
[PMID: 11299738]

[107]    Zhang T, Li Y, Park KA, *et al.* Cucurbitacin induces autophagy through mitochondrial ROS production which counteracts to limit caspase-dependent apoptosis. Autophagy 2012; 8(4): 559-76.
[http://dx.doi.org/10.4161/auto.18867] [PMID: 22441021]

[108]    Gao Y, Islam MS, Tian J, Lui VWY, Xiao D. Inactivation of ATP citrate lyase by Cucurbitacin B: A bioactive compound from cucumber, inhibits prostate cancer growth. Cancer Lett 2014; 349(1): 15-25.
[http://dx.doi.org/10.1016/j.canlet.2014.03.015] [PMID: 24690568]

[109]    Piao XM, Gao F, Zhu JX, *et al.* Cucurbitacin B inhibits tumor angiogenesis by triggering the mitochondrial signaling pathway in endothelial cells. Int J Mol Med 2018; 42(2): 1018-25.
[http://dx.doi.org/10.3892/ijmm.2018.3647] [PMID: 29717773]

[110]    Kong J, Wang L, Ren L, Yan Y, Cheng Y, Huang Z, *et al.* Triptolide induces mitochondria-mediated apoptosis of Burkitt's lymphoma cell *via* deacetylation of GSK-3β by increased SIRT3 expression.

Toxicol Appl Pharmacol 2017; 2018(342): 1-13.

[111]　Li R, Zhang Z, Wang J, *et al.* Triptolide suppresses growth and hormone secretion in murine pituitary corticotroph tumor cells *via* NF-kappaB signaling pathway. Biomed Pharmacother 2017; 95(August): 771-9.
[http://dx.doi.org/10.1016/j.biopha.2017.08.127] [PMID: 28892788]

[112]　Kumar A, Corey C, Scott I, Shiva S, D'Cunha J. Minnelide/Triptolide impairs mitochondrial function by regulating SIRT3 in P53-dependent manner in non-small cell lung cancer. PLoS One 2016; 11(8): e0160783.
[http://dx.doi.org/10.1371/journal.pone.0160783] [PMID: 27501149]

[113]　Chan SF, Chen YY, Lin JJ, *et al.* Triptolide induced cell death through apoptosis and autophagy in murine leukemia WEHI-3 cells *in vitro* and promoting immune responses in WEHI-3 generated leukemia mice *in vivo*. Environ Toxicol 2017; 32(2): 550-68.
[http://dx.doi.org/10.1002/tox.22259] [PMID: 26990902]

[114]　Borlinghaus J, Albrecht F, Gruhlke M, Nwachukwu I, Slusarenko A. Allicin: chemistry and biological properties. Molecules 2014; 19(8): 12591-618.
[http://dx.doi.org/10.3390/molecules190812591] [PMID: 25153873]

[115]　Chu YL, Ho CT, Chung JG, Rajasekaran R, Sheen LY. Allicin induces p53-mediated autophagy in Hep G2 human liver cancer cells. J Agric Food Chem 2012; 60(34): 8363-71.
[http://dx.doi.org/10.1021/jf301298y] [PMID: 22860996]

[116]　Xu L, Yu J, Zhai D, Zhang D, Shen W, Bai L, *et al.* Role of JNK activation and mitochondrial Bax translocation in allicin-induced apoptosis in human ovarian cancer SKOV3 cells. Evidence-based Complement Altern Med 2014.
[http://dx.doi.org/10.1155/2014/378684]

[117]　Zhang J, Wang Y, Zhou Y, He QY. Jolkinolide B induces apoptosis of colorectal carcinoma through ROS-ER stress-Ca$^{2+}$-mitochondria dependent pathway. Oncotarget 2017; 8(53): 91223-37.
[http://dx.doi.org/10.18632/oncotarget.20077] [PMID: 29207638]

[118]　Gao C, Yan X, Wang B, *et al.* Jolkinolide B induces apoptosis and inhibits tumor growth in mouse melanoma B16F10 cells by altering glycolysis. Sci Rep 2016; 6(1): 36114.
[http://dx.doi.org/10.1038/srep36114] [PMID: 27796318]

[119]　Takasugi M, Nagao S, Masamune T, Shirata A, Takahashi K. Chalcomoracin, a natural Diels–Alder Adduct from diseased mulberry. Chem Lett 1980; 9(12): 1573-6.
[http://dx.doi.org/10.1246/cl.1980.1573]

[120]　Zhang QJ, Tang YB, Chen RY, Yu DQ. Three new cytotoxic Diels-Alder-type adducts from Morus australis. Chem Biodivers 2007; 4(7): 1533-40.
[http://dx.doi.org/10.1002/cbdv.200790133] [PMID: 17638335]

[121]　Han H, Chou CC, Li R, *et al.* Chalcomoracin is a potent anticancer agent acting through triggering Oxidative stress *via* a mitophagy- and paraptosis-dependent mechanism. Sci Rep 2018; 8(1): 9566.
[http://dx.doi.org/10.1038/s41598-018-27724-3] [PMID: 29934599]

# Bioactive Natural Compounds as Inhibitors of Signal Transducer and Activator of Transcription 3: Prospects in Anti-Cancer Therapeutics

Praveen Deepak[1,*]

[1] *PG Department of Zoology, Swami Sahajanand College, Jehanabad-804417, Bihar, India*

**Abstract:** STAT3 is regarded as a latent transcription factor, which is activated by tyrosine phosphorylation at position 705 by non-receptor tyrosine kinase, leading to its dimerization, nuclear translocation, DNA binding, and activation of gene transcription. Activation of STAT3 is important for the transcription of genes related to cell cycle, growth, proliferation, migration, and angiogenesis. Under normal physiological conditions, its upstream signaling that leads to its activation is tightly regulated, but in cancer, the activation of STAT3 is dysregulated. Studies on various cancer models suggest that it is constitutively activated in cancer cells and plays a crucial role in the growth, progression, and metastasis of cancer. It is involved in the induced expression of procarcinogenic cytokines, such as interleukin-13, and suppressed expression of Anti-cancer cytokines, such as interleukin-12, indicating shifting of the balancer of tumor immunity toward tumor growth and progression. Thus it appears to be a potential target for cancer therapeutics. Several bioactive compounds from natural sources have been found to interfere with the signaling leading to deregulated STAT3 activation in cancer cells and subsequent cancer suppression/rejection. This chapter discusses a wide range of natural bioactive compounds that show antitumor effects by inhibiting STAT3 activation both *in vitro* and *in vivo*, as well as their future perspectives in anti-cancer therapeutics.

**Keywords:** Apoptosis, Anticancer therapeutics, Cell cycle, Cell proliferation, Cell migration, Lignans, Flavonoids, Metastasis, Polyphenols, STAT3, Tumor growth, Triterpenes.

## INTRODUCTION

Transcription factors (TFs) are protein molecules that bind to the DNA-regulatory sequence of the genes and regulate gene expression. Its binding to regulatory

* **Corresponding author Praveen Deepak:** PG Department of Zoology, Swami Sahajanand College, Jehanabad-804417, Bihar, India: Email: deepakpraveen@sscollegejehanabad.org

**Ashok Kumar Pandurangan (Ed.)**

sequence, *i.e.*, enhancers and silencers, upstream to target genes may result in increased or decreased gene expression and protein synthesis, and subsequent altered cellular function. Several families of transcription factors exist and members of each family may share structural characteristics. Signal transducer and activator of transcription (STAT) proteins are a distinct type of latent cytoplasmic transcription factors consisting of seven mammalian members, *viz.* STAT1, STAT2, STAT3, STAT4, STAT5A, STAT5B, and STAT6 [1]. They mediate many aspects of cellular immunity, cell proliferation, apoptosis, and differentiation in a tightly controlled way with finite kinetics in normal physiological conditions [2]. Initially, STAT3 has been identified as a transcription factor bound with interleukin-6 responsive element downstream to IL-6/gp130/JAK pathway in response to IL-6 [3]. It has been found to be expressed in response to several other cytokine growth factors, such as epidermal growth factor (EGF) [4], platelet-derived growth factor [5], hepatocyte growth factor (HGF) [6], transforming growth factor-alpha (TGF-α) [7], granulocyte-macrophage-colony stimulating factor (GM-CSF) [8], fibrocyte growth factor-1 (FGF-1) [9], *etc.*, cytokines, such as IL-6, IL-7, IL-9, IL-10, IL-11, IL-15, IL-22, IFN-α/β, Leukemia inhibitory factor (LIF), oncostatin M (OSM), leptin, and growth hormone (GH) [3, 10, 11]. The activation of STAT3 proteins downstream to signaling in response to cytokines and growth factors regulates the expression of a multitude of genes related to cell proliferation, survival, differentiation, apoptosis, inflammation, *etc.*, like other STAT proteins [12]. Notably, it has been found that STAT3 is also activated to induce gene expression in response to many environmental factors, including carcinogens, sunlight, infection, tobacco consumption, cigarette smoking, and stress (Fig. **1**) [13 - 15].

It has been noted that the deregulated signaling results in constitutive activation of these STAT proteins in the cell that results in aberrated control of cellular machinery. Constitutive or unregulated activation of STAT proteins, particularly STAT3 and STAT5, has been found to be associated with many tumor cell types. It shows that aberrant signaling associated with these STATs has some crucial role in oncogenesis and the process of malignant transformation [16]. Aberrant STAT3 signaling has been found to promote uncontrolled growth and survival of cells through dysregulated expression of various genes associated with cell cycle, survival, and apoptosis, such as cyclin D1, cMyc, B-cell lymphoma-extra-large (Bcl-xL), myeloid cell leukemia-1 (Mcl-1), and survivin. Moreover, aberrant/constitutive activation of STAT3 has been found to induce the expression of vascular endothelial growth factors that contribute to tumor angiogenesis and promote immune evasion of tumor cells or metastasis [17, 18]. These findings indicate that STAT3 may be a new target for cancer therapy [19]. Thus these studies provided the rationale for designing and developing small molecules that could interfere with the signaling cascade that might otherwise lead to STAT3 activation.

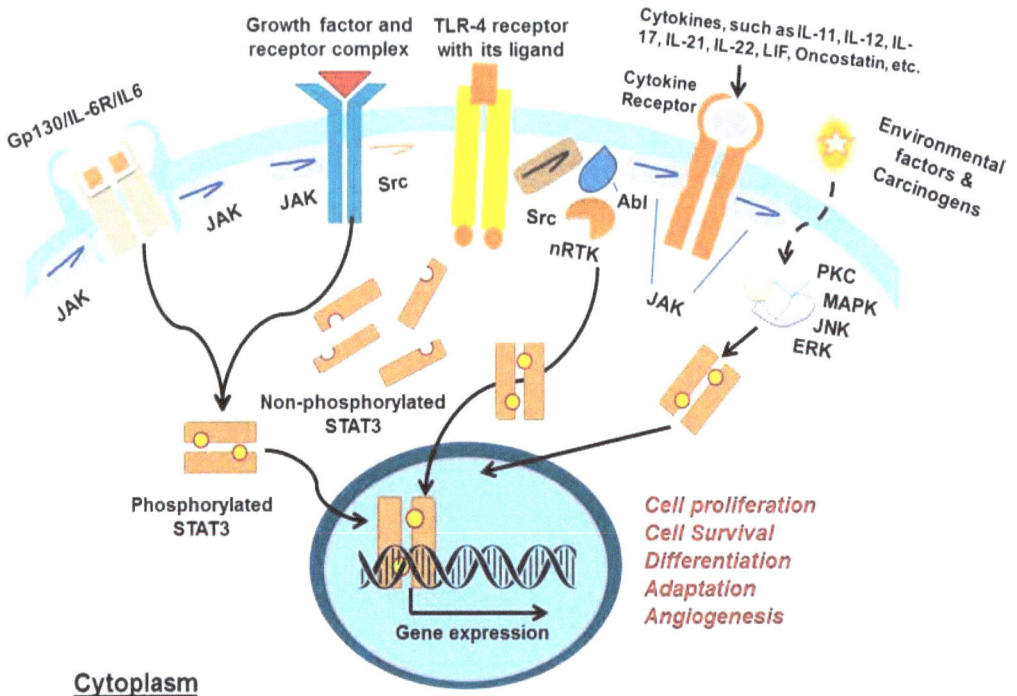

**Fig. (1).** Signaling pathway activating STAT3 in the cell. STAT3 is activated by a diverse array of molecules comprising both endogenous as well as exogenous origin. Different cytokines and growth factors bind to their corresponding receptor and activate receptor tyrosine kinase, such as JAK, which results in the phosphorylation of STAT monomer. STAT proteins then dimerise and translocate to the nucleus where they bind to the promoter region of the STAT3-inducible gene leading to the expression of a number of proteins involved in cell proliferation, survival, differentiation, adaptation, and angiogenesis. Upon internal stimuli, some serine/threonine kinases, such as Src and Abl with JNK activate cytoplasmic STAT3. Some environmental factors and carcinogens are able to activate STAT3 molecules through the activation of PKC/MAPK/ERK/JNK molecules.

## THERAPEUTIC TARGETING OF STAT3 SIGNALING IN CANCER

The downstream signaling cascade that leads to STAT3 activation indicates several target points that can lead to disruption of the signaling pathway. There may therefore be several strategies to regulate or eliminate STAT3 signaling, like strategies to prevent the activation of STAT3 by preventing receptor-ligand interaction or by inhibiting kinases, to block the protein-protein molecule interaction of the signaling pathway, to block the nuclear translocation of STAT3 proteins, and further to block/inhibit binding of STAT3 with a promoter region of the genes.

## Targeting of STAT3 to Prevent Activation

One of the potential strategies that have gained much attention in recent times is to prevent STAT3 activation. Preventing STAT3 from activation can be achieved by applying various approaches. One potential approach may be to inhibit the activation of kinases, like JAK (Janus Kinase), JNK (c-Jun N-terminal kinase), SFK (Src family of protein tyrosine kinase), *etc.*, that have been activated upon coupling of various cytokines and growth factors to their receptors. The inhibition of receptor protein tyrosine kinase (RTKs) by some small molecules, such as Gefitinib, Erlotinib, Lapatinib, Ruxolitinib, Dasatinib, and Lestaurtinib has been extensively studied and found effective in limiting the growth and progression of tumor cells in different tumor models [20 - 24]. Out of these small inhibitors, Ruxolitinib and Dasatinib that inhibit JAK and Src/Abl, respectively, have been approved by the FDA for cancer therapy. In this line, one monoclonal antibody Siltuximab that targets IL-6 has also been approved for cancer therapy [25]. Other molecules that target gp-130-associated JAKs (*i.e.*, JAK1, JAK2, and Tyk2) in the IL-6/IL-6R signaling cascade are AG490, LS-104, ICNB18424, and CEP701 (Table **1**), which are extensively studied and tested in several tumor xenograft models [20, 23, 24]. JAK2 small molecule inhibitor AG490 has been reported to inhibit STAT3 activation and thereby significantly block STAT3 from nuclear translocation and subsequently growth of leukemia cells by disrupting gene expression [20]. Similarly, other small-molecule inhibitors of JAKs, LS-104 (JAK2 inhibitor) and INCB1824 (inhibits both JAK1 and JAK2) inhibited the phosphorylation of STAT3 and thus reduced the level of activated STAT3 in cells and now they are under clinical trials [20]. Some kinases, such as ERK (extracellular-signal-regulated kinase), and MAPK (mitogen-activated protein kinase) that have been activated in response to environmental factors can also be targeted in the environmental factor-induced tumor. However, studies indicate that targeting kinases is not feasible as it has several challenges and it may lead to the development of resistance, kinase selectivity, and GI toxicity as well as cardiovascular toxicity [26].

Another approach may be to block the interaction of ligands with their receptor by employing monoclonal antibodies (mAbs) that effectively bind to target molecules through their extracellular domain. In line with this rationale, mAbs, namely Cetuximab (ICM-225, Erbitux™) [27] and Panitumumab (Formerly ABX-EGF, Vecitibix®) [28] that bind to the extracellular domain III of EGFR preventing EGF from binding, have been developed and studied for their anti-cancer potential in different cancer types [29 - 33]. Despite the observation that the patient is refractory to RGFR-targeted therapy, the FDA granted approval for the clinical use of these mAbs for the treatment of colorectal cancer and head and neck squamous cell carcinomas (HNSCC) [34 - 36].

**Table 1. Different approaches to targeting STAT3 transcription factor for anticancer therapy.**

| Types of Targeting | Molecules | | Targets |
|---|---|---|---|
| *Indirect directing of STAT3* | Monoclonal antibodies | Monoclonal antibodies, such as Cetuximab (ICM-225, Erbitux™)* and Panitumumab (Vecitibix®)* | Target extracellular domain of receptor EGFR. |
| | | Siltuximab* | Targets IL-6 |
| | Small molecules | Gefitinib, Erlotinib, Lapatinib,, Dasatinib* Ruxolitinib (INCB018424)*, and Lestaurtinib (CEP-701) | Inhibit receptor tyrosine kinase (RTKs) and SFKs (Src family kinases). |
| | | AG490*, LS-104*, ICNB18424*, and CEP701* | Inhibit gp-130 associated JAKs, such as JAK1, JAK2, and Tyk2. |
| | Double-stranded oligodeoxy-nucleotides (dsODN) | GQ-ODN | Target STAT3 DNA binding by disrupting its homodimerization (interacts with residues Q643, Q644, N646, and N647 of the SH2 domain). |
| *Direct directing of STAT3* | Small molecules | Karyostatin 1A | Target nuclear translocation of STAT3. |
| | Peptide | PpYLKTK-mts, SS-610, PM-73 and LLL12B | Targets SH2 domain of STAT proteins. |
| | dsODN | 5'-CATTTCCCGTAA ATC-3' | Target STAT3 binding to promoter. |
| | | CpG-STAT3 decoy fusion molecule | Target STAT3 binding to promoter. |
| | | AZD9150 and CpG-coupled STAT3 | Neutralize STAT3 mRNA to prevent them from expression. |

Star (*) indicates molecules that are either in clinical trials or clinical use.

## Targeting Protein-Protein Interactions in the STAT3 Signaling Pathway

It has been well noted that the SH2 (Src homology 2) domain of STAT3 binds to the tyrosine-phosphorylated sequence of other STAT3 proteins to form STAT3 dimer, enabling them to translocate to the nucleus and initiate the expression of STAT3-responsive genes [37]. The SH2 domain of STAT3 can be blocked by using a peptide sequence that includes tyrosine (Y) residues making them available for activated kinases in the cells. The phosphorylation of tyrosine residues of Y1068 and Y1086 within the EGFR has already been demonstrated to be essential for the recruitment of monomeric STAT3 to the intracellular domain of the activated EGFR [38]. Such peptides have been designed by several groups and found to effectively inhibit homodimerization and thus binding of STAT3 to DNA [39]. Some such peptides are PpYLKTK-mts, SS-160, PM-73, and LLL12B, which have been extensively studied in several tumor models [40 - 42]. Recently, the binding of STAT3 with the DNA has been targeted by designing specific double-stranded oligonucleotide decoy, *e.g.* Quartet Oligodeoxy-nucleotides (GQ-ODNs) have been tested in different tumors and found exciting results [43]. In a recent study on an ovarian cancer model, LLL12B has been found to be a potent inhibitor and found promising in combinatorial cancer chemotherapy with cisplatin and paclitaxel [42]. However these peptide inhibitors have largely been found to exhibit poor cell permeability and metabolic stability, and therefore the work on the prospect of STAT3 peptide inhibitor as a potential therapeutic tool has not gained much impetus.

## Targeting Nuclear Translocation of STAT3

One potential approach may be to block the nuclear translocation of STAT3, which involves the translocation of STAT3 homodimer through the nuclear pore complex from the periphery of the cell. Nuclear translocation of STAT3 has been found to be steady-state process independent of phosphorylation of its SH2 domain. However, phosphorylated STAT3 has been found to enter the nucleus faster through the nuclear pore complex than non-phosphorylated STAT3. The nuclear translocation of STAT3 is facilitated by two multi-subunit proteins of the nuclear pore complex, namely importin (importin-α and importin-β family proteins) and exportin (mainly, exportin-1) [44, 45]. The involvement of importin family of proteins in the translocation of STAT3 indicates that the translocation of STAT3 can be disrupted by blocking or inhibiting importin proteins. However, no small-molecule inhibitors of importin-α family proteins have been identified to date. Though an inhibitor of importin-β, Karyostatin 1A has been reported, it has not been properly studied in relation to STAT3 translocation and therefore not in the position to validate its role in cancer therapy [44]. However, it is not feasible and seems to be impractical to use such inhibitors that can also block the general nuclear translocation through the nuclear pore and hence may prove to be deleterious.

## Targeting Binding of STAT3 to the Promoter Region of DNA

An approach may also be possible where the binding of STAT3 (STAT3 dimer) could be inhibited by the use of small molecules that specifically bind to the STAT3-binding promoter sequence on DNA, thus preventing its binding to cognate DNA binding sites within STAT3-responsive genes [46, 47]. The oligonucleotide decoy, such as 5'-CATTTCCCGTAAATC-3' [48] and CpG-STAT3 decoy fusion molecule [49, 50] act as competitive inhibitors of STAT3 transcription factors capable of inhibiting the expression of STAT3-responsive genes [51]. In another approach, oligonucleotides have been designed that directly neutralize STAT3 mRNA and thus block its expression in the cells. These anti-sense ODNs, which are AZD9150 [52, 53] and CpG-coupled STAT3 siRNA [54], have been tested in many cancer models. The binding of these antisense ODNs results in readily cleavage of the target *via* RNAse H, alteration of post-transcriptional RNA splicing, or arrest of translation, leading to down-regulated expression of STAT3 [53]. The use of CpG-coupled STAT3 siRNA additionally leads to the activation of the immune system and consequent release of pro-inflammatory cytokines as well as the presentation of tumor-specific antigens to immune cells [55], however, the activation of CpG is evanescent and it is soon abrogated by STAT3 mRNA neutralization. Compelling evidence suggests that the use of ODNs to control tumor growth and progression may be a potential anti-cancer approach that may represent a new treatment strategy for 'undruggable' cancer targets with no or minimal side effects [56].

## TARGETING STAT3 BY NATURAL BIOACTIVE COMPOUNDS

A number of bioactive compounds derived from natural sources have been shown to possess anti-cancer properties and are capable of suppressing the growth and progression both *in vitro* and *in vivo* in a variety of tumor cell lines. These bioactive natural molecules not only have cytotoxic effects on tumor cells by activating apoptosis or direct toxicity but also stimulate an antitumor immune response. However, whether these natural bioactive molecules also have an effect on STAT3 activation is not much debated. Studies suggest that a number of natural products, such as guggulsterone [57], honokiol [58], curcumin [59], resveratrol, flavopiridol, cucurbitacin [26], etc. are capable of suppressing STST3 activation and thus able to inhibit/suppress the growth of tumor cells. These natural compounds having immunomodulatory as well as anti-cancer properties are mostly polyphenols containing flavonoids and other polyphenols. However other types of natural compounds have also been found to be promising.

### Polyphenols as Inhibitors of STAT3

Anti-cancer effects of phytochemicals have been debated for a long time and are gaining attention as one of the easily available and promising anti-cancer therapeutics. In this line of investigation, a study has been conducted to assess the possible association between green tea consumption and cancer and mortality due to cancer and found that green tea consumption has beneficial effects on cancer patients [60]. These cohort studies led to the belief that natural or dietary polyphenolic compounds may be a good candidate for cancer therapeutics. These dietary polyphenols were later found to exert a regulatory effect on a variety of cellular functions regulating the growth and progression of tumor. Increasing evidence suggests that dietary polyphenols have a regulatory/inhibitory role in signaling pathways that might otherwise lead to the activation of STAT3 and consequently the growth and progression of tumor cells [61, 62].

### Flavonoids as STAT3 Inhibitors

Flavonoids are hydroxylated polyphenolic compounds with variable phenolic structures naturally found in fruits, vegetables, grains, bark, roots, stems, flowers, tea, and wine (Table **2**). Chemically, they have the general structure of a 15-carbon skeleton consisting of two phenyl rings (ring A and ring B) and a heterocyclic ring (ring C having oxygen in the ring) with a general carbon structure of C6-C3-C6. The degree of oxidation in pyran ring, and hydroxylation and alkylation in benzene rings result in the formation of different types of flavonoid compounds that have slightly varied effects on the physiology. On the basis of structural modification, flavonoids can be classified into 6 major classes that are flavones, flavonones, flavanols, flavonols, isoflavonols, and anthocyanidins [63, 64]. These flavonoids have been studied for their anti-cancer role, emphasizing the effect on STAT3 activation (Fig. **2**).

**Table 2. Overview of polyphenols and other compounds that inhibit STAT3 (Adapted from Deepak P, Unpublished) [155].**

| Polyphenols | | |
|---|---|---|
| **Flavonoid Subclass** | **Flavonoid Compounds** | **Vegetal Sources** |
| Flavones | Apigenin, Chrysin, Diosmetin, Luteolin, Rutin, Tricin, Wogonin | Fruits, fruit skins, tomato skins, red wine, red pepper (*Capsicum annuum*), buckwheat (*Fagopyrum esculentum*) and some medicinal plants and others such as *Aloe vera* (Luteolin), *Bacopa moneirra* (Luteolin), *Mentha longifolia* (Luteolin-7-O-glycoside), *Momordica charantia* (Luteolin), *Oroxylum indicum* (Chrysin), *Scutellaria baicalensis* (Wogonin), Rice bran (Tricin) |
| Flavanones | Abyssinones, Hesperidin, Naringenin, Pinocembrin, Taxifolin, Xanthohumol | *Erythrina droogmansiana* (Fabaceae) (abyssinoones), Citrus fruits such as oranges, lemons, grapefruits, *Citrus medica* (hesperidin), Waste *Larix olgensis* roots (taxifolin), female inflorescences of *Humulus lupulus* (Hops) (xanthohumol), and *Eucalyptus sieberi* leaves (pinacembrin) |

*(Table 2) cont.....*

| Polyphenols | | |
|---|---|---|
| Flavanol | (+)-Catechins, (-)-Epicatechin, Epigallocatechin, Epicatechin gallate, Epigallocatechin--gallate (ECGC), Theaflavin | Tea (*Camellia sinensis*), Bananas (*Musa paradisiaca*), Apples (*Malus domestica*), Blueberries (*Cyanococcus*), Peaches (*Prunus persica*), and Pears (*Pyrus sps*) |
| Flavonol | Fisetin, Galangin, Kaempferol, Myricetin, Quercetin | Vegetables such as onion (*Allium cepa*), fruits such as berries and grapefruit (*Citrus paradisi*), red wine, olive oil (Olea europaea) and some medicinal plants such as Indian copperleaf (*Acalypha indica* – Kaempferol glycosides), Aparajita (*Clitoria ternatea* - Kaempferol-3-neohesperidoside), Neem (*Azadirachta indica* – Quercetin), Common silver birch (*Betula pendula* – Quercetrin), Hemp (*Cannabis sativa* – Quercetin), *Alpinia officinarum* (Lesser Galangal) |
| Anthocyanidin | Cyanidin, Delphinidin, Malvidin, Pelargonidin, Peonidin, Petunidin | Fruits such as cherry (*Prunus avium*), black currants (*Ribes nigrum*), red grapes (*Vitis vinifera*), blueberries (*Cyanococcus*), blackberries (*Rubus fruticosus*), raspberry (*Rubus idaeus*) and strawberry (*Fragaria ananassa*), vegetables such as bell peppers (*Capsicum annuum*), *etc.*, some nuts and dried fruits |
| Isoflavonone | Biochanin, Daidzein, Daidzin, Genistin, Genistein, Glycitein | Soyabeans (*Glycine max*) and some other legumes such as chick pea (*Cicer arietinum*), lupin seeds (*Lupinus sps*), *etc.*, and some medicinal plants such as flame of the forest (*Butea monosperma* – Genistein), |
| Chalcones | Arbutin, Chardomonin, Phloridzin, Phloretin | Tomatoes (*Solanum lycopersicum*), pears (*Pyrus sps*), strawberries (*Fragaria ananassa*), bearberries (*Arctostaphylos uva-ursi*) and certain wheat varieties |
| **Other Polyphenols** | **Types of Compounds** | **Vegetal sources** |
| Xanthohumol | Prenylated flavonoid | Found in the female inflorescences of *Humulus lupulus*, also known as hops. |
| Curcumin | Beta-diketone Polyphenol (Flavonoid) | Found in plants of the *Curcuma longa* species, a member of the ginger family, Zingiberaceae. |
| Resveratrol | Polyphenols | Found in the skin of grapes, blueberries, raspberries, mulberries, knotweed (*Polygonum cuspidatum*) and peanuts. |
| 6-shogaol | Polyphenols | Found prominently in *Zingiber officinale*. |
| Berberine | Alkaloid | Found in *Berberis vulgaris* (barberry), *Berberis aristata* (tree turmeric), *Mahonia aquifolium* (Oregon grape), *Hydrastis Canadensis* (goldenseal), Coptis chinensis (Chinese goldthread), *Tinospora cardifolia* (Guduchi), *Argemone mexicana* (prickly poppy), *etc.* |
| Honokiol | Lignan | Found prominently in the bark, seed cones, and leaves of trees belonging to the genus *Magnolia*. |
| Sesamin | Lignan | Found mainly in *Cinnamomum camphora* (Cinnamon) |

*(Table 2) cont.....*

| Polyphenols | | |
|---|---|---|
| Silibinin | Flavonolignan | Found mainly in milk thistle, *Silybum marianum*. It is presented as a mixture of two diastereomers, silybin A and silybin B, found in an approximately equimolar ratio. |
| **Non-polyphenol Compounds** | | |
| Guggulsterone | Phytosteroid | Found in the resin of the guggul plant, *Commiphora mukul*. |
| Cucurbitacin | Triterpenes | Found in the plants of the family Cucurbitaceae such as pumpkins, gourds, and cucumbers. |

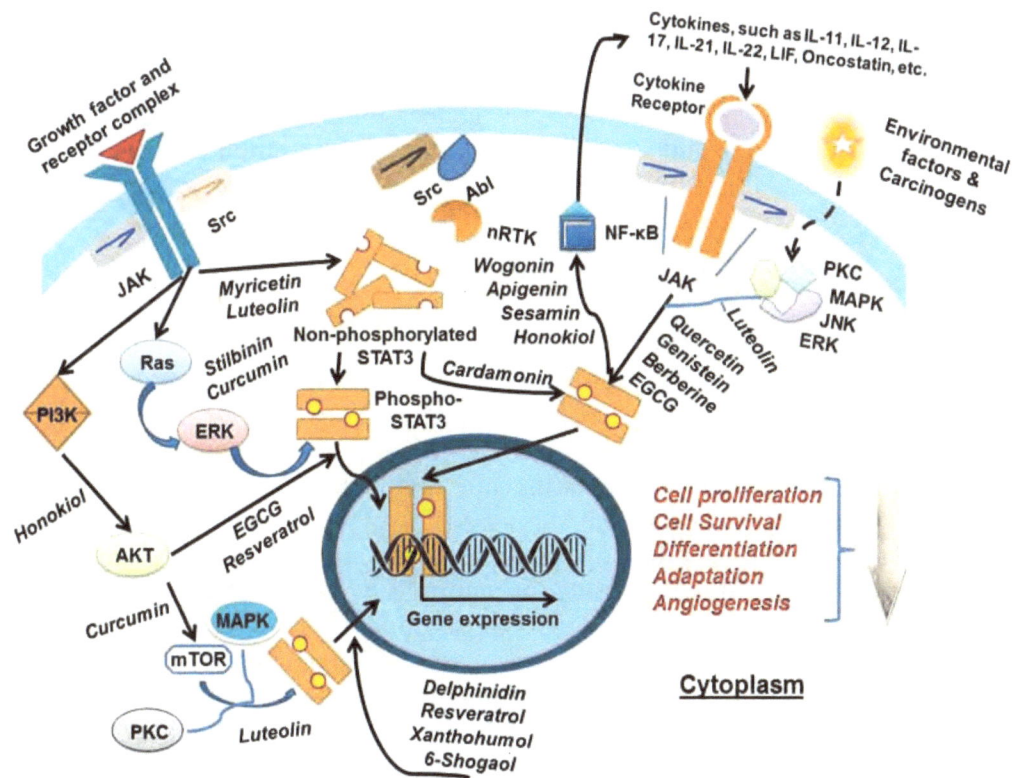

**Fig. (2).** Dietary polyphenols and other natural compounds in the targeting of STAT3 signaling (Adapted from Aziz *et al.*, 2021) [155].

## Flavones in the Regulation of STAT3

Flavones are a group of pale yellow flavonoids that have been found to exhibit diverse biological activities both *in vitro* and *in vivo*. In a recent study, it has been found that Manuka honey (MH), which contains flavones, like chrysin and luteolin, binds to IL-6Rα and inhibits p-STAT3 in a dose-dependent manner with an estimated IC50 of 3.5-70 μM range [65]. Further luteolin has been observed to decrease the levels of S100A7, phosphorylated Src (p-Src), and p-STAT3 in the human squamous carcinoma A431-III cell line [66]. Apigenin has been found to effectively suppress the phosphorylation of STAT3, thereby decreasing its nuclear translocation and expression of STAT3 target genes, such as MMP-2 (Matrix-metalloproteinase-2), MMP-9, VEGF (Vascular Endothelial Growth Factor) and TWIST 1 (Twist-related protein 1) and melanoma cells, which are involved in tumor cell migration and invasion [67]. Furthermore *in vitro* study on the BT-474 tumor cell line indicates that it effectively suppresses the growth and progression of tumor cells by regulating cell proliferation and inducing apoptosis by regulating STAT3 activation [68]. Correspondingly, other flavones, such as rutin [69], tricin [70, 71], diosmetin [72], and wogonin [73, 74] have been found to either directly interact with STAT3 protein or inhibit the JAK (Janus Kinase) or AMPK (AMP-activated protein kinase) to ultimately inhibit STAT3 phosphorylation and subsequent STAT3 nuclear translocation in various tumor cell lines leading to the suppression of tumor cell proliferation and induction in cell apoptosis in addition to the inhibition of cell evasion, which emphasize the role of flavones in controlling tumor growth in cancer patients.

## Flavanones in the Regulation of STAT3

Flavanones are an important group of flavonoids studied for their anti-cancer properties. Most studied flavanone naringenin is richly found in grapefruit that has been found very effective in inhibiting STAT3 activation by attenuating STAT3 phosphorylation directly in MDA-MB-231 breast cancer cells [75]. Further, it has been observed that naringenin inhibits STAT3 activation indirectly by inducing the expression of the suppressor of cytokine signaling 3 (SOCS3) genes in endothelial cells [76], suggesting that it suppresses the expression of the STAT3 target gene by interfering at multiple points in STAT3 signaling. Hesperidin isolated from oranges has been found to significantly reduce cell viability, proliferation, migration, and invasion, and induce programmed cell death by abrogating STAT3 phosphorylation in various cancer cell lines including oral cancer cells HN6 and HN15 [77, 78]. Abysinone, another flavanone, has also been found to be effective in inhibiting STAT3 activation, however, its study is limited to SARS-CoV-2 infection [79], both *in vitro* and *in vivo* in cancer is lacking. Other flavanones such as taxifolin was extracted from *Larix olgensis* roots [80], xanthohumol was extracted from female inflorescences of *Humulus lupulus* (Hops) [81], and pinacembrin was extracted from *Eucalyptus sieberi* leaves [82].

## Flavanol in the Regulation of STAT3

Flavanols are flavan-3-ols as the hydroxyl group is always bound to position 3 of ring C. It has no double bond between positions 2 and 3 of ring C. Dihydroflavanols, also referred to as flavanonols, are called catechins, which are most studied flavanols as anti-oxidant, anti-inflammatory, and anti-cancer agents in different tumor models. Catechins in green tea have been found to inhibit cell migration and vascular endothelial growth factor (VEGF) induces neovascularization *in vivo* by inhibiting STAT3 phosphorylation and homodimerization *in vivo* in MDA-MB231 breast cancer cells [83]. Epigallocatechin-3-gallate (ECGC) has been demonstrated to abrogate the STAT3 pathway and thus attenuate tumor formation in tumor-initiating cells of nasopharyngeal carcinoma [84] and *via* AMPK modulation in lung carcinoma [85]. Theaflavin inhibits STAT3 activation and therefore reduces the level of STAT3 and STAT3-responsive gene products thereby suppressing the growth, progression, and evasion of tumor cells [86]. Likewise, other flavanols, such as (−)-epicatechin, epigallocatechin, and epicatechin gallate from green tea extract have also been found to be very effective in cancer chemoprevention through the active modulation of the STAT3 signaling pathway [87], indicating flavanols as a potential candidate for cancer chemoprevention and anti-cancer therapeutics.

## Flavonol in the Regulation of STAT3

Flavonols are a class of flavonoids that contain a ketone group at position 3 of ring C, and a hydroxyl group, which may be glycosylated and usually found in dark-colored fruits and vegetables. The most studied flavonoids are kaempferol, quercetin, myricetin and fisetin. Kaempferol has been shown to inhibit the STAT3 activation both directly by suppressing STAT3 phosphorylation and indirectly by regulating the PI3K/AKT signaling pathway [88, 89]. Other flavonols have also been found to exert anti-cancer effects on various tumor cells both directly and indirectly suppressing the STAT3 activation. Galangin induces the production of reactive oxygen species (ROS) through the modulation of STAT3 activation and the growth of tumors in gastric cancer [90], and suppresses the growth of lung cancer through the inhibition of STAT3--regulated nuclear factor-kappa B in a combinatorial study with galangin and cisplatin (NF-κB) [91]. Quercetin has been observed to decrease the levels of S100A7, phosphorylated Src (p-Src), and p-STAT3 in human squamous carcinoma A431-III cell line [65], abrogate the JAK2/STAT3 signaling pathway in LM3 hepatocellular carcinoma cells [92], and IL-6/STAT3 signaling in glioblastoma cell line and other tumor cell lines [93, 94] to halt the growth and progression of tumor cells. Another flavonol myricetin extracted from nuts, berries, and other herbs has been found to suppress STAT3 activation by directly targeting STAT3 phosphorylation [95] or JAK1 in STAT3 signaling pathway and ameliorates cell transformation in several tumor models [96]. Myricetin can augment autophagy and cell cycle arrest by inhibiting STAT3 phosphorylation in Hep3B and HepG2 human hepatocyte cancer cells [97] and fisetin induces apoptosis *via* JAK/STAT3 signaling in human thyroid TPC1 cells [98], that further emphasizes the importance of flavonoids in general and flavonols in particular in the cancer chemotherapeutic regimen.

## Anthocyanidin in the Regulation of STAT3

Anthocyanidins are pigments that are responsible for the bluish-red color of the skin of red grapes and berries. It contains a pyrrole heterocycle having a positive charge at the oxygen atom of the ring C of the basic flavonoid structure. The major anthocyanidins are cyanidins and delphinidins, which have a reddish-purple color and a blue-violet color, respectively. Studies suggest that anthocyanidins, like other flavonoids, have anti-cancer properties. In this line, Ding *et al.*, have observed that cyanidin-3-glucoside (C3G) inhibits UVB- and TPA-induced transactivation of NF-B and AP-1 through the inhibition of MAPK activity resulting in the inhibition of migration and invasion of JB6 and A549 cells [99], which is suggestive of its possible link with the regulation of STAT3 activation. The C3G has been found to curtail cell transformation, tumor growth, and progression by inducing cell-cycle arrest, apoptosis, angiogenesis, and suppression of cell migration and invasion by modulating the activation of STAT3 in various tumor cell lines [100, 101]. Other anthocyanidin molecules, *viz.* delphinidin, malvidin, pelargonidin, peonidin and petunidin have also been found to inhibit cell cycle progression, and angiogenesis, and induce mitochondrial-mediated apoptosis by modulating JAK/STAT3 signaling pathway in various tumor cell lines [102 - 106]. Delphinidin, pelargonidin, and petunidin also repress growth factor-activated NF-κB transcription by inhibiting the phosphorylation of IKKα/β and IκBα resulting in suppressing NF-κB activation and nuclear translocation [102, 105, 106], while peonidin downregulates MAPK pathway that indirectly modulates the STAT3 activation [104].

## Isoflavonone as STAT3 Inhibitors

Isoflavonones are a type of flavonoid having a 3-phenylchromen-4-one backbone unlike another flavonoid that has a 2-phenylchromen-4-one backbone in their chemical structure. They are similar to 17-β-estradiol and therefore they are also known as phytoestrogen. It has diverse biological effects, such as anti-oxidant, anti-microbial, anti-inflammatory, and anti-cancer effects in the body when taken with a diet. Among them, genistein is the most studied isoflavonoid for its anti-cancer properties and has been demonstrated to inhibit constitutive expression of STAT3 in pancreatic cancer cells directly [107], through downregulating the activity of JNK [108, 109] thus inducing cell cycle arrest, angiogenesis, and mitochondrial apoptosis in various tumor cell lines. Other isoflavonones, such as daidzin [110], biochanin [111, 112], and glycitenin [113] inhibit cytokines as well as growth factor-mediated STAT3 activation by directly interfering with the STAT3 phosphorylation or by upregulating p38δ MAPK phosphorylation in tumor cells. Biochanin A has been found to activate retinoic acid-related orphan receptor-gamma (RORγ)-dependent IL-17 transcription, which is a pro-inflammatory cytokine that activates NF-κB, through the enhancement of STAT3 phosphorylation and STAT3-mediated recruitment of NCOAI (nuclear-receptor coactivator 1) to RORγ [113], showing the duality of its function as well.

**Chalcones as STAT3 Inhibitors**

Chalcones are flavonoids that are characterized by the absence of ring C from the basic flavan skeleton. They are linked with antiviral, anti-inflammatory, anti-oxidant, and anti-cancer activities. They have also been demonstrated to modulate the activation of STAT3 in tumor cell lines. Chalcone cardamonin has been found to repress proliferation, and invasion, and cause apoptosis through the modulation of STAT3 activation in prostate cancer [114] and glioblastoma stem cells [115], and epigenetically by inhibiting LncRNA-PVT1-STAT3 axis [116]. Phloridzin and phloretin antagonize the JAK2/STAT3 signaling pathway to inhibit the growth and progression of esophageal cancer [117], while it attenuates STAT3 activation *via* SHP (Src homology 2 domain-containing protein tyrosine phosphatase)-1-mediated inhibition of STAT3 and AKT/mTOR/JAK2/VEGF2 pathway in hepatocellular carcinoma [118]. Although another chalcone arbutin has been found to suppress STAT3 activation by ameliorating the JAK2 signaling pathway in the murine colitis model [119], it shows that it might be effective in curtailing tumor growth and progression as well.

**Other Polyphenols Targeting STAT3**

Xanthohumol is a prenylated flavonoid isolated from female inflorescence of plants *Humulus lupulus,* which inhibits STAT3 activation leading to the suppression of cell growth and induction of apoptosis of tumor cells in the human cholangiocarcinoma tumor model [81] and other tumor cells both *in vitro* and *in vivo* as reviewed by Harish *et al.* [120]. Furthermore, prenylation has been reported to restrain immune response by inhibiting Rac1 effector interactions with its target molecules of PI3K/AKT signaling [121] that may also lead to the inhibition of STAT3 molecule and subsequent expression of STAT3-responsive genes leading to suppressed growth and evasion of tumor.

Curcumin, which is extensively studied with reference to its anti-tumor role, is a beta-diketone polyphenol, a flavonoid, that can also inhibit STAT3 in various tumor models and lead to induction of cell cycle arrest and apoptosis by downregulating the expression of surviving/BIRC5 gene as well as mitochondrial apoptosis in various tumor cell lines [122 - 124]. Interestingly it directly interacts with the cysteine 259 residue of STAT3 and hampers the access of the phosphorylation site to the kinases of upstream STAT3 signaling [125], however, it is an unstable compound and its bioavailability is very low.

The next most studied polyphenol for its anti-cancer properties is resveratrol, which is abundantly found in red wine. Resveratrol inhibits STAT3 activation indirectly by interfering with other intermediate molecules upstream to the STAT3 signaling, such as by inhibiting Src protein [126], inducing SOCS-1 protein [127], and sirtuin-1 protein [128] or through JAK2 inhibition [129] and thus inducing tumor cell growth and evasion in many tumor models.

(6)-Shogaol, which is mono methoxy benzene, is a kind of polyphenol, that exerts anti-proliferative and pro-apoptotic effects on various tumors. It induces cell cycle arrest and apoptosis by inhibiting activation and nuclear translocation of STAT3 through the modulation of STAT3 and MAPK signaling pathways [130]. It also reduces IL-6-induced STAT3 activation both *in vitro* and *in vivo* [131].

An alkaloid berberine has also been found to exhibit the anti-cancer property that mediates its effect by modulating the activation of STAT3. It suppresses tumorigenicity and growth of tumors by inducing cell cycle arrest and apoptosis by inhibiting STAT3 activation in human nasopharyngeal carcinoma [132]. It also suppresses the invasion and metastasis of tumor cells *via* COX-2/PGE2 involving JAK2/STAT3 signaling pathway in colorectal cancer [133]. These findings suggest that berberine can target STAT3 activation and inhibit nuclear translocation as well.

Another class of polyphenols, lignans, is gaining importance as anticancer agents attributing to its ability to inhibit tumor growth and progression. Among them, honokiol extracted from *Magnolia grandiflora* (Magnolia), and silibinin extracted from *Silybum marianaum* (Milk thistle) are major anti-cancer lignans, which have been found to inhibit STAT3 in tumor cells and result in the suppression of tumor growth, invasion and metastasis through reducing epithelial-mesenchymal transition due to diminished E-cadherin expression in breast cancer cells and caspase-dependent apoptotic death of human prostate carcinoma DU145 and other tumor cells [134 - 137]. In addition, honokiol also activates tumor suppressor LKB1 (Liver kinase B1, also known as STK11 or serine/threonine kinase 11) *via* inhibition of oncogenic STAT3 in cancer stem cell-like phenotype in breast cancer leading to growth inhibition [138]. Evidently, silibinin is also known to be a direct activator of STAT3 [139]. Another lignin sesamin has been found to directly inhibit STAT3 [140], and indirectly through modulating p38/C-Jun N-terminal kinase mitogen-activated protein kinase (JNK-MAPK) [141], and activation of tumor suppressor PTEN (phosphatase and tensin homolog) expression [142] in different tumor cell lines.

## Non-Polyphenolic Compounds as Inhibitors of STAT3

Although bioactive compounds that have anti-cancer properties are polyphenolic in chemical nature, however, some compounds that are not polyphenols have also been very effective in controlling the growth and progression of tumor. Guggulsterone, which is a phytosteroid having a comparable structure with 17---estradiol, inhibits tumor cell proliferation by inducing S-phase arrest and promotes apoptosis by activating intrinsic mitochondrial apoptotic pathway or by downregulating anti-apoptotic gene products through the activation of JNK in the PI3K/AKT signaling pathway [143, 144]. This ultimately inhibits STAT3 phosphorylation by upregulating the expression of MET (Mesenchymal Epithelial Transition) [145]. Furthermore, guggulsterone inhibits constitutive as well as inducible activation of STAT3 protein through the induction of a SHP-1 protein [146] and inhibits angiogenesis by blocking STAT3-induced VEGF expression in tumor cells [147].

Another potent non-polyphenolic compound with potent anti-cancer properties is cucurbitacin which is a very diverse group of triterpene compounds. Nearly all types of cucurbitacin inhibit the proliferation of tumor cells by inducing cell cycle arrest, and promoting apoptosis *via* inhibition of STAT3 signaling pathway in various tumor cell lines like A549 lung cancer cell line [148], Sézary cells [149], SH-SY5Y human neuroblastoma cells [152], human breast cancer cells [153], and other [150, 151]. It has also been reported to inhibit the growth of tumor cells and induce apoptosis by inhibiting JAK2 in the JAK2/STAT3 signaling pathway leading to suppressed activation of STAT3 [152]. Furthermore, it has been demonstrated to induce G2/M phase arrest in tumor cells through STAT3/p53/p21 signaling and promotes apoptosis *via* Fas/CD95 and mitochondria-dependent pathways in human bladder cancer T24 cells [154]. Thus, cucurbitacin has also proved to be a triterpene of major importance in anticancer therapy.

## CONCLUSION

Natural polyphenols are secondary metabolites of plant origin that have been shown to confer defense against different types of stress, infections, and cancer. Natural polyphenols are abundantly found in fruits and vegetables. The dietary intake of polyphenols naturally could reduce the risk of cancers. Apigenin, resveratrol, curcumin, genistein, epigallocatechin gallate (EGCG), and cucurbitacin are among the most extensively studied polyphenols in various tumor models. Although, most of their anti-cancer effects are attributed to their anti-bacterial, anti-oxidant, and anti-inflammatory properties; it has been observed that they equally inhibit the STAT3 transcription receptor and thus suppress the expression of STAT3 responsive genes leading to the cell cycle arrest and outcome of apoptosis in multiple ways. However, there has been only sporadic work on some of the natural polyphenols and hence despite very low bioavailability, extensive work is needed to validate the preliminary evidence in the anti-cancer therapeutic regimen. Evidence from combinatorial therapy with polyphenols also suggests that they may be a new possibility in combinatorial cancer therapeutics having less or minimal side effects on the overall health of cancer patients.

Thus, in a nutshell, it can be concluded that the use of natural polyphenols either alone or in a mixture of multiple polyphenolic compounds or in combinatorial therapy with other drugs has immense prospects in anti-cancer measures. However, further studies are needed to deeply evaluate the mechanisms of action in the different types of tumor cells and their effect on other normal physiological processes of cancer patients, which, if carried out with a scientific approach, could lead to a new potential therapeutic approach.

## ACKNOWLEDGEMENTS

The author would like to acknowledge Dr. Sudhir Kumar Mishra, Principal, Swami Sahajanand College, Jehanabad for his constant support and encouragement.

## REFERENCES

[1]    O'Shea JJ, Holland SM, Staudt LM. JAKs and STATs in immunity, immunodeficiency, and cancer. N Engl J Med 2013; 368(2): 161-70.
[http://dx.doi.org/10.1056/NEJMra1202117] [PMID: 23301733]

[2]    Lim CP, Cao X. Structure, function, and regulation of STAT proteins. Mol Biosyst 2006; 2(11): 536-50.
[http://dx.doi.org/10.1039/b606246f] [PMID: 17216035]

[3]    Akira S, Nishio Y, Inoue M, *et al.* Molecular cloning of APRF, a novel IFN-stimulated gene factor 3 p91-related transcription factor involved in the gp130-mediated signaling pathway. Cell 1994; 77(1): 63-71.
[http://dx.doi.org/10.1016/0092-8674(94)90235-6] [PMID: 7512451]

[4]    Cao X, Tay A, Guy GR, Tan YH. Activation and association of Stat3 with Src in v-Src-transformed cell lines. Mol Cell Biol 1996; 16(4): 1595-603.
[http://dx.doi.org/10.1128/MCB.16.4.1595] [PMID: 8657134]

[5]    Vignais ML, Sadowski HB, Watling D, Rogers NC, Gilman M. Platelet-derived growth factor induces phosphorylation of multiple JAK family kinases and STAT proteins. Mol Cell Biol 1996; 16(4): 1759-69.
[http://dx.doi.org/10.1128/MCB.16.4.1759] [PMID: 8657151]

[6]     Boccaccio C, Andò M, Tamagnone L, *et al.* Induction of epithelial tubules by growth factor HGF depends on the STAT pathway. Nature 1998; 391(6664): 285-8.
[http://dx.doi.org/10.1038/34657] [PMID: 9440692]

[7]     Shao H, Cheng HY, Cook RG, Tweardy DJ. Identification and characterization of signal transducer and activator of transcription 3 recruitment sites within the epidermal growth factor receptor. Cancer Res 2003; 63(14): 3923-30.
[PMID: 12873986]

[8]     Gu L, Chiang KY, Zhu N, Findley HW, Zhou M. Contribution of STAT3 to the activation of survivin by GM-CSF in CD34+ cell lines. Exp Hematol 2007; 35(6): 957-66.
[http://dx.doi.org/10.1016/j.exphem.2007.03.007] [PMID: 17533050]

[9]     Udayakumar TS, Stratton MS, Nagle RB, Bowden GT. Fibroblast growth factor-1 induced promatrilysin expression through the activation of extracellular-regulated kinases and STAT3. Neoplasia 2002; 4(1): 60-7.
[http://dx.doi.org/10.1038/sj.neo.7900207] [PMID: 11922392]

[10]    Mizoguchi A. Animal models of inflammatory bowel disease. Progress in Molecular Biology and Translational Science 2012; 105: 263-320.
[http://dx.doi.org/10.1016/B978-0-12-394596-9.00009-3]

[11]    Nguyen PM, Putoczki TL, Ernst M. STAT3-activating cytokines: A therapeutic opportunity for inflammatory bowel disease? J Interferon Cytokine Res 2015; 35(5): 340-50.
[http://dx.doi.org/10.1089/jir.2014.0225] [PMID: 25760898]

[12]    Qi Q-R, Yang Z-M. Regulation and function of signal transducer and activator of transcription 3. World J Biol Chem 2014; 5(2): 231-9.
[PMID: 24921012]

[13]    Arredondo J, Chernyavsky AI, Jolkovsky DL, Pinkerton KE, Grando SA. Receptor-mediated tobacco toxicity: cooperation of the Ras/Raf-1/MEK1/ERK and JAK-2/STAT-3 pathways downstream of a7 nicotinic receptor in oral keratinocytes. FASEB J 2006; 20(12): 2093-101.
[http://dx.doi.org/10.1096/fj.06-6191com] [PMID: 17012261]

[14]    Aziz MH, Manoharan HT, Verma AK. Protein kinase C epsilon, which sensitizes skin to sun's UV radiation-induced cutaneous damage and development of squamous cell carcinomas, associates with Stat3. Cancer Res 2007; 67(3): 1385-94.
[http://dx.doi.org/10.1158/0008-5472.CAN-06-3350] [PMID: 17283176]

[15]    Bronte-Tinkew DM, Terebiznik M, Franco A, *et al. Helicobacter pylori* cytotoxin-associated gene A activates the signal transducer and activator of transcription 3 pathway *in vitro* and *in vivo*. Cancer Res 2009; 69(2): 632-9.
[http://dx.doi.org/10.1158/0008-5472.CAN-08-1191] [PMID: 19147578]

[16]    Bowman T, Garcia R, Turkson J, Jove R. STATs in oncogenesis. Oncogene 2000; 19(21): 2474-88.
[http://dx.doi.org/10.1038/sj.onc.1203527] [PMID: 10851046]

[17]    Wang Y, Shen Y, Wang S, Shen Q, Zhou X. The role of STAT3 in leading the crosstalk between human cancers and the immune system. Cancer Lett 2018; 415: 117-28.
[http://dx.doi.org/10.1016/j.canlet.2017.12.003] [PMID: 29222039]

[18]    Rébé C, Végran F, Berger H, Ghiringhelli F. STAT3 activation. JAK-STAT 2013; 2(1): e23010.
[http://dx.doi.org/10.4161/jkst.23010] [PMID: 24058791]

[19]    Turkson J. STAT proteins as novel targets for cancer drug discovery. Expert Opin Ther Targets 2004; 8(5): 409-22.
[http://dx.doi.org/10.1517/14728222.8.5.409] [PMID: 15469392]

[20]    Wilks AF. The JAK kinases: Not just another kinase drug discovery target. Semin Cell Dev Biol 2008; 19(4): 319-28.
[http://dx.doi.org/10.1016/j.semcdb.2008.07.020] [PMID: 18721891]

[21]   Sen B, Saigal B, Parikh N, Gallick G, Johnson FM. Sustained Src inhibition results in signal transducer and activator of transcription 3 (STAT3) activation and cancer cell survival *via* altered Janus-activated kinase-STAT3 binding. Cancer Res 2009; 69(5): 1958-65.
       [http://dx.doi.org/10.1158/0008-5472.CAN-08-2944] [PMID: 19223541]

[22]   Lee SH, Lee H, Kwon YJ, Kim SK, Seo EB, Sohn JO, Kim BH, Park JY, Ye SK. Chalcone-9: a novel inhibitor of the JAK-STAT pathway with potent anti-cancer effects in triple-negative breast cancer cells. Pharmacol Rep. 2025.
       [http://dx.doi.org/10.1007/s43440-025-00721-w]

[23]   Santos FPS, Kantarjian HM, Jain N, *et al*. Phase 2 study of CEP-701, an orally available JAK2 inhibitor, in patients with primary or post-polycythemia vera/essential thrombocythemia myelofibrosis. Blood 2010; 115(6): 1131-6.
       [http://dx.doi.org/10.1182/blood-2009-10-246363] [PMID: 20008298]

[24]   Verstovsek S, Kantarjian H, Mesa RA, *et al*. Safety and efficacy of INCB018424, a JAK1 and JAK2 inhibitor, in myelofibrosis. N Engl J Med 2010; 363(12): 1117-27.
       [http://dx.doi.org/10.1056/NEJMoa1002028] [PMID: 20843246]

[25]   Zou S, Tong Q, Liu B, Huang W, Tian Y, Fu X. Targeting STAT3 in cancer immunotherapy. Mol Cancer 2020; 19(1): 145.
       [http://dx.doi.org/10.1186/s12943-020-01258-7] [PMID: 32972405]

[26]   Johnston PA, Grandis JR. STAT3 signaling: anticancer strategies and challenges. Mol Interv 2011; 11(1): 18-26.
       [http://dx.doi.org/10.1124/mi.11.1.4] [PMID: 21441118]

[27]   Brand TM, Iida M, Wheeler DL. Molecular mechanisms of resistance to the EGFR monoclonal antibody cetuximab. Cancer Biol Ther 2011; 11(9): 777-92.
       [http://dx.doi.org/10.4161/cbt.11.9.15050] [PMID: 21293176]

[28]   Sickmier EA, Kurzeja RJM, Michelsen K, *et al*. The panitumumab EGFR complex reveals a binding mechanism that overcomes cetuximab induced resistance. PLoS One 2016; 11:e0163366.
       [http://dx.doi.org/10.1371/journal.pone.0163366]

[29]   Vermorken JB, Mesia R, Rivera F, *et al*. Platinum-based chemotherapy plus cetuximab in head and neck cancer. N Engl J Med 2008; 359(11): 1116-27.
       [http://dx.doi.org/10.1056/NEJMoa0802656] [PMID: 18784101]

[30]   Specenier P, Vermorken JB. Cetuximab: its unique place in head and neck cancer treatment. Biologics 2013; 7: 77-90.
       [PMID: 23723688]

[31]   Ishiki H, Iwase S, Shimada N, Chiba T, Imai K. Panitumumab for locally advanced head and neck squamous-cell carcinoma. Lancet Oncol 2015; 16(4): e156.
       [http://dx.doi.org/10.1016/S1470-2045(15)70101-4] [PMID: 25846092]

[32]   Siano M, Molinari F, Martin V, *et al*. Multicenter phase II study of panitumumab in platinum penetrated advanced head and neck squamous cell cancer. Oncologist 2017; 22(7): 782-e70.
       [http://dx.doi.org/10.1634/theoncologist.2017-0069] [PMID: 28592616]

[33]   Bharadwaj U, Kasembeli M, Eckols T, *et al*. Monoclonal antibodies specific for STAT3β receal its contribution to constitutive STAT3 phophorylation in breast cancer. Cancers (Basel) 2014; 6(4): 2012-34.
       [http://dx.doi.org/10.3390/cancers6042012] [PMID: 25268166]

[34]   Egloff AM, Grandis JR. Improving response rates to EGFR-targeted therapies for head and neck squamous cell carcinoma: Candidate predictive biomarkers and combination treatment with Src inhibitors. J Oncol 2009; 2009: 1-12.
       [http://dx.doi.org/10.1155/2009/896407] [PMID: 19636423]

[35]   Chen LF, Cohen EEW, Grandis JR. New strategies in head and neck cancer: understanding resistance

to epidermal growth factor receptor inhibitors. Clin Cancer Res 2010; 16(9): 2489-95.
[http://dx.doi.org/10.1158/1078-0432.CCR-09-2318] [PMID: 20406834]

[36]    Quesnelle KM, Boehm AL, Grandis JR. STAT-mediated EGFR signaling in cancer. J Cell Biochem 2007; 102(2): 311-9.
[http://dx.doi.org/10.1002/jcb.21475] [PMID: 17661350]

[37]    Zhang T, Kee WH, Seow KT, Fung W, Cao X. The coiled-coil domain of Stat3 is essential for its SH2 domain-mediated receptor binding and subsequent activation induced by epidermal growth factor and interleukin-6. Mol Cell Biol 2000; 20(19): 7132-9.
[http://dx.doi.org/10.1128/MCB.20.19.7132-7139.2000] [PMID: 10982829]

[38]    Leeman RJ, Lui VWY, Grandis JR. STAT3 as a therapeutic target in head and neck cancer. Expert Opin Biol Ther 2006; 6(3): 231-41.
[http://dx.doi.org/10.1517/14712598.6.3.231] [PMID: 16503733]

[39]    Fletcher S, Drewry JA, Shahani VM, Page BDG, Gunning PT. Molecular disruption of oncogenic signal transducer and activator of transcription 3 (STAT3) protein. Biochem Cell Biol 2009; 87(6): 825-33.
[http://dx.doi.org/10.1139/O09-044] [PMID: 19935868]

[40]    Turkson J, Kim JS, Zhang S, *et al.* Novel peptidomimetic inhibitors of signal transducer and activator of transcription 3 dimerization and biological activity. Mol Cancer Ther 2004; 3(3): 261-9.
[http://dx.doi.org/10.1158/1535-7163.261.3.3] [PMID: 15026546]

[41]    Mandal PK, Gao F, Lu Z, *et al.* Potent and selective phosphopeptide mimetic prodrugs targeted to the Src homology 2 (SH2) domain of signal transducer and activator of transcription 3. J Med Chem 2011; 54(10): 3549-63.
[http://dx.doi.org/10.1021/jm2000882] [PMID: 21486047]

[42]    Zhang R, Yang X, Roque DM, Li C, Lin J. A novel small molecule LLL12B inhibits STAT3 signaling and sensitizes ovarian cancer cell to paclitaxel and cisplatin. PLoS One 2021; 16(4): e0240145.
[http://dx.doi.org/10.1371/journal.pone.0240145] [PMID: 33909625]

[43]    Zhu Q, Jing N. Computational study on mechanism of G-quartet oligonucleotide T40214 selectively targeting Stat3. J Comput Aided Mol Des 2007; 21(10-11): 641-8.
[http://dx.doi.org/10.1007/s10822-007-9147-6] [PMID: 18034310]

[44]    Liu L, McBride KM, Reich NC. STAT3 nuclear import is independent of tyrosine phosphorylation and mediated by importin-α3. Proc Natl Acad Sci USA 2005; 102(23): 8150-5.
[http://dx.doi.org/10.1073/pnas.0501643102] [PMID: 15919823]

[45]    Herrmann A, Vogt M, Mönnigmann M, *et al.* Nucleocytoplasmic shuttling of persistently activated STAT3. J Cell Sci 2007; 120(18): 3249-61.
[http://dx.doi.org/10.1242/jcs.03482] [PMID: 17726064]

[46]    Zhang X, Zhang J, Wang L, Wei H, Tian Z. Therapeutic effects of STAT3 decoy oligodeoxynucleotide on human lung cancer in xenograft mice. BMC Cancer 2007; 7(1): 149.
[http://dx.doi.org/10.1186/1471-2407-7-149] [PMID: 17683579]

[47]    Njatcha C, Farooqui M, Kornberg A, Johnson DE, Grandis JR, Siegfried JM. STAT3 cyclic decoy demonstrates robust antitumor effects in non-small cell lung cancer. Mol Cancer Ther 2018; 17(9): 1917-26.
[http://dx.doi.org/10.1158/1535-7163.MCT-17-1194] [PMID: 29891486]

[48]    Wagner BJ, Hayes TE, Hoban CJ, Cochran BH. The SIF binding element confers sis/PDGF inducibility onto the c-fos promoter. EMBO J 1990; 9(13): 4477-84.
[http://dx.doi.org/10.1002/j.1460-2075.1990.tb07898.x] [PMID: 2176154]

[49]    Zhang Q, Hossain DMS, Duttagupta P, *et al.* Serum-resistant CpG-STAT3 decoy for targeting survival and immune checkpoint signaling in acute myeloid leukemia. Blood 2016; 127(13): 1687-700.
[http://dx.doi.org/10.1182/blood-2015-08-665604] [PMID: 26796361]

[50]   Zhao X, Zhang Z, Moreira D, *et al.* B cell lymphoma immunotherapy using TLR9-targeted oligonucleotide STAT3 inhibitors. Mol Ther 2018; 26(3): 695-707.
       [http://dx.doi.org/10.1016/j.ymthe.2018.01.007] [PMID: 29433938]

[51]   Lau YK, Ramaiyer M, Johnson DE, Grandis JR. Targeting STAT3 in cancer with nucleotide therapeutics. Cancers (Basel) 2019; 11(11): 1681.
       [http://dx.doi.org/10.3390/cancers11111681] [PMID: 31671769]

[52]   Engelhard HH. Antisense oligodeoxynucleotide technology: potential use for the treatment of malignant brain tumors. Cancer Contr 1998; 5(2): 163-70.
       [http://dx.doi.org/10.1177/107327489800500207] [PMID: 10761027]

[53]   Dean NM, Bennett CF. Antisense oligonucleotide-based therapeutics for cancer. Oncogene 2003; 22(56): 9087-96.
       [http://dx.doi.org/10.1038/sj.onc.1207231] [PMID: 14663487]

[54]   Kortylewski M, Swiderski P, Herrmann A, *et al. In vivo* delivery of siRNA to immune cells by conjugation to a TLR9 agonist enhances antitumor immune responses. Nat Biotechnol 2009; 27(): 925-32.
       [http://dx.doi.org/10.1038/nbt.1564]

[55]   Kortylewski M, Kuo YH. Push and release. OncoImmunology 2014; 3(2): e27441.
       [http://dx.doi.org/10.4161/onci.27441] [PMID: 24800162]

[56]   Sen M, Tosca PJ, Zwayer C, *et al.* Lack of toxicity of a STAT3 decoy oligonucleotide. Cancer Chemother Pharmacol 2009; 63(6): 983-95.
       [http://dx.doi.org/10.1007/s00280-008-0823-6] [PMID: 18766340]

[57]   Leeman-Neill RJ, Wheeler SE, Singh SV, *et al.* Guggulsterone enhances head and neck cancer therapies *via* inhibition of signal transducer and activator of transcription-3. Carcinogenesis 2009; 30(11): 1848-56.
       [http://dx.doi.org/10.1093/carcin/bgp211] [PMID: 19762335]

[58]   Leeman-Neill RJ, Cai Q, Joyce SC, *et al.* Honokiol inhibits epidermal growth factor receptor signaling and enhances the antitumor effects of epidermal growth factor receptor inhibitors. Clin Cancer Res 2010; 16(9): 2571-9.
       [http://dx.doi.org/10.1158/1078-0432.CCR-10-0333] [PMID: 20388852]

[59]   Zhang C, Li B, Zhang X, Hazarika P, Aggarwal BB, Duvic M. Curcumin selectively induces apoptosis in cutaneous T-cell lymphoma cell lines and patients' PBMCs: potential role for STAT-3 and NF-kappaB signaling. J Invest Dermatol 2010; 130(8): 2110-9.
       [http://dx.doi.org/10.1038/jid.2010.86] [PMID: 20393484]

[60]   Filippini T, Malavolti M, Borrelli F, *et al.* Green tea (Camellia sinensis) for the prevention of cancer. Cochrane Database Syst Rev 2020; 3(3): CD005004.
       [PMID: 32118296]

[61]   Momtaz S, Niaz K, Maqbool F, Abdollahi M, Rastrelli L, Nabavi SM. STAT3 targeting by polyphenols: Novel therapeutic strategy for melanoma. Biofactors 2017; 43(3): 347-70.
       [http://dx.doi.org/10.1002/biof.1345] [PMID: 27896891]

[62]   Aziz MA, Sarwar MS, Akter T, *et al.* Polyphenolic molecules targeting STAT3 pathway for the treatment of cancer. Life Sci 2021; 268: 118999.
       [http://dx.doi.org/10.1016/j.lfs.2020.118999] [PMID: 33421525]

[63]   Panche AN, Diwan AD, Chandra SR. Flavonoids: an overview. J Nutr Sci 2016; 5: e47.
       [http://dx.doi.org/10.1017/jns.2016.41] [PMID: 28620474]

[64]   Durazzo A, Lucarini M, Souto EB, *et al.* Polyphenols: A concise overview on the chemistry, occurrence, and human health. Phytother Res 2019; 33(9): 2221-43.
       [http://dx.doi.org/10.1002/ptr.6419] [PMID: 31359516]

[65]    Aryappalli P, Shabbiri K, Masad RJ, *et al.* Inhibition of tyrosine-phophorylated STAT3 in human breast and lung cancer cells by Manuka Honey is mediated by selective antagonism of the IL-6 receptor. In J Mol Sci 2019; 20(18): 4340.

[66]    Fan JJ, Hsu WH, Lee KH, *et al.* Dietary flavonoids luteolin and quercetin inhibit migration and invasion of squamous carcinoma through reduction of Src/STAT3/S100A7 signaling. Antioxidants 2019; 8(11): 557.
[http://dx.doi.org/10.3390/antiox8110557] [PMID: 31731716]

[67]    Cao HH, Chu JH, Kwan HY, *et al.* Inhibition of the STAT3 signaling pathway contributes to apigenin-mediated anti-metastatic effect in melanoma. Sci Rep 2016; 6(1): 21731.
[http://dx.doi.org/10.1038/srep21731] [PMID: 26911838]

[68]    Seo HS, Jo JK, Ku JM, *et al.* Induction of caspase-dependent extrinsic apoptosis by apigenin through inhibition of signal transducer and activator of transcription 3 (STAT3) signalling in HER2-overexpressing BT-474 breast cancer cells. Biosci Rep 2015; 35(6): e00276.
[http://dx.doi.org/10.1042/BSR20150165] [PMID: 26500281]

[69]    Perk AA, Shatynska-Mytsyk I, Gerçek YC, *et al.* Rutin mediated targeting of signaling machinery in cancer cells. Cancer Cell Int 2014; 14(1): 124.
[http://dx.doi.org/10.1186/s12935-014-0124-6] [PMID: 25493075]

[70]    Henderson AJ, Ollila CA, Kumar A, *et al.* Chemopreventive properties of dietary rice bran: current status and future prospects. Adv Nutr 2012; 3(5): 643-53.
[http://dx.doi.org/10.3945/an.112.002303] [PMID: 22983843]

[71]    Shalini V, Jayalekshmi A, Helen A. Mechanism of anti-inflammatory effect of tricin, a flavonoid isolated from Njavara rice bran in LPS induced hPBMCs and carrageenan induced rats. Mol Immunol 2015; 66(2): 229-39.
[http://dx.doi.org/10.1016/j.molimm.2015.03.004] [PMID: 25839778]

[72]    Ning R, Chen G, Fang R, Zhang Y, Zhao W, Qian F. Diosmetin inhibits cell proliferation and promotes apoptosis through STAT3/c-Myc signaling pathway in human osteosarcoma cells. Biol Res 2021; 54(1): 40.
[http://dx.doi.org/10.1186/s40659-021-00363-1] [PMID: 34922636]

[73]    Xiao W, Wu K, Yin M, *et al.* Wogonin inhibits tumor-derived regulatory molecules by suppressing STAT3 signaling to promote tumor immunity. J Immunother 2015; 38(5): 167-84.
[http://dx.doi.org/10.1097/CJI.0000000000000080] [PMID: 25962106]

[74]    Tan H, Li X, Yang WH, Kang Y. A flavone, Wogonin from Scutellaria baicalensis inhibits the proliferation of human colorectal cancer cells by inducing of autophagy, apoptosis and G2/M cell cycle arrest *via* modulating the PI3K/AKT and STAT3 signalling pathways. J BUON 2019; 24(3): 1143-9.
[PMID: 31424673]

[75]    Noori S, Rezaei Tavirani M, Deravi N, Mahboobi Rabbani MI, Zarghi A. Naringenin enhances the anti-cancer effect of cyclophosphamide against MDA-MB-231 breast cancer cells *via* targeting the STAT3 signaling pathway. Iran J Pharm Res 2020; 19(3): 122-33.
[PMID: 33680016]

[76]    Wiejak J, Dunlop J, Mackay SP, Yarwood SJ. Flavanoids induce expression of the suppressor of cytokine signalling 3 ( SOCS3 ) gene and suppress IL-6-activated signal transducer and activator of transcription 3 (STAT3) activation in vascular endothelial cells. Biochem J 2013; 454(2): 283-93.
[http://dx.doi.org/10.1042/BJ20130481] [PMID: 23782265]

[77]    Aggarwal V, Tuli HS, Thakral F, *et al.* Molecular mechanisms of action of hesperidin in cancer: Recent trends and advancements. Exp Biol Med (Maywood) 2020; 245(5): 486-97.
[http://dx.doi.org/10.1177/1535370220903671] [PMID: 32050794]

[78]    Wudtiwai B, Makeudom A, Krisanaprakornkit S, Pothacharoen P, Kongtawelert P. Anticancer

activities of hesperidin *via* suppression of up-regulated programmed death-ligand 1 expression in oral cancer cells. Molecules 2021; 26(17): 5345.
[http://dx.doi.org/10.3390/molecules26175345] [PMID: 34500779]

[79]    Shawan MMAK, Halder SK, Hasan MA. Luteolin and abyssinone II as potential inhibitors of SARS-CoV-2: an *in silico* molecular modeling approach in battling the COVID-19 outbreak. Bull Natl Res Cent 2021; 45(1): 27.
[http://dx.doi.org/10.1186/s42269-020-00479-6] [PMID: 33495684]

[80]    Wang R, Zhu X, Wang Q, *et al.* The anti-tumor effect of taxifolin on lung cancer *via* suppressing stemness and epithelial-mesenchymal transition *in vitro* and oncogenesis in nude mice. Ann Transl Med 2020; 8(9): 590.
[http://dx.doi.org/10.21037/atm-20-3329] [PMID: 32566617]

[81]    Dokduang H, Yongvanit P, Namwat N, *et al.* Xanthohumol inhibits STAT3 activation pathway leading to growth suppression and apoptosis induction in human cholangiocarcinoma cells. Oncol Rep 2016; 35(4): 2065-72.
[http://dx.doi.org/10.3892/or.2016.4584] [PMID: 26794001]

[82]    Aryappalli P, Shabbiri K, Masad RJ, *et al.* Inhibition of tyrosine-phosphorylated STAT3 human breast and lung cancer cells by Manuka Honey is mediated by selective antagonism of the IL-6 receptor. Int J Mol Sci 2019; 20(18): 4340.
[http://dx.doi.org/10.3390/ijms20184340] [PMID: 31491838]

[83]    Leong H, Mathur PS, Greene GL. Green tea catechins inhibit angiogenesis through suppression of STAT3 activation. Breast Cancer Res Treat 2009; 117(3): 505-15.
[http://dx.doi.org/10.1007/s10549-008-0196-x] [PMID: 18821062]

[84]    Lin CH, Chao LK, Hung PH, Chen YJ. EGCG inhibits the growth and tumorigenicity of nasopharyngeal tumor-initiating cells through attenuation of STAT3 activation. Int J Clin Exp Pathol 2014; 7(5): 2372-81.
[PMID: 24966947]

[85]    Chen BH, Hsieh CH, Tsai SY, Wang CY, Wang CC. Anticancer effects of epigallocatechin-3-gallate nanoemulsion on lung cancer cells through the activation of AMP-activated protein kinase signaling pathway. Sci Rep 2020; 10(1): 5163.
[http://dx.doi.org/10.1038/s41598-020-62136-2] [PMID: 32198390]

[86]    O'Neill EJ, Termini D, Albano A, Tsiani E. Anti-cancer properties of theaflavins. Molecules 2021; 26(4): 987.
[http://dx.doi.org/10.3390/molecules26040987] [PMID: 33668434]

[87]    Hou Z, Lambert JD, Chin KV, Yang CS. Effects of tea polyphenols on signal transduction pathways related to cancer chemoprevention. Mutat Res 2004; 555(1-2): 3-19.
[http://dx.doi.org/10.1016/j.mrfmmm.2004.06.040] [PMID: 15476848]

[88]    Cao HH, Chu JH, Kwan HY, *et al.* Inhibition of the STAT3 signaling pathway contributes to apigenin-mediated anti-metastatic effect in melanoma. Sci Rep 2016; 6(1): 21731.
[http://dx.doi.org/10.1038/srep21731] [PMID: 26911838]

[89]    Li Q, Wei L, Lin S, Chen Y, Lin J, Peng J. Synergistic effect of kaempferol and 5-fluorouracil on the growth of colorectal cancer cells by regulating the PI3K/Akt signaling pathway. Mol Med Rep 2019; 20(1): 728-34.
[http://dx.doi.org/10.3892/mmr.2019.10296] [PMID: 31180555]

[90]    Liang X, Wang P, Yang C, *et al.* Galangin inhibits gastric cancer growth through enhancing STAT3 mediated ROS production. Front Pharmacol 2021; 12: 646628.
[http://dx.doi.org/10.3389/fphar.2021.646628] [PMID: 33981228]

[91]    Yu S, Gong L, Li N, Pan Y, Zhang L. Galangin (GG) combined with cisplatin (DDP) to suppress human lung cancer by inhibition of STAT3-regulated NF-κB and Bcl-2/Bax signaling pathways. Biomed Pharmacother 2018; 97: 213-24.

[http://dx.doi.org/10.1016/j.biopha.2017.10.059] [PMID: 29091869]

[92]    Wu L, Li J, Liu T, *et al.* Quercetin shows anti-tumor effect in hepatocellular carcinoma LM3 cells by abrogating JAK2/STAT3 signaling pathway. Cancer Med 2019; 8(10): 4806-20.
[http://dx.doi.org/10.1002/cam4.2388] [PMID: 31273958]

[93]    Michaud-Levesque J, Bousquet-Gagnon N, Béliveau R. Quercetin abrogates IL-6/STAT3 signaling and inhibits glioblastoma cell line growth and migration. Exp Cell Res 2012; 318(8): 925-35.
[http://dx.doi.org/10.1016/j.yexcr.2012.02.017] [PMID: 22394507]

[94]    Vafadar A, Shabaninejad Z, Movahedpour A, *et al.* Quercetin and cancer: new insights into its therapeutic effects on ovarian cancer cells. Cell Biosci 2020; 10(1): 32.
[http://dx.doi.org/10.1186/s13578-020-00397-0] [PMID: 32175075]

[95]    Senggunprai L, Tuponchai P, Kukongviriyapan V, Prawan A, Kongpetch S. Myricetin ameliorates cytokine-induced migration and invasion of cholangiocarcinoma cells *via* suppression of STAT3 pathway. J Cancer Res Ther 2019; 15(1): 157-63.
[http://dx.doi.org/10.4103/jcrt.JCRT_287_17] [PMID: 30880773]

[96]    Kumamoto T, Fujii M, Hou DX. Myricetin directly targets JAK1 to inhibit cell transformation. Cancer Lett 2009; 275(1): 17-26.
[http://dx.doi.org/10.1016/j.canlet.2008.09.027] [PMID: 18995957]

[97]    Yang W, Su J, Li M, *et al.* Myricetin induces autophagy and cell cycle arrest of HCC bu inhibiting MARCH1-regulated STAT3 and p38 MAPK signaling pathways. Front Pharmacol 2021; 12: 709526.
[http://dx.doi.org/10.3389/fphar.2021.709526] [PMID: 34733155]

[98]    Liang Y, Kong D, Zhang Y, *et al.* Fisetin inhibits cell proliferation and induces apoptosis *via* JAk/STAt3 signaling pathways in human thyroid TPC1 cancer cells. Biotechnol Bioprocess Eng; BBE 2020; 25(2): 197-205.
[http://dx.doi.org/10.1007/s12257-019-0326-9]

[99]    Ding M, Feng R, Wang SY, *et al.* Cyanidin-3-glucoside, a natural product derived from blackberry, exhibits chemopreventive and chemotherapeutic activity. J Biol Chem 2006; 281(25): 17359-68.
[http://dx.doi.org/10.1074/jbc.M600861200] [PMID: 16618699]

[100]   Liu X, Zhang D, Hao Y, *et al.* Cyanidin curtails renal cell carcinoma tumorigenesis. Cell Physiol Biochem 2018; 46(6): 2517-31.
[http://dx.doi.org/10.1159/000489658] [PMID: 29742507]

[101]   Ma X, Ning S. Cyanidin-3-glucoside attenuates the angiogenesis of breast cancer *via* inhibiting STAT3/VEGF pathway. Phytother Res 2019; 33(1): 81-9.
[http://dx.doi.org/10.1002/ptr.6201] [PMID: 30251280]

[102]   Syed DN, Afaq F, Sarfaraz S, *et al.* Delphinidin inhibits cell proliferation and invasion *via* modulation of Met receptor phosphorylation. Toxicol Appl Pharmacol 2008; 231(1): 52-60.
[http://dx.doi.org/10.1016/j.taap.2008.03.023] [PMID: 18499206]

[103]   Baba AB, Nivetha R, Chattopadhyay I, Nagini S. Blueberry and malvidin inhibit cell cycle progression and induce mitochondrial-mediated apoptosis by abrogating the JAK/STAT-3 signalling pathway. Food Chem Toxicol 2017; 109(Pt 1): 534-43.
[http://dx.doi.org/10.1016/j.fct.2017.09.054] [PMID: 28974439]

[104]   Ho ML, Chen PN, Chu SC, *et al.* Peonidin 3-glucoside inhibits lung cancer metastasis by downregulation of proteinases activities and MAPK pathway. Nutr Cancer 2010; 62(4): 505-16.
[http://dx.doi.org/10.1080/01635580903441261] [PMID: 20432172]

[105]   Limtrakul P, Yodkeeree S, Pitchakarn P, Punfa W. Suppression of inflammatory responses by black rice extract in RAW 164.7 macrophage cells *via* downregulation of NF-κB and AP-1 signaling pathways. Asian Pac J Cancer Prev 2015; 16(10): 4277-83.
[http://dx.doi.org/10.7314/APJCP.2015.16.10.4277] [PMID: 26028086]

[106]   Yin Q, Wang L, Yu H, Chen D, Zhu W, Sun C. Pharmacological effects of polyphenol phytochemicals

on the JAK-STAT signaling pathway. Front Pharmacol 2021; 12: 716672.
[http://dx.doi.org/10.3389/fphar.2021.716672] [PMID: 34539403]

[107]   Lian JP, Word B, Taylor S, Hammons GJ, Lyn-Cook BD. Modulation of the constitutive activated STAT3 transcription factor in pancreatic cancer prevention: effects of indole-3-carbinol (I3C) and genistein. Anticancer Res 2004; 24(1): 133-7.
[PMID: 15015587]

[108]   Bi Y, Min M, Shen W, Liu Y. Genistein induced anticancer effects on pancreatic cancer cell lines involves mitochondrial apoptosis, $G_0$/$G_1$ cell cycle arrest and regulation of STAT3 signalling pathway. Phytomedicine 2018; 39: 10-6.
[http://dx.doi.org/10.1016/j.phymed.2017.12.001] [PMID: 29433670]

[109]   Cheng WX, Huang H, Chen JH, *et al.* Genistein inhibits angiogenesis developed during rheumatoid arthritis through the IL-6/JAK2/STAT3/VEGF signalling pathway. J Orthop Translat 2020; 22: 92-100.
[http://dx.doi.org/10.1016/j.jot.2019.07.007] [PMID: 32440504]

[110]   Yang MH, Jung SH, Chinnathambi A, *et al.* Attenuation of STAT3 signaling cascade by daidzin can enhance the apoptotic potential of bortezomib against multiple myeloma. Biomolecules 2019; 10(1): 23.
[http://dx.doi.org/10.3390/biom10010023] [PMID: 31878046]

[111]   Basu A, Das AS, Borah PK, Duary RK, Mukhopadhyay R. Biochanin A impedes STAT3 activation by upregulating p38δ MAPK phosphorylation in IL-6-stimulated macrophages. Inflamm Res 2020; 69(11): 1143-56.
[http://dx.doi.org/10.1007/s00011-020-01387-1] [PMID: 32852592]

[112]   Takahashi M, Muromoto R, Kojima H, *et al.* Biochanin A enhances RORγ activity through STAT3-mediated recruitment of NCOA1. Biochem Biophys Res Commun 2017; 489(4): 503-8.
[http://dx.doi.org/10.1016/j.bbrc.2017.05.181] [PMID: 28579428]

[113]   Zang YQ, Feng YY, Luo YH, *et al.* Glycitein induces reactive oxygen species-dependent apoptosis and G0/G1 cell cycle arrest through the MAPK/STAT3/NF-κB pathway in human gastric cancer cells. Drug Dev Res 2019; 80(5): 573-84.
[http://dx.doi.org/10.1002/ddr.21534] [PMID: 30916421]

[114]   Wu N, Liu J, Zhao X, *et al.* Cardamonin induces apoptosis by suppressing STAT3 signaling pathway in glioblastoma stem cells. Tumour Biol 2015; 36(12): 9667-76.
[http://dx.doi.org/10.1007/s13277-015-3673-y] [PMID: 26150336]

[115]   Zhang J, Sikka S, Siveen KS, *et al.* Cardamonin represses proliferation, invasion, and causes apoptosis through the modulation of signal transducer and activator of transcription 3 pathway in prostate cancer. Apoptosis 2017; 22(1): 158-68.
[http://dx.doi.org/10.1007/s10495-016-1313-7] [PMID: 27900636]

[116]   Wang Z, Tang X, Wu X, *et al.* Cardamonin exerts anti-gastric cancer activity *via* inhibiting LncRNA-PVT1-STAT3 axis. Biosci Rep 2019; 39(5): BSR20190357.
[http://dx.doi.org/10.1042/BSR20190357] [PMID: 31028131]

[117]   Jia Z, Xie Y, Wu H, *et al.* Phlorizin from sweet tea inhibits the progress of esophageal cancer by antagonizing the JAK2/STAT3 signaling pathway. Oncol Rep 2021; 46(1): 137.
[http://dx.doi.org/10.3892/or.2021.8088] [PMID: 34036398]

[118]   Saraswati S, Alhaider A, Abdelgadir AM, Tanwer P, Korashy HM. Phloretin attenuates STAT-3 activity and overcomes sorafenib resistance targeting SHP-1–mediated inhibition of STAT3 and Akt/VEGFR2 pathway in hepatocellular carcinoma. Cell Commun Signal 2019; 17(1): 127.
[http://dx.doi.org/10.1186/s12964-019-0430-7] [PMID: 31619257]

[119]   Wang L, Feng Y, Wang J, *et al.* Arbutin ameliorates murine colitis by inhibiting JAk2 signaling pathway. Front Pharmacol 2021; 12: 683818.
[http://dx.doi.org/10.3389/fphar.2021.683818] [PMID: 34594215]

[120] Harish V, Haque E, Śmiech M, *et al.* Xanthohumol for human malignancies: Chemistry, pharmacokinetics and molecular targets. Int J Mol Sci 2021; 22(9): 4478.
[http://dx.doi.org/10.3390/ijms22094478] [PMID: 33923053]

[121] Akula MK, Ibrahim MX, Ivarsson EG, *et al.* Protein prenylation restrains innate immunity by inhibiting Rac1 effector interactions. Nat Commun 2019; 10(1): 3975.
[http://dx.doi.org/10.1038/s41467-019-11606-x] [PMID: 31484924]

[122] Alexandrow MG, Song LJ, Altiok S, Gray J, Haura EB, Kumar NB. Curcumin. Eur J Cancer Prev 2012; 21(5): 407-12.
[http://dx.doi.org/10.1097/CEJ.0b013e32834ef194] [PMID: 22156994]

[123] Glienke W, Maute L, Wicht J, Bergmann L. Curcumin inhibits constitutive STAT3 phosphorylation in human pancreatic cancer cell lines and downregulation of survivin/BIRC5 gene expression. Cancer Invest 2009; 28(2): 166-71.
[http://dx.doi.org/10.3109/07357900903287006] [PMID: 20121547]

[124] Liu Y, Wang X, Zeng S, *et al.* The natural polyphenol curcumin induces apoptosis by suppressing STAT3 signaling in esophageal squamous cell carcinoma. J Exp Clin Cancer Res 2018; 37(1): 303.
[http://dx.doi.org/10.1186/s13046-018-0959-0] [PMID: 30518397]

[125] Hahn YI, Kim SJ, Choi BY, *et al.* Curcumin interacts directly with the Cysteine 259 residue of STAT3 and induces apoptosis in H-*Ras* transformed human mammary epithelial cells. Sci Rep 2018; 8(1): 6409.
[http://dx.doi.org/10.1038/s41598-018-23840-2] [PMID: 29686295]

[126] Kotha A, Sekharam M, Cilenti L, *et al.* Resveratrol inhibits Src and Stat3 signaling and induces the apoptosis of malignant cells containing activated Stat3 protein. Mol Cancer Ther 2006; 5(3): 621-9.
[http://dx.doi.org/10.1158/1535-7163.MCT-05-0268] [PMID: 16546976]

[127] Baek SH, Ko JH, Lee H, *et al.* Resveratrol inhibits STAT3 signaling pathway through the induction of SOCS-1: Role in apoptosis induction and radiosensitization in head and neck tumor cells. Phytomedicine 2016; 23(5): 566-77.
[http://dx.doi.org/10.1016/j.phymed.2016.02.011] [PMID: 27064016]

[128] Chao SC, Chen YJ, Huang KH, *et al.* Induction of sirtuin-1 signaling by resveratrol induces human chondrosarcoma cell apoptosis and exhibits antitumor activity. Sci Rep 2017; 7(1): 3180.
[http://dx.doi.org/10.1038/s41598-017-03635-7] [PMID: 28600541]

[129] Quoc Trung L, Espinoza JL, Takami A, Nakao S. Resveratrol induces cell cycle arrest and apoptosis in malignant NK cells *via* JAK2/STAT3 pathway inhibition. PLoS One 2013; 8(1): e55183.
[http://dx.doi.org/10.1371/journal.pone.0055183] [PMID: 23372833]

[130] Kim SM, Kim C, Bae H, *et al.* 6-Shogaol exerts anti-proliferative and pro-apoptotic effects through the modulation of STAT3 and MAPKs signaling pathways. Mol Carcinog 2015; 54(10): 1132-46.
[http://dx.doi.org/10.1002/mc.22184] [PMID: 24962868]

[131] Saha A, Blando J, Silver E, Beltran L, Sessler J, DiGiovanni J. 6-Shogaol from dried ginger inhibits growth of prostate cancer cells both *in vitro* and *in vivo* through inhibition of STAT3 and NF-κB signaling. Cancer Prev Res (Phila) 2014; 7(6): 627-38.
[http://dx.doi.org/10.1158/1940-6207.CAPR-13-0420] [PMID: 24691500]

[132] Tsang CM, Cheung YC, Lui VWY, *et al.* Berberine suppresses tumorigenicity and growth of nasopharyngeal carcinoma cells by inhibiting STAT3 activation induced by tumor associated fibroblasts. BMC Cancer 2013; 13(1): 619.
[http://dx.doi.org/10.1186/1471-2407-13-619] [PMID: 24380387]

[133] Liu X, Ji Q, Ye N, *et al.* Berberine inhibits invasion and metastasis of colorectal cancer cells *via* COX-2/PGE$_2$ mediated JAK2/STAT3 signaling pathway. PLoS One 2015; 10(5): e0123478.
[http://dx.doi.org/10.1371/journal.pone.0123478] [PMID: 25954974]

[134] Pan J, Lee Y, Zhang Q, *et al.* Honokiol decreases lung cancer metastasis through inhibition of the

STAT3 signaling pathway. Cancer Prev Res (Phila) 2017; 10(2): 133-41.
[http://dx.doi.org/10.1158/1940-6207.CAPR-16-0129] [PMID: 27849557]

[135]   Avtanski DB, Nagalingam A, Bonner MY, Arbiser JL, Saxena NK, Sharma D. Honokiol inhibits epithelial—mesenchymal transition in breast cancer cells by targeting signal transducer and activator of transcription 3/Zeb1/E-cadherin axis. Mol Oncol 2014; 8(3): 565-80.
[http://dx.doi.org/10.1016/j.molonc.2014.01.004] [PMID: 24508063]

[136]   Bosch-Barrera J, Menendez JA. Silibinin and STAT3: A natural way of targeting transcription factors for cancer therapy. Cancer Treat Rev 2015; 41(6): 540-6.
[http://dx.doi.org/10.1016/j.ctrv.2015.04.008] [PMID: 25944486]

[137]   Agarwal C, Tyagi A, Kaur M, Agarwal R. Silibinin inhibits constitutive activation of Stat3, and causes caspase activation and apoptotic death of human prostate carcinoma DU145 cells. Carcinogenesis 2007; 28(7): 1463-70.
[http://dx.doi.org/10.1093/carcin/bgm042] [PMID: 17341659]

[138]   Sengupta S, Nagalingam A, Muniraj N, *et al.* Activation of tumor suppressor LKB1 by honokiol abrogates cancer stem-like phenotype in breast cancer *via* inhibition of oncogenic Stat3. Oncogene 2017; 36(41): 5709-21.
[http://dx.doi.org/10.1038/onc.2017.164] [PMID: 28581518]

[139]   Verdura S, Cuyàs E, Llorach-Parés L, *et al.*  Silibinin is a direct inhibitor of STAT3. Food Chem Toxicol 2018; 116(Pt B): 161-72.
[http://dx.doi.org/10.1016/j.fct.2018.04.028]

[140]   Deng P, Wang C, Chen L, *et al.* Sesamin induces cell cycle arrest and apoptosis through the inhibition of signal transducer and activator of transcription 3 signalling in human hepatocellular carcinoma cell line HepG2. Biol Pharm Bull 2013; 36(10): 1540-8.
[http://dx.doi.org/10.1248/bpb.b13-00235] [PMID: 24088253]

[141]   Kuo TN, Lin CS, Li GD, Kuo CY, Kao SH. Sesamin inhibits cervical cancer cell proliferation by promoting p53/PTEN-mediated apoptosis. Int J Med Sci 2020; 17(15): 2292-8.
[http://dx.doi.org/10.7150/ijms.48955] [PMID: 32922194]

[142]   Kong X, Ma M, Zhang Y, *et al.* Differentiation therapy: sesamin as an effective agent in targeting cancer stem-like side population cells of human gallbladder carcinoma. BMC Complement Altern Med 2014; 14(1): 254.
[http://dx.doi.org/10.1186/1472-6882-14-254] [PMID: 25038821]

[143]   Shi JJ, Jia X-L, Li M, *et al.* Guggulsterone induces apoptosis of human hepatocellular carcinoma cells through intrinsic mitochondrial pathway. World J Gastroenterol 2015; 21(47): 13277-87.
[http://dx.doi.org/10.3748/wjg.v21.i47.13277] [PMID: 26715810]

[144]   Shishodia S, Sethi G, Ahn KS, Aggarwal BB. Guggulsterone inhibits tumor cell proliferation, induces S-phase arrest, and promotes apoptosis through activation of c-Jun N-terminal kinase, suppression of Akt pathway, and downregulation of antiapoptotic gene products. Biochem Pharmacol 2007; 74(1): 118-30.
[http://dx.doi.org/10.1016/j.bcp.2007.03.026] [PMID: 17475222]

[145]   Bian C, Liu Z, Li D, Zhen L. PI3K/AKT inhibition induces compensatory activation of the MET/STAT3 pathway in non-small cell lung cancer. Oncol Lett 2018; 15(6): 9655-62.
[http://dx.doi.org/10.3892/ol.2018.8587] [PMID: 29928341]

[146]   Ahn KS, Sethi G, Sung B, Goel A, Ralhan R, Aggarwal BB. Guggulsterone, a farnesoid X receptor antagonist, inhibits constitutive and inducible STAT3 activation through induction of a protein tyrosine phosphatase SHP-1. Cancer Res 2008; 68(11): 4406-15.
[http://dx.doi.org/10.1158/0008-5472.CAN-07-6696] [PMID: 18519703]

[147]   Kim ES, Hong SY, Lee HK, *et al.* Guggulsterone inhibits angiogenesis by blocking STAT3 and VEGF expression in colon cancer cells. Oncol Rep 2008; 20(6): 1321-7.
[PMID: 19020709]

[148] Zhang M, Bian ZG, Zhang Y, *et al.* Cucurbitacin B inhibits proliferation and induces apoptosis *via* STAT3 pathway inhibition in A549 lung cancer cells. Mol Med Rep 2014; 10(6): 2905-11.
[http://dx.doi.org/10.3892/mmr.2014.2581] [PMID: 25242136]

[149] van Kester MS, Out-Luiting JJ, von dem Borne PA, Willemze R, Tensen CP, Vermeer MH. Cucurbitacin I inhibits Stat3 and induces apoptosis in Sézary cells. J Invest Dermatol 2008; 128(7): 1691-5.
[http://dx.doi.org/10.1038/sj.jid.5701246] [PMID: 18200050]

[150] Guo H, Kuang S, Song Q, Liu M, Sun X, Yu Q. Cucurbitacin I inhibits STAT3, but enhances STAT1 signaling in human cancer cells *in vitro* through disrupting actin filaments. Acta Pharmacol Sin 2018; 39(3): 425-37.
[http://dx.doi.org/10.1038/aps.2017.99] [PMID: 29119966]

[151] Sun J, Blaskovich MA, Jove R, Livingston SK, Coppola D, Sebti SM. Cucurbitacin Q: a selective STAT3 activation inhibitor with potent antitumor activity. Oncogene 2005; 24(20): 3236-45.
[http://dx.doi.org/10.1038/sj.onc.1208470] [PMID: 15735720]

[152] Zheng Q, Liu Y, Liu W, *et al.* Cucurbitacin B inhibits growth and induces apoptosis through the JAK2/STAT3 and MAPK pathways in SH-SY5Y human neuroblastoma cells. Mol Med Rep 2014; 10(1): 89-94.
[http://dx.doi.org/10.3892/mmr.2014.2175] [PMID: 24789581]

[153] Ku JM, Hong SH, Kim HI, *et al.* Cucurbitacin D exhibits its anti-cancer effect in human breast cancer cells by inhibiting STAT3 and AKT signaling. Eur J Inflamm 2018; 16: 1-9.
[http://dx.doi.org/10.1177/2058739218777300]

[154] Huang WW, Yang JS, Lin MW, *et al.* Cucurbitacin E induces G2/M phase arrest through STAT3/p53/p21 signaling and provokes apoptosis *via* Fas/CD95 and mitochondria-dependent pathways in human bladder cancer T24 cells. Evid Based Complement Alternat Med 2012; 2012: 1-11.
[http://dx.doi.org/10.1155/2012/952762] [PMID: 22272214]

# CHAPTER 5

# Targeting Cancer Stemness by Exosomes as a Therapeutic Approach against Ovarian Cancer

**Kaumudi Pande**[1,2] and **Anbarasu Kannan**[1,2,*]

[1] *Department of Biochemistry, CSIR-Central Food Technological Research Institute, Mysuru-570020, India*

[2] *Academy of Scientific and Innovative Research (AcSIR), Ghaziabad-201002, India*

**Abstract:** Early detection and effective treatment are daunting challenges in the field of cancer biology. Ovarian cancer has emerged as a third-ranked health issue among women worldwide. In recent decades, there have been numerous pieces of evidence regarding ovarian cancer depicting a high-grade cellular transformation leading to self-renewal, defining cancer stemness, aggressive growth, and distribution to other organs. Deregulated biological processes are activated, including the Wnt pathway, AKT/MAPK, and STAT3, in typical cells that turn down the governed cell division into uncontrolled expansion through cancer stem cell markers SOX2, CD133, CD44, CD117, and Aldehyde dehydrogenase, thereby suppressing the cell immune system and apoptotic activity. Currently, there has been the advent of innovative therapy for cancer known as "Exosomes," which are nanovesicles secreted by all cells conveying nucleic acids, proteins, lipids, and carbohydrates to the recipient cells. The upper-hand use of exosomes is marked by their immune tolerability, stability, and systemic delivery to target cells, which will contribute to cancer therapy. In this analysis, we will focus on the behavior of cancer stem cells in the EMT mechanism that promotes ovarian cancer and discusses exosome-based therapeutic applications that require further research to prevent tumor growth.

**Keywords:** Nanovesicles, Ovarian cancer, Wnt pathway.

## INTRODUCTION

Ovarian cancer is classified as a leading gynecological carcinoma, with over 25,000 cases and an incidence rate between 5-8/100,000 in India. As stated by the WHO in the year 2020, there were 45,701 new cases of ovarian cancer with a mortality of 32,077 cases, thereby exhibiting lower chances of survival in India (Fig. **1**) [1].

* **Corresponding author Anbarasu Kannan:** Department of Biochemistry, CSIR-Central Food Technological Research Institute, Mysuru-570020, India and Academy of Scientific and Innovative Research (AcSIR), Ghaziabad-201002, India; Tel: +91-8870795252; E-mail: anbarasu@cftri.res.in

Ashok Kumar Pandurangan (Ed.)

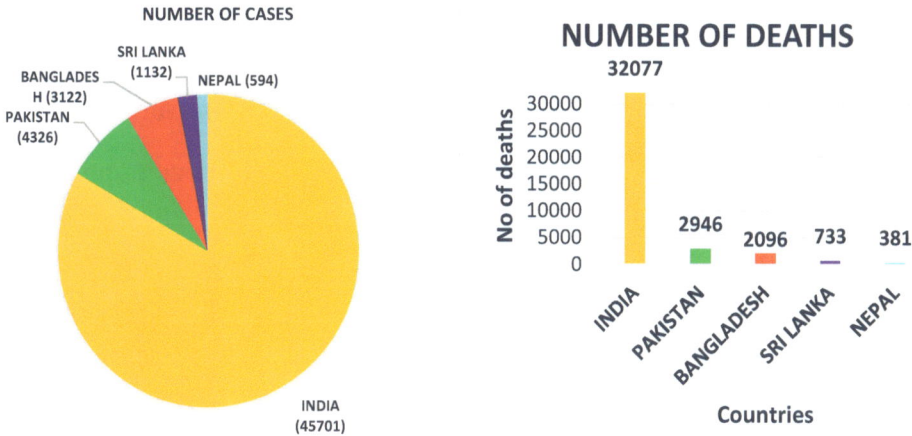

**Fig. (1).** Ovarian cancer cases statistics in India and its neighboring countries in the year 2020.

Ovarian cancer emanates from a single or both ovaries in its primary stage and dissipates through the fallopian tube to the uterine tract towards distant organs. Ovarian malignancies are of three types: the first is an epithelial tumor covering the ovarian membrane, which is categorized as serous epithelial cancer found in younger people (low grade) with altered KRAS and BRAF genes as well as in older age (high grade) populations with altered p53 and BRCA1/2 genes in the majority of cases. Mucinous epithelial cancer comprises solid tumor masses with mutated KRAS and HER2 genes' higher reoccurrence rate, and endometrial cancer results from mutations of PI3KCA, PTEN gene, and Clear-Cell Carcinomas, which are unusually early age conditions that give rise to solid tumor formation in the abdominal region and increased calcium content in the blood, which weakens the bones due to the alteration of ARID1A and PI3KCA gene expression [2]. The second type is Stromal Cell ovarian cancer regulated by hormone-producing granulosa cells and theca cells, resulting in anomalous vaginal bleeding, abdominal distress, and growth of facial hair at the juvenile age expressing a polycystic mass [3]. Genetic modifications of DICER1 at its RNase IIIb domain and of FOXL2 at its c.402C> G (p.C134W) site result in Sertoli-Leydig cell ovarian tumors [4]. The third is germ-cell ovarian malignancy originating from reproductive cells reported at the age of 10 to 30 years, with a higher expression of alpha-fetoprotein, b-hCG, and lactic dehydrogenase isoenzyme-1, which were examined in the majority of patients. Unilateral nodules with necrosis and hemorrhage were confirmed by computed tomography and could be eliminated through Surgery, Hysterectomy, and bilateral salpingo-oophorectomy in the second and third stages. Furthermore, surgery along with platinum-based chemotherapy or adjuvant chemotherapy is recommended for the fourth stage of cancer [5]. Therefore, typical tumor germ cells exhibiting increased telomerase activity and aggressive growth caused by a certain set of genes typically expressed in progenitor cells were found to be overexpressed in tumor germ cells, resulting in genomic instability and DNA impairment [6].

Advancing ovarian tumor cells by means of ascetic fluid communicate with specific cell types, including stromal cells, fibroblasts, and adipocyte cells, which activate certain metabolic pathways that promote tumor growth. Ovarian cancer ascitic fluid is composed of lysophosphatidic acid, interleukin-6, VEGF, TNF-alpha, and TGF, which enables new blood vessel formation, chemoresistance, and epithelial-mesenchymal transition, and prevents cell death [7].

Cancer stem cells are young masses of uncontrolled growing cells with specialized competency for regeneration and dynamic division and possess oncogenic characteristics for their survival (Fig. **2**). They can reform themselves into a heterogeneous variety of cells and have significant variation in their gene expression compared to normal embryonic stem cells (ESCs) and adult stem cells. The foremost breakthrough in the discipline of stem cells was the transmission of human acute myeloid leukemia stem cells to severely immune-deficient mice with a higher expression of CD34 [8]. Notably, ovarian high-grade serous adenocarcinoma cells develop clones acquiring cancer stem cell characteristics and exhibit anchorage-independent growth by upregulating vimentin, slug, snail, and metastatic behavior by dispersing to the omentum, stomach, liver, pancreas, intestines, and heart [9]. Ovarian cancer stem cells (OCSC) were identified using biological markers, particularly CD133, CD44, CD117, CD24, and aldehyde dehydrogenase (ALDH), which trigger the NF-κB signaling mechanism for cellular proliferation [10].

Exosomes are cup-shaped double-layer nanovesicles that are constitutively released from all cells for intercellular communication. Their structure measures around 40-150 nm in diameter with zeta potential, and cargo varying from exosome sources exhibiting diversification; therefore, this variegation in exosomes helps simplify the identification of distinct types of cancer in comparison with the exosome-derived healthy population. Exosomes transport their conventional constituents, namely, lipids, nucleic acids, proteins, carbohydrates, and certain metabolites that are either present in their lumen or embedded in a lipid bilayer with the intention of delivering to the target cells for development [11]. Exosome biosynthesis is eventuated by the endosomal sorting complex required for transport (ESCRT) complexes, beginning from endosomes forming in the cytoplasm followed by the stepwise incorporation of specific molecules in the intraluminal vesicles (ILVs) through the Vps27–Hse1 complex assembled together in the multivesicular body (MVB) that is combined with the plasma membrane and released outside the extracellular space [12, 13]. The classical biomarkers found in exosomes are tetraspanins (CD9, CD63, and CD81), ALIX, MUC13, TSG101, actin, EpCAM, annexin V, Rab, Hsp 70, Hsp 90, and RNAs (miRNAs and lncRNAs) [14]. Exosomes are regarded as excellent media for conveying a broad range of molecules that can be further utilized in cancer therapeutics. Exosomes were harvested using different techniques, such as ultracentrifugation, size exclusion chromatography, immunoaffinity capture-based, and exosome precipitation kits [15], for experimentation in a good yield to incorporate anti-cancer drugs, such as paclitaxel, through electroporation and sonication, and further showed cytotoxicity in lung cancer cell lines targeting free drug resistance [16]. Similarly, exosomes loaded with curcumin act as inhibitors of tumor cell growth, leading to their degradation by suppressing various oncogenes in breast, cervical, and pancreatic cancers [17]. The goal of the current study was to understand the transformation mechanism of normal stem cells into cancerous cells and their role in metastasis advancement, as well as the role of exosomes in countering cancer stem cell multiplication, resulting in their apoptosis.

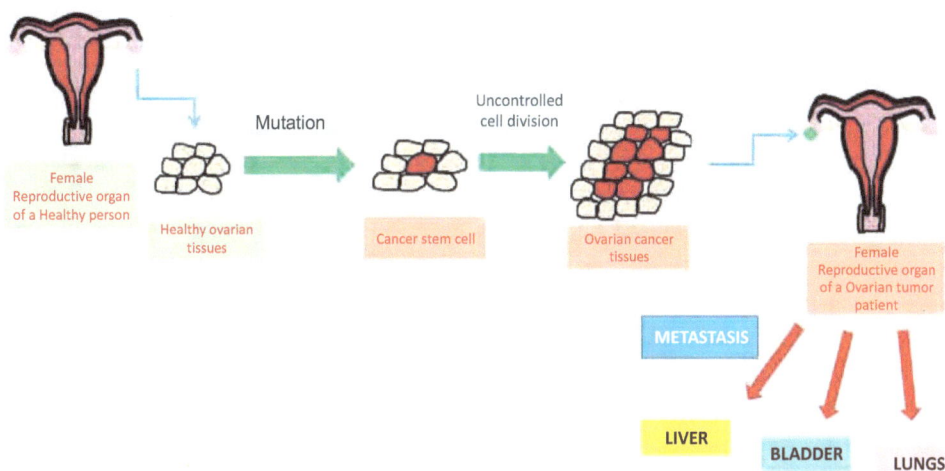

**Fig. (2).** Growth of Cancer Stem Cells in Ovarian Tissues.

## MECHANISM OF CANCER STEM CELLS LEADING TO OVARIAN CANCER AND ITS METASTATIC SITES

A crucial turning point in this investigation was the discovery of precise molecules and their downstream signaling pathways that lead to the transition of healthy stem cells into cancer stem cells. The cancer-clone evolution system is caused by the genetic alteration of reproductive cells arising from alcohol, smoking, drug consumption, and UV radiation exposure. Aggregation of these transformations occurring in reproductive cells in the course of existence lengthened the time interval exerting the dominant influence resulting in cancer [18]. The notion behind the cancer stem cell model in which the beginning of cancer stem cell production occurred is still indefinable. The ungoverned self-renewal process to maintain a subpopulation of tumorigenic cells arises when self-renewal normal stem cells are exposed to carcinogenic agents that allow modification in normal stem cell niches to evolve differentiated cells into cancer stem cells (Fig. **2**). These parent cancer stems have advanced to form further varied phenotypic malignant cells [19, 20].

Various metabolic pathways are involved in the mutagenesis of progenitor and normal stem cells into benign tumor stem cells, which undergo clonal evolution and differentiation to form malignant tumor stem cells. The solid mass of ovarian cancer stem cells observed with the measurement of 5 μm on the ovarian cortex tissue leads to borderline ovarian cancer confirmed after the surgery with the higher expression of SOX2, OCT4, NANOG, and STELLA along with SOX17, FOXQ1, and CA125 indicators of ovarian cancer [21]. Studies have revealed that OCT4 (Octamer-binding transcription factor 4) is involved in the cell cycle transition from G1 to S phase; however, doxycycline treatment upregulates cyclin-dependent kinase inhibitor 1 (p21) expression for cell proliferation [22]. OCT4 promotes drug resistance and tumor infiltration by elevating JAK1 and STAT3 levels, as well as cyclin D1, Bcl-2, and c-Myc, which are crucial for tumor advancement [23, 24] (Fig. **3**). In addition, SRY-box 2 (SOX2) aids in the pluripotency of embryonic stem cells by triggering the JAK-STAT signaling mechanism under normal conditions, despite its role as an oncogene in malignancy, with a low survival rate in high-grade serous ovarian carcinoma. SOX9 usually participates in the morphogenesis of stem cells, ovary-testis transition, and skeletal development, whereas patients show resistance to chemotherapy due to the high expression of LINC00115, which determines CD133, NANOG, CD44, and SOX9 levels. The effect of LINC00115 on SOX9 stimulates the Wnt/β-cateninpathway and suppresses caspase 3 apoptotic function [25, 26]. CD166 glycoprotein governs spheroid formation, which is one of the hallmarks of ovarian cancer stemness, and exhibits drug resistance by activating ABC transporters (ABCB1, ABCG2, and ABCC6) to suppress drug absorption and its toxicity to tumor cells [27]. Cancer stem cells are identified as the "Cancer initiating cells" with an increased stemness related to aldehyde dehydrogenase 1 and fibroblast growth factor 4 (FGF4) resulting in enhanced tumor volume [28]. High expression levels of aldehyde dehydrogenase (ALDH1A1, ALDH1A3, ALDH1L1, ALDH2, ALDH6A1, and ALDH9A1) were noted after platinum-taxane combination therapy, resulting in a poor survival rate [29]. CD133 was detected as a cancer stem cell marker due to its sphere-producing potential by cisplatin and paclitaxel chemoresistance, resulting in structural modification in

SKOV3 cells and the development of a solid tumor mass in the mouse xenograft model. CD133 is associated with the phosphatidylinositol 3-kinase (PI3K)/AKT signaling pathway along with chemokine and Wnt signaling by the subjugation of focal adhesion kinase and stimulation of LRP5/6, TCF/LEF for cell cycle progression, G-protein-coupled receptor (GPCR), cAMP response element-binding protein (CREB), and Bcl2 for tumor cell viability [30]. CD133$^+$ ovarian tumor cells exhibit a 4.7-fold increase in primary colony-forming efficiency and can be regarded as a biomarker for the majority of patients with primary ovarian cancer [31] (Table **1**).

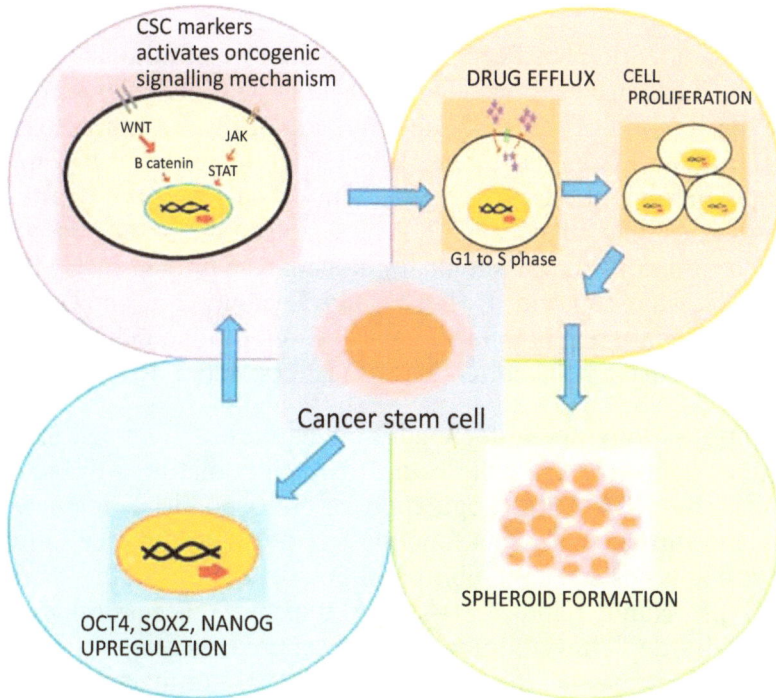

**Fig. (3).** Mechanism of cancer stemness in ovarian tissues.

**Table 1. List of Cancer Stemness molecules in ovarian cancer.**

| Sl. No. | Name | Function | References |
|---|---|---|---|
| 1 | SOX2 | Increased spheroid formation and tumorigenicity. | [21] |
| 2 | CD44 | Related to glutamine deficiency in chemoresistance. | [39] |
| 3 | CD117 | Activates NFκB pathway | [10] |
| 4 | CD24 | Activates NFκB pathway, detected in patients' blood samples. | [10] |
| 5 | ALDH | This lead to platinum resistance, surpasses cell cycle checkpoints. | [29] |

*(Table 1) cont.....*

| Sl. No. | Name | Function | References |
|:---:|:---:|:---|:---:|
| 6 | CD133 | Aggressive cell proliferation by triggering PI3K/AKT signaling pathway. | [31] |
| 7 | NANOG | Highly expressed in tumor mass by upregulating EMT markers. | [21] |
| 8 | OCT4 | Cell cycle progression from G1 to S phase, enhance JAK1, STAT3 levels | [22 - 24] |
| 9 | CD166 | Tumorsphere formation prevents drug incorporation in cells. | [27] |
| 10 | SOX9 | Resistance to chemotherapy by activating the Wnt/β-catenin pathway. | [25, 26] |

## MITOCHONDRIAL & EMT MECHANISMS ON OVARIAN CANCER AND ITS METASTATIC SITES

Recently, much attention has been focused on the role of mitochondrial dynamics in maintaining a balanced cell metabolism. Mitochondrial dynamics deals with the equitable coordination of the union and division of mitochondria to sustain their count, structure, and arrangement in cells. The conjugation of two mitochondria into a single mitochondrion is governed by mitofusins 1 and 2 (Mfn1 and Mfn2, respectively) and optic atrophy 1 (OPA1), enabling membrane association. The segmentation of mitochondria into dual mitochondria piloted by GTPase proteins dynamin-related/-like protein 1 (Drp1) and Dynamin2 (Dnm2) gives rise to compression at certain points followed by excision. Mitochondrial dynamic fusion and fission factors have been correlated with cell evolution [32].

In stem cell physiology, the mitochondrial dynamics of stem cell markers play a vital role in cell survival and cell death. It is known that growth factor erv1-like (Gfer) is associated with the regulation of mitochondrial characteristics and mitophagy and further widens its function in embryonic stem cell mitochondrial dynamics and apoptosis. The inhibition of Gfer at exon 2 and its 3' untranslated region lessens Nanog and Oct-4 and improves accessibility inside the mitochondria by depleting its membrane potential, resulting in mitophagy and apoptosis. Gfer prevents the activity of DRP1 mitochondrial fission by suppressing mitochondrial fragmentation in embryonic stem cells [33]. An essential question to ask is how cancer stem cells are involved in mitochondrial dynamics to promote tumor growth and metastasis. DRP1 phosphorylation at serine (S616) residue by CDK1/cyclin B with the aid of phosphorylated RALA and RALBP1 triggered by Aurora A further allows cell duplication from G1 to S phase [34]. DRP1 mitochondrial fission facilitates cancer stem cell propagation and tumorsphere formation and imparts metastatic properties in melanoma, breast, and lung cancer cells [35]. Likewise, cancer stem cells show a high expression ratio of DRP1/MFN2 in Pancreatic ductal adenocarcinoma patients, followed by the aggregation of many small defective mitochondria, consequently elevating reactive oxygen species and oncogenicity [36]. Brain tumor-initiating cells reflect similarity with neural progenitor cells in terms of self-renewal behavior; however, the tumorsphere environment in these tumor-initiating cells promotes mitochondrial fragmentation and tubular appearance with the major presence of CD133, SOX2, OLIG2, CD15, OCT4, and POUF3F2 stem cell markers. It is cyclin-dependent kinase 5 (CDK5), which allows the activation of DRP1. Nevertheless, we noticed that the suppression of DRP1 using shRNA or its inhibitor Mdivi-1 decreased cell viability along with AMP-activated protein kinase (AMPK) stimulation by its phosphorylation, which promotes caspase activity [37]. To our knowledge, single-cell metrics for measuring mitochondrial dynamics utilize mito-PSmO2 fluorescence and the Mitotracker-633 detection system. The mito-SinCe2 analysis conducted on ovarian tumor-initiating cells overexpressing ALDH and mitochondrial membrane potential repressed fusion and promoted the fission process [38]. It is well accepted that a lack of nourishment promotes cancer stemness and glucose metabolism for ATP generation, which is essential for tumor cell expansion. Amino acid glutamine insufficiency in ovarian cancer stem cells raises CD44 and CD117 expression, thereby causing reactive oxygen species generation and influencing MAPK-ERK1/2 to activate DRP1. Glutamine is concerned with the TCA cycle and drives STAT3 and mTORC1 to bring about the fast increase of tumor cells (Fig. **4**). In addition, phosphorylated DRP1 was detected after 24 h of glutamine inadequacy and upregulated SOX2, NANOG OCT4, and ABCG2, supporting cancer stemness and drug resistance [39].

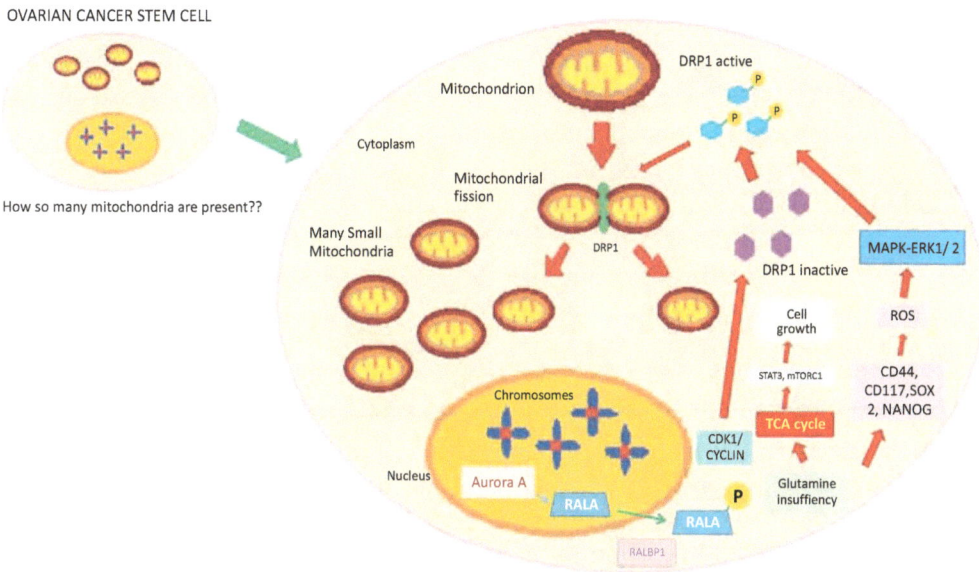

**Fig. (4).** Cancer stemness signalling mechanism related to mitochondrial dynamics.

## NATURAL AND SMALL MOLECULES TARGETING OVARIAN CANCER

Ovarian cancer treatment comprises novel strategies that should be reviewed for challenges including relapse, chemoresistance, and metastasis. Many reports have suggested that the specific or collective repression of cancer stem cell markers, along with clonogenic ability, can be used to treat cancer. Food-derived molecules such as 7-difluoromethoxyl-5,4'-di-n-octylygenistein (DFOG) modulate cell metabolism by preventing the activation of FoxM1, AKT, NFκB, and ERK1/2 proteins. DFOG allows the interdiction of not only CD133, CD44, and ALDH1 but also prevents spheroid and colony formation [40]. miR-199a restrains CD44 by binding to its 3'-UTR region, interferes with the cell cycle at the G2/M phase, and eradicates multidrug resistance of ovarian cancer cells towards cisplatin, paclitaxel, and adriamycin [42]. Many studies have indicated that Chinese bayberry leaf proanthocyanidins (BLPs) comprised of epigallocatechin-3-O-gallate focused on cancer stemness by minimizing the expression of OCT4, SOX2, and ALDH, and controlling tumor cell proliferation from 81.4 ± 2.0% to 44.4 ± 0.7%, thereby preventing the Wnt/β-catenin pathway from strengthening metastasis [43]. Cancer stemness is controlled by 1α,25-dihydroxy vitamin D, which impedes the activity of SOX2, CD44, NANOG, and Krüppel-like factor 4 (KLF4) and, inhibits cell survival by downregulating cyclin, and D1.,Xenograft experiments indicated that vitamin D3 also suppressed tumor growth *in vivo* [45]. Platinum-based therapy is carried out by the flavonoid compound (E)-1-4(4-aminophenyl)-3-(2,4-methoxyphenyl)prop-2-en-1-one or methoxyphenyl chalcone (MTC), which restricts the cell cycle at the G2/M checkpoint by subjugating autophagy-related protein 5 (Atg-5), SOX2, Oct4, KLF4, and elevating p-BAD and caspase activity [46]. Tumor relapse and chemo resistance in CD44+/MyD88+ ovarian cancer cells were surpassed by TRX-E-002-1, causing phosphorylation of c-Jun by Jun N-terminal kinase and blocking of cyclic ERK activation. TRX-E-002-1 facilitates apoptosis by triggering caspases and regressing tumor volume and kinetics [48]. Theasaponin E1 isolated from tea is recognized as an anti-cancer stemness molecule that eliminates tumor sphere formation; consequently, A2780 with around 51.29% and OVCAR3 with around 47.99% cell viability, respectively [49]. Co-adjuvant therapy with cisplatin and eugenol resulted in cell death in 87% and 82.5% of OV2774 and SKOV3 cells, respectively. Eugenol promotes cisplatin sensitivity, prevents spheroid formation, and simultaneously inhibits Hes Family BHLH Transcription Factor 1 (Hes1), CD44, and ALDH, which eventually suppress c-Myc, phospho-Akt, and other subsequent factors of the Notch pathway. Collectively, they counter the γ-secretase complex *in vitro* and reduce tumor cell multiplication by lowering the expression of Ki-67 and PAX8 *in vivo*, which may be a viable option for human ovarian carcinoma treatment [50]. Trimebutine maleate (TM) is apparent for ovarian cancer therapy because of its half-maximal growth inhibitory concentration (GI50) around 0.4 μM in A2780 sphere-forming cells, obstructing $Na^+$ and large-conductance voltage- and Ca2+-activated K+ channel (BKCa), which is active in ovarian cancer stem cells. It targets the Wnt/β-catenin pathway by preventing the phosphorylation of β-catenin at the serine residue 552, thereby diminishing the growth and metastatic traits of cancer stem cells [53]. It has been reported that the cell plasticity of tumor stem cells is significantly reduced by simvastatin, which causes depletion of CD44 expression to minimize spheroid volume, N-cadherin, and RhoA to limit EMT and the Hippo/YAP/TAZ pathway accompanied by the activation of PARP for apoptosis [55]. The synergistic effects of ursolic acid and cisplatin subdue hypoxia-inducible factor-1α (HIF-1α) and ABCG2 molecules are involved in hypoxia-induced resistance. HIF-1α levels were elevated in SKOV3 cells at 48 h and increased cell viability and cancer stemness (CD44, CD133, OCT4, and NANOG). In contrast, ursolic acid and cisplatin inhibited cell growth with a lower IC50 value in comparison with the individual treatments, along with a reduction in the level of PI3K affecting the PI3K/ Akt signaling mechanism [57] (Table **2**).

**Table 2. Drug molecules inhibiting ovarian cancer stemness.**

| Sl. No. | Molecules | Isolation Sources | Its Function | References |
|---|---|---|---|---|
| 1 | 7-difluoromethoxyl-5,4'-di-n-octylygenistein | Genistein analogues prepared by difluoromethylation and alkylation | Suppresses spheroid formation and cell growth by countering CD133, CD44, and ALDH1. | [40, 41] |
| 2 | miR-199a | highly conserved miRNA family present in cells. | Targets CD44, CD117, and prevents multidrug resistance. | [42] |
| 3 | Bayberry leaves proanthocyanidins | Chinese bayberry (*Myrica rubra* Sieb. et Zucc.) | Suppress OCT4, SOX2, ALDH, and target the Wnt/β-catenin pathway. | [43, 44] |
| 4 | Methoxyphenyl chalcone (MTC) | 1-(3,4,5-trimethoxyphenyl)propan-1-one and 4-methoxybenzaldehyde | Inhibits autophagy-related protein 5 (Atg-5), SOX2 and prevents cell migration. | [46, 47] |

*(Table 2) cont.....*

| Sl. No. | Molecules | Isolation Sources | Its Function | References |
|---|---|---|---|---|
| 5 | 1α,25-dihydroxyvitamin D3 | Kidney, intestine | KLF4, NANOG, and cyclin D1 stem cell-like phenotype inhibition. | [45] |
| 6 | TRX-E-002-1 | Benzopyran molecule | Enhanced expression of c-Jun for apoptosis. | [48] |
| 7 | Theasaponin E1 | Green tea seeds | Prevents cell growth of ALDH+ cells. | [49] |
| 8 | Co-adjuvant therapy of Eugenol and cisplatin | Eugenol from clove, cinnamon, basil leaf Cisplatin from Magnus' green salt | CD44, ALDH, and Hes1 suppression related to Notch pathway. | [50 - 52] |
| 9 | Trimebutine maleate | 3,4,5-trimethoxybenzoic acid [2-(dimethylamino)-2-phenylbutyl] ester | Block BKCa channel, therefore, reduces SOX2, OCT4, and β-catenin. | [53, 54] |
| 10 | Simvastatin | Fungus *Aspergillus terreus* and direct alkylation of lovastatin | Reduces CD44, N-cadherin, and RhoA to affect stem cell plasticity. | [55, 56] |
| 11 | Co-adjuvant therapy of Ursolic acid and cisplatin | Ursolic Acid from the peels of fruits, apples, cranberries, prunes | Reduction in HIF-1α and chemo resistance | [57, 58] |
| 12 | All-trans retinoic acid | Vitamin A sources, like, cereals and fish oils | Downregulates ALDH1, FoxM1 and Notch1 signalling. | [59] |
| 13 | Co-adjuvant therapy of Poziotinib and Manidipine | Poziotinib from 4-chloro-7-hydroxyquinazolin-6-yl pivalate with *d3*-methyliodide and 3,4-dichloro-2-fluoroaniline reaction Manidipine from dihydropyridine | Targets CD133, KLF4, and NANOG, thereby, decreasing β-catenin activity of cell survival and proliferation. | [60 - 62] |
| 13 | Salinomycin | *Streptomyces albus* | Inhibits SOX2, OCT3/4, CD44 and enhances apoptosis. | [63, 64] |

(Table 2) cont.....

| Sl. No. | Molecules | Isolation Sources | Its Function | References |
|---|---|---|---|---|
| 14 | Interleukin-21 by Human umbilical cord mesenchymal stem cells | Pleiotropic cytokine formed in Human umbilical cord mesenchymal stem cells. | Decreases the expression of β-catenin and cyclin-D1. | [65] |
| 15 | Metformin | Biguanide compound of goat's rue plants or French Lilac (*Galega officinalis*). | Suppresses PI3K/Akt/mTOR pathway. | [66, 67] |
| 16 | Verrucarin J | Trichothecene family is present in wheat, oats or maize. | ALDH1, LGR5, NANOG and OCT4 inhibit Notch1 and Wnt1 signaling pathways. | [68, 69] |

Taken together, these potential therapeutic drugs have been identified as major contributors to the prevention of ovarian cancer relapse and drug elimination. However, there is still a need for improved therapies that effectively target cancer stem cells.

## EXOSOMES-BASED DELIVERY OF DRUGS AND OTHER MOLECULES TARGETING OVARIAN

The comprehension of the synthesis, delivery, and intake of exosomes proceeds to develop, and consequently, these nanovesicles are an effective tumor-specific medium for cancer treatment (Fig. **5**). Exosomes effortlessly merge with the plasma membrane, thus ensuring a steady microenvironment for the incorporation of specific drug molecules into the cells for efficient delivery. One study utilized mesenchymal stem cell-derived exosomes with (96.5% ± 2.8% positive) TRAIL expression, which exhibited cytotoxicity towards adenocarcinoma cells along with resistant cells [70]. Human adipose-derived mesenchymal stem cell-derived exosomes prompt caspase, and p53, elevate the BAX/BCL2 ratio, and lower the cell plating ability by up to 30% to 35% in A2780 and SKOV-3 ovarian cancer cells. The presence of hsa-miR-124-3p in these exosomes along with many cytokines causes the suppression of CDKs, insulin-like growth factor 1, transforming growth factor-beta receptor I, and CD29, and targets the KEGG pathway molecules RAS (K-RAS, N-RAS), MAPK1, STAT3, PIK3R3, and AKT3, thereby preventing ovarian cancer progression [71]. The impact of exosome-encapsulated miRNAs on tumor therapy has been explored in human umbilical cord mesenchymal stem cells conveying anti-inflammatory miR-146a, which was found to alleviate chemo resistance as well as drug resistance to Taxane and Docetaxel in A2780 and SKOV3 cell lines, respectively. It was then investigated whether the miR-146a influences Laminin subunit gamma-2, which is involved in tumor proliferation in ovarian cells, modifies its expression by attaching to the 3'UTR of LAMC2 and further, impeding phosphorylation of PI3K and Akt for their activation holding back cell cycle advancement [72].

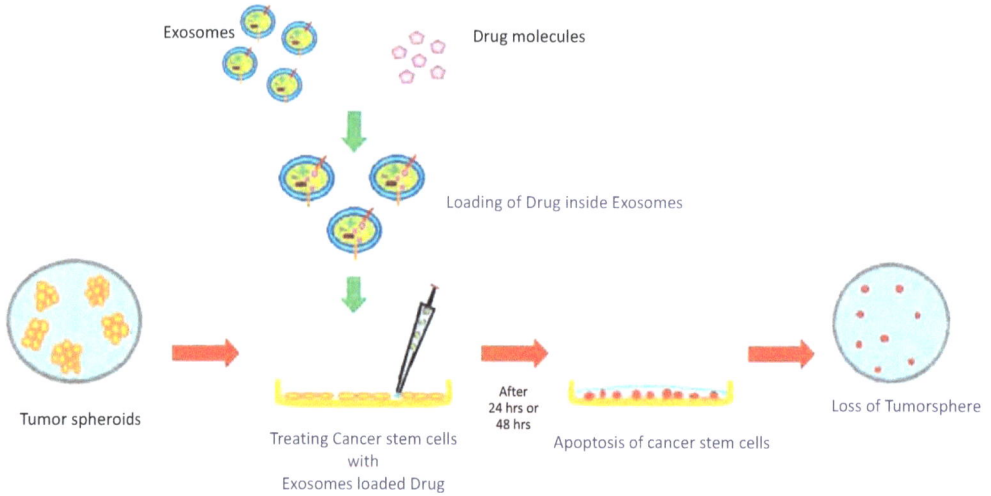

**Fig. (5).** Exosomes-based drug delivery targeting ovarian cancer stemness.

In a tumor-targeting study of exosomes, the role of mesenchymal stem cell exosomes MSC544 was augmented by transporting anti-tumor drugs to curb tumor growth. MSC544 exosomes cargoes Taxol in its lumen proved to limit the cell growth of SK-OV3$^{GFP}$ ovarian cancer cells by $75.1 \pm 1.0\%$ and shrinkage of tumor size in other cancers [73]. Owing to the characteristics of exosomes of a particular cell origin, low immunogenicity, high endurance, and convenient delivery, they have shown promising results in therapeutic and diagnostic approaches.

## CONCLUSION

An increasing number of recent studies have revealed the evolutionary system of cancer and have proposed different procedures for potent tumor inhibition. The conventional characteristics of stem cells are their self-renewal and maintenance of their population. However, cancer stem cells exhibit aggressive proliferation, metastasis, chemo resistance, and drug rejection. The involvement of distinct oncogenic signaling mechanisms boosts CSC features and imparts resistance to chemotherapy.

One limitation of this study is the early detection of ovarian cancer stemness in patients, which can be achieved by analyzing the molecular and functional profiles of cancer exosomes in human serum samples for the identification of a set of CSC molecules. The use of exosomes derived from food sources with coadjuvant therapy can contribute to enhancing the anti-cancer effect, thereby allowing a new window of opportunity for cancer stemness therapy.

## LIST OF ABBREVIATIONS

**ALDH**   Aldehyde Dehydrogenase

**ESCs**   Embryonic Stem Cells

**ESCRT**  Endosomal Sorting Complex Required for Transport

**EMT**    Epithelial to Mesenchymal Transition

**ILVs**   Intraluminal Vesicles

**MVB**    Multivesicular Body

**OCSC**   Ovarian Cancer Stem Cells

## REFERENCES

[1]    Ovarian Cancer landscape in Asia-Pacific 2021.

[2]    Kossaï M, Leary A, Scoazec JY, Genestie C. Ovarian cancer: A heterogeneous disease. Pathobiology 2018; 85(1-2): 41-9.
[http://dx.doi.org/10.1159/000479006] [PMID: 29020678]

[3]    Horta M, Cunha TM. Sex cord-stromal tumors of the ovary: a comprehensive review and update for radiologists. Diagn Interv Radiol 2015; 21(4): 277-86.
[http://dx.doi.org/10.5152/dir.2015.34414] [PMID: 26054417]

[4]    Karnezis AN, Wang Y, Keul J, *et al.* DICER1 and FOXL2 mutation status correlates with clinicopathologic features in ovarian sertoli-leydig cell tumors. Am J Surg Pathol 2019; 43(5): 628-38.
[http://dx.doi.org/10.1097/PAS.0000000000001232] [PMID: 30986800]

[5]    Shaaban AM, Rezvani M, Elsayes KM, *et al.* Ovarian malignant germ cell tumors: cellular classification and clinical and imaging features. Radiographics 2014; 34(3): 777-801.
[http://dx.doi.org/10.1148/rg.343130067] [PMID: 24819795]

[6]    Hashimoto H, Sudo T, Mikami Y, *et al.* Germ cell specific protein VASA is over-expressed in epithelial ovarian cancer and disrupts DNA damage-induced G2 checkpoint. Gynecol Oncol 2008; 111(2): 312-9.
[http://dx.doi.org/10.1016/j.ygyno.2008.08.014] [PMID: 18805576]

[7]    Thibault B, Castells M, Delord JP, Couderc B. Ovarian cancer microenvironment: implications for cancer dissemination and chemoresistance acquisition. Cancer Metastasis Rev 2014; 33(1): 17-39.
[http://dx.doi.org/10.1007/s10555-013-9456-2] [PMID: 24357056]

[8]    Lapidot T, Sirard C, Vormoor J, *et al.* A cell initiating human acute myeloid leukaemia after transplantation into SCID mice. Nature 1994; 367(6464): 645-8.
[http://dx.doi.org/10.1038/367645a0] [PMID: 7509044]

[9]    Bapat SA, Mali AM, Koppikar CB, Kurrey NK. Stem and progenitor-like cells contribute to the aggressive behavior of human epithelial ovarian cancer. Cancer Res 2005; 65(8): 3025-9.
[http://dx.doi.org/10.1158/0008-5472.CAN-04-3931] [PMID: 15833827]

[10]   Burgos-Ojeda D, Rueda BR, Buckanovich RJ. Ovarian cancer stem cell markers: Prognostic and therapeutic implications. Cancer Lett 2012; 322(1): 1-7.
[http://dx.doi.org/10.1016/j.canlet.2012.02.002] [PMID: 22334034]

[11] Makler A, Asghar W. Exosomal biomarkers for cancer diagnosis and patient monitoring. Expert Rev Mol Diagn 2020; 20(4): 387-400.
[http://dx.doi.org/10.1080/14737159.2020.1731308] [PMID: 32067543]

[12] Hurley JH. ESCRT complexes and the biogenesis of multivesicular bodies. Curr Opin Cell Biol 2008; 20(1): 4-11.
[http://dx.doi.org/10.1016/j.ceb.2007.12.002] [PMID: 18222686]

[13] Hessvik NP, Llorente A. Current knowledge on exosome biogenesis and release. Cell Mol Life Sci 2018; 75(2): 193-208.
[http://dx.doi.org/10.1007/s00018-017-2595-9] [PMID: 28733901]

[14] Villarroya-Beltri C, Baixauli F, Gutiérrez-Vázquez C, Sánchez-Madrid F, Mittelbrunn M. Sorting it out: Regulation of exosome loading. Semin Cancer Biol 2014; 28: 3-13.
[http://dx.doi.org/10.1016/j.semcancer.2014.04.009] [PMID: 24769058]

[15] Li P, Kaslan M, Lee SH, Yao J, Gao Z. Progress in exosome isolation techniques. Theranostics. 2017; 7(3): 789-804.
[http://dx.doi.org/10.7150/thno.18133]

[16] Kim MS, Haney MJ, Zhao Y, *et al.* Development of exosome-encapsulated paclitaxel to overcome MDR in cancer cells. Nanomedicine 2016; 12(3): 655-64.
[http://dx.doi.org/10.1016/j.nano.2015.10.012] [PMID: 26586551]

[17] Oskouie MN, Aghili Moghaddam NS, Butler AE, Zamani P, Sahebkar A. Therapeutic use of curcumin-encapsulated and curcumin-primed exosomes. J Cell Physiol 2019; 234(6): 8182-91.
[http://dx.doi.org/10.1002/jcp.27615] [PMID: 30317632]

[18] Greaves M, Maley CC. Clonal evolution of cancer cells Nature. 2012;481(7381):306-313.
[http://dx.doi.org/10.1038/nature10762]

[19] Bjerkvig R, Tysnes BB, Aboody KS, Najbauer J, Terzis AJA. The origin of the cancer stem cell: current controversies and new insights. Nat Rev Cancer 2005; 5(11): 899-904.
[http://dx.doi.org/10.1038/nrc1740] [PMID: 16327766]

[20] Kreso A, Dick JE. Evolution of the cancer stem cell model. Cell Stem Cell 2014; 14(3): 275-91.
[http://dx.doi.org/10.1016/j.stem.2014.02.006] [PMID: 24607403]

[21] Virant-Klun I, Stimpfel M. Novel population of small tumour-initiating stem cells in the ovaries of women with borderline ovarian cancer. Sci Rep. 2016; 6: 34730.
[http://dx.doi.org/10.1038/srep34730]

[22] Lee J, Go Y, Kang I, Han YM, Kim J. Oct-4 controls cell-cycle progression of embryonic stem cells. Biochem J. 2010; 426(2): 171-181.
[http://dx.doi.org/10.1042/BJ20091439]

[23] Ruan Z, Yang X, Cheng W. OCT4 accelerates tumorigenesis through activating JAK/STAT signaling in ovarian cancer side population cells. Cancer Manag Res. 2018; 11: 389-399.
[http://dx.doi.org/10.2147/CMAR.S180418]

[24] Samardzija C, Quinn M, Findlay JK, Ahmed N. Attributes of Oct4 in stem cell biology: perspectives on cancer stem cells of the ovary. J Ovarian Res. 2012; 5(1): 37.
[http://dx.doi.org/10.1186/1757-2215-5-37]

[25] Sherman-Samis M, Onallah H, Holth A, Reich R, Davidson B. SOX2 and SOX9 are markers of clinically aggressive disease in metastatic high-grade serous carcinoma. Gynecol Oncol 2019; 153(3): 651-60.
[http://dx.doi.org/10.1016/j.ygyno.2019.03.099] [PMID: 30904337]

[26] Hou R, Jiang L. RETRACTED ARTICLE: LINC00115 promotes stemness and inhibits apoptosis of ovarian cancer stem cells by upregulating SOX9 and inhibiting the Wnt/β-catenin pathway through competitively binding to microRNA-30a. Cancer Cell Int 2021; 21(1): 360.

[http://dx.doi.org/10.1186/s12935-021-02019-2] [PMID: 34238293]

[27] Kim DK, Ham MH, Lee SY, *et al.* CD166 promotes the cancer stem-like properties of primary epithelial ovarian cancer cells. BMB Rep 2020; 53(12): 622-7.
[http://dx.doi.org/10.5483/BMBRep.2020.53.12.102] [PMID: 32843129]

[28] Yasuda K, Torigoe T, Mariya T, *et al.* Fibroblasts induce expression of FGF4 in ovarian cancer stem-like cells/cancer-initiating cells and upregulate their tumor initiation capacity. Lab Invest 2014; 94(12): 1355-69.
[http://dx.doi.org/10.1038/labinvest.2014.122] [PMID: 25329002]

[29] Kaipio K, Chen P, Roering P, *et al.* ALDH1A1-related stemness in high-grade serous ovarian cancer is a negative prognostic indicator but potentially targetable by EGFR/mTOR-PI3K/aurora kinase inhibitors. J Pathol 2020; 250(2): 159-69.
[http://dx.doi.org/10.1002/path.5356] [PMID: 31595974]

[30] Liu CL, Chen YJ, Fan MH, Liao YJ, Mao TL. Characteristics of cd133-sustained chemoresistant cancer stem-like cells in human ovarian carcinoma. Int J Mol Sci. 2020; 21(18): 6467.
[http://dx.doi.org/10.3390/ijms21186467]

[31] Ferrandina G, Bonanno G, Pierelli L, *et al.* Expression of CD133-1 and CD133-2 in ovarian cancer. Int J Gynecol Cancer 2008; 18(3): 506-14.
[http://dx.doi.org/10.1111/j.1525-1438.2007.01056.x] [PMID: 17868344]

[32] Maycotte P, Marín-Hernández A, Goyri-Aguirre M, Anaya-Ruiz M, Reyes-Leyva J, Cortés-Hernández P. Mitochondrial dynamics and cancer. Tumour Biol 2017; 39: 5.
[http://dx.doi.org/10.1177/1010428317698391] [PMID: 28468591]

[33] Todd LR, Gomathinayagam R, Sankar U. A novel Gfer-Drp1 link in preserving mitochondrial dynamics and function in pluripotent stem cells. Autophagy 2010; 6(6): 821-2.
[http://dx.doi.org/10.4161/auto.6.6.12625] [PMID: 20581476]

[34] Chen H, Chan DC. Mitochondrial dynamics in regulating the unique phenotypes of cancer and stem cells. Cell Metab 2017; 26(1): 39-48.
[http://dx.doi.org/10.1016/j.cmet.2017.05.016] [PMID: 28648983]

[35] Peiris-Pagès M, Bonuccelli G, Sotgia F, Lisanti MP. Mitochondrial fission as a driver of stemness in tumor cells: mDIVI1 inhibits mitochondrial function, cell migration and cancer stem cell (CSC) signalling. Oncotarget. 2018; 9(17): 13254-13275.
[http://dx.doi.org/10.18632/oncotarget.24285]

[36] Courtois S, de Luxán-Delgado B, Penin-Peyta L, *et al.* Inhibition of mitochondrial dynamics preferentially targets pancreatic cancer cells with enhanced tumorigenic and invasive potential. Cancers (Basel). 2021; 13(4): 698.
[http://dx.doi.org/10.3390/cancers13040698]

[37] Xie Q, Wu Q, Horbinski CM, *et al.* Mitochondrial control by DRP1 in brain tumor initiating cells. Nat Neurosci 2015; 18(4): 501-10.
[http://dx.doi.org/10.1038/nn.3960] [PMID: 25730670]

[38] Spurlock B, Gupta P, Basu MK, *et al.* New quantitative approach reveals heterogeneity in mitochondrial structure-function relations in tumor-initiating cells. J Cell Sci. 2019; 132(9): jcs230755.
[http://dx.doi.org/10.1242/jcs.230755]

[39] Prasad P, Ghosh S, Roy SS. Glutamine deficiency promotes stemness and chemoresistance in tumor cells through DRP1-induced mitochondrial fragmentation. Cell Mol Life Sci 2021; 78(10): 4821-45.
[http://dx.doi.org/10.1007/s00018-021-03818-6] [PMID: 33895866]

[40] Ning Y, Xu M, Cao X, Chen X, Luo X. Inactivation of AKT, ERK and NF-κB by genistein derivative, 7-difluoromethoxyl-5,4′-di-n-octylygenistein, reduces ovarian carcinoma oncogenicity. Oncol Rep 2017; 38(2): 949-58.

[http://dx.doi.org/10.3892/or.2017.5709] [PMID: 28627607]

[41]   Xiang HL, Liu F, Quan MF, Cao JG, Lv Y. 7-difluoromethoxyl-5,4′-di-n-octylgenistein inhibits growth of gastric cancer cells through downregulating forkhead box M1. World J Gastroenterol 2012; 18(33): 4618-26.
[http://dx.doi.org/10.3748/wjg.v18.i33.4618] [PMID: 22969238]

[42]   Cheng W, Liu T, Wan X, Gao Y, Wang H. MicroRNA-199a targets *CD44* to suppress the tumorigenicity and multidrug resistance of ovarian cancer-initiating cells. FEBS J 2012; 279(11): 2047-59.
[http://dx.doi.org/10.1111/j.1742-4658.2012.08589.x] [PMID: 22498306]

[43]   Zhang Y, Chen S, Wei C, Rankin GO, Ye X, Chen YC. Dietary compound proanthocyanidins from Chinese bayberry ( *Myrica rubra* Sieb. et Zucc.) leaves attenuate chemotherapy-resistant ovarian cancer stem cell traits *via* targeting the Wnt/β-catenin signaling pathway and inducing G1 cell cycle arrest. Food Funct 2018; 9(1): 525-33.
[http://dx.doi.org/10.1039/C7FO01453H] [PMID: 29256569]

[44]   Shi L, Cao S, Chen X, Chen W, Zheng Y, Yang Z. Proanthocyanidin synthesis in chinese bayberry (*Myrica rubra* Sieb. et Zucc.) fruits. Front Plant Sci 2018; 9: 212.
[http://dx.doi.org/10.3389/fpls.2018.00212] [PMID: 29541082]

[45]   Ji M, Liu L, Hou Y, Li B. 1α,25-Dihydroxyvitamin D3 restrains stem cell-like properties of ovarian cancer cells by enhancing vitamin D receptor and suppressing CD44. Oncol Rep 2019; 41(6): 3393-403.
[http://dx.doi.org/10.3892/or.2019.7116] [PMID: 31002352]

[46]   Su Y, Huang WC, Lee WH, *et al.* Methoxyphenyl chalcone sensitizes aggressive epithelial cancer to cisplatin through apoptosis induction and cancer stem cell eradication. Tumour Biol 2017; 39: 5.
[http://dx.doi.org/10.1177/1010428317691689] [PMID: 28466786]

[47]   Zhang Y, Srinivasan B, Xing C, Lü. J new chalcone derivative (E)-3-(4-methoxyphenyl)-2-me-hyl-1-(3,4,5-trimethoxyphenyl)prop-2-en-1-one suppresses prostate cancer involving p53-mediated cell cycle arrests and apoptosis. Anticancer Res 2012; 32(9): 3689-98.
[PMID: 22993307]

[48]   Alvero AB, Heaton A, Lima E, *et al.* TRX-E-002-1 induces c-jun–dependent apoptosis in ovarian cancer stem cells and prevents recurrence *in vivo*. Mol Cancer Ther 2016; 15(6): 1279-90.
[http://dx.doi.org/10.1158/1535-7163.MCT-16-0005] [PMID: 27196760]

[49]   Jia LY, Xia HL, Chen ZD, *et al.* Anti-proliferation effect of theasaponin $E_1$ on the ALDH-positive ovarian cancer stem-like cells. Molecules. 2018;23(6):1469.
[http://dx.doi.org/10.3390/molecules23061469]

[50]   Islam SS, Aboussekhra A. Sequential combination of cisplatin with eugenol targets ovarian cancer stem cells through the Notch-Hes1 signalling pathway. J Exp Clin Cancer Res. 2019;38(1):382.
[http://dx.doi.org/10.1186/s13046-019-1360-3]

[51]   Paidi RK, Jana M, Raha S, *et al.* Eugenol, a Component of holy basil (tulsi) and common spice clove, inhibits the interaction between SARS-CoV-2 Spike S1 and ACE2 to induce therapeutic responses. J Neuroimmune Pharmacol 2021; 16(4): 743-55.
[http://dx.doi.org/10.1007/s11481-021-10028-1] [PMID: 34677731]

[52]   Kauffman GB, Pentimalli R, Doldi S, Hall MD. Michele peyrone (1813-1883), discoverer of cisplatin. Platin Met Rev 2010; 54(4): 250-6.
[http://dx.doi.org/10.1595/147106710X534326]

[53]   Lee H, Kwon OB, Lee JE, *et al.* Repositioning trimebutine maleate as a cancer treatment targeting ovarian cancer stem cells. Cells. 2021;10(4):918.
[http://dx.doi.org/10.3390/cells10040918]

[54]   National Center for Biotechnology Information. PubChem Compound Summary for CID 51066575.

Available from: https://pubchem.ncbi.nlm.nih.gov/compound/51066575

[55]  Kato S, Liberona MF, Cerda-Infante J, *et al.* Simvastatin interferes with cancer 'stem-cell' plasticity reducing metastasis in ovarian cancer. Endocr Relat Cancer 2018; 25(10): 821-36.
[http://dx.doi.org/10.1530/ERC-18-0132] [PMID: 29848667]

[56]  Subhan M, Faryal R, Macreadie I. Exploitation of aspergillus terreus for the production of natural statins. J Fungi (Basel). 2016; 2(2): 13.
[http://dx.doi.org/10.3390/jof2020013]

[57]  Wang WJ, Sui H, Qi C, *et al.* Ursolic acid inhibits proliferation and reverses drug resistance of ovarian cancer stem cells by downregulating ABCG2 through suppressing the expression of hypoxia-inducible factor-1α *in vitro.* Oncol Rep 2016; 36(1): 428-40.
[http://dx.doi.org/10.3892/or.2016.4813] [PMID: 27221674]

[58]  Frighetto RTS, Welendorf RM, Nigro EN, Frighetto N, Siani AC. Isolation of ursolic acid from apple peels by high speed counter-current chromatography. Food Chem 2008; 106(2): 767-71.
[http://dx.doi.org/10.1016/j.foodchem.2007.06.003]

[59]  Young MJ, Wu YH, Chiu WT, Weng TY, Huang YF, Chou CY. All-trans retinoic acid downregulates ALDH1-mediated stemness and inhibits tumour formation in ovarian cancer cells. Carcinogenesis 2015; 36(4): 498-507.
[http://dx.doi.org/10.1093/carcin/bgv018] [PMID: 25742746]

[60]  Lee H, Kim JW, Lee DS, Min SH. Combined poziotinib with manidipine treatment suppresses ovarian cancer stem-cell proliferation and stemness. Int J Mol Sci. 2020; 21(19): 7379.
[http://dx.doi.org/10.3390/ijms21197379]

[61]  Ma S, Wang L, Ouyang B, Bai X, Ji Q, Yao L. The design, synthesis and preliminary pharmacokinetic evaluation of d3-poziotinib hydrochloride. Biol Pharm Bull 2019; 42(6): 873-6.
[http://dx.doi.org/10.1248/bpb.b19-00153] [PMID: 31155586]

[62]  McKeage K, Scott LJ. Manidipine. Drugs 2004; 64(17): 1923-40.
[http://dx.doi.org/10.2165/00003495-200464170-00011] [PMID: 15329044]

[63]  Lee HG, Shin SJ, Chung HW, *et al.* Salinomycin reduces stemness and induces apoptosis on human ovarian cancer stem cell. J Gynecol Oncol 2017; 28(2): e14.
[http://dx.doi.org/10.3802/jgo.2017.28.e14] [PMID: 27894167]

[64]  Zhang X, Lu C, Bai L. Mechanism of salinomycin overproduction in Streptomyces albus as revealed by comparative functional genomics. Appl Microbiol Biotechnol 2017; 101(11): 4635-44.
[http://dx.doi.org/10.1007/s00253-017-8278-5] [PMID: 28401259]

[65]  Zhang Y, Wang J, Ren M, *et al.* Gene therapy of ovarian cancer using IL-21-secreting human umbilical cord mesenchymal stem cells in nude mice. J Ovarian Res. 2014; 7:8.
[http://dx.doi.org/10.1186/1757-2215-7-8]

[66]  Gadducci A, Biglia N, Tana R, Cosio S, Gallo M. Metformin use and gynecological cancers: A novel treatment option emerging from drug repositioning. Crit Rev Oncol Hematol 2016; 105: 73-83.
[http://dx.doi.org/10.1016/j.critrevonc.2016.06.006] [PMID: 27378194]

[67]  Witters LA. The blooming of the French lilac. J Clin Invest 2001; 108(8): 1105-7.
[http://dx.doi.org/10.1172/JCI14178] [PMID: 11602616]

[68]  Carter K, Rameshwar P, Ratajczak MZ, Kakar SS. Verrucarin J inhibits ovarian cancer and targets cancer stem cells. Oncotarget. 2017; 8(54): 92743-92756.
[http://dx.doi.org/10.18632/oncotarget.21574]

[69]  Foroud NA, Baines D, Gagkaeva TY, *et al.* Trichothecenes in cereal grains - an update. Toxins (Basel). 2019; 11(11): 634.
[http://dx.doi.org/10.3390/toxins11110634]

[70]  Yuan Z, Kolluri KK, Gowers KH, Janes SM. TRAIL delivery by MSC-derived extracellular vesicles is

an effective anticancer therapy. J Extracell Vesicles. 2017; 6(1): 1265291.
[http://dx.doi.org/10.1080/20013078.2017.1265291]

[71]   Reza AMMT, Choi YJ, Yasuda H, Kim JH. Human adipose mesenchymal stem cell-derived exosomal-miRNAs are critical factors for inducing anti-proliferation signaling to A2780 and SKOV-3 ovarian cancer cells. Sci Rep. 2016; 6: 38498.
[http://dx.doi.org/10.1038/srep38498]

[72]   Qiu L, Wang J, Chen M, Chen F, Tu W. Exosomal microRNA-146a derived from mesenchymal stem cells increases the sensitivity of ovarian cancer cells to docetaxel and taxane *via* a LAMC2-mediated PI3K/Akt axis. Int J Mol Med 2020; 46(2): 609-20.
[http://dx.doi.org/10.3892/ijmm.2020.4634] [PMID: 32626953]

[73]   Melzer C, Ohe JV, Hass R. Anti-tumor effects of exosomes derived from drug-incubated permanently growing human MSC. Int J Mol Sci. 2020; 21(19): 7311.
[http://dx.doi.org/10.3390/ijms21197311]

CHAPTER 6

# Sphingosine Kinase as a Target to Treat Gastrointestinal Cancers

**Mit Joshi**[1] and **Bhoomika M. Patel**[2,*]

[1] *Institute of Pharmacy, Nirma University, Ahmedabad, India*

[2] *National Forensic Science University, Gujarat, India*

**Abstract:** Gastrointestinal cancer is a malignant condition of the gastrointestinal tract including the esophagus, stomach, small and large intestine, rectum, and anus. About 4.8 million new cases of gastrointestinal cancer were recorded in 2020. Current treatment options of gastrointestinal cancers have failed to treat the disease condition and newer approaches are under investigation. One such approach includes targeting the sphingosine kinase, a critical enzyme in sphingolipid metabolism. Known as structural molecules of the cellular membrane, sphingolipids, and their metabolism have emerged as important components of cellular functions like cell proliferation, cell survival, and cell apoptosis. Over the last few years, most of the enzymes involved in the metabolism of sphingolipids have been extensively studied, which has enlightened the primary roles of these metabolic enzymes in the sphingolipid metabolic pathway. Ceramide and sphingosine are synthesized mainly by oxidative stress, and chemotherapy/radiation which mediates apoptosis, and cell cycle arrest, while sphingosine-1-phosphate (S1P) converted from ceramide, has proliferation and anti-apoptotic properties. Findings regarding the nature of ceramide and/or S1P lead to evaluating the potential target enzymes, which are involved in the metabolism of ceramide and S1P. Sphingosine kinase HK1 (SPHK1) and sphingosine kinase HK2 (SPHK2) are diacylglycerol kinase family which converts ceramide into S1P. The overexpression of SPHK1 and SPHK2 has been documented in various cancers. Many *in vitro* and *in vivo* studies have been carried out to evaluate the role of sphingosine kinase in cancer. Based on the findings, few pharmacological interventions are under clinical study. This chapter includes sphingolipid metabolism and its essential enzymes, the role of sphingolipids and metabolic enzymes in cancer, potential enzyme targets for the treatment of cancer, and molecules under investigation.

**Keywords:** Ceramide, Ceramidase, Gastrointestinal tract, Gastrointestinal cancer, Sphingosine kinase.

---

* **Corresponding author Bhoomika M. Patel:** National Forensic Science University, Gujarat, India;
E-mail: drbhoomikampatel@gmail.com

## INTRODUCTION

Gastrointestinal cancer is a broad term that includes cancer of the upper gastrointestinal (GI) tract and lower GI tract. Upper GI tract cancer mainly includes esophagus cancer, stomach cancer, pancreatic cancer, gallbladder, and small intestine cancer while lower GI tract cancer includes colon cancer, rectal cancer, and gastrointestinal carcinoid cancer. Out of all types of cancer, colon, stomach, rectum, and esophageal cancer accounts for 6.1%, 5.7%, 3.9%, and 3.2% respectively. In 2018, over 1.8 million new colorectal cancer cases were registered and 881,000 deaths were estimated around the world. Colorectal cancer lines are second regarding mortality and third regarding incidence. The incidence of colorectal cancer is higher in developed countries compared to developing countries although the scenario is changing dramatically. For stomach cancer, over 1,000,000 new cases in 2018 were reported with an estimated number of deaths of 783,000 persons, making it the fifth most frequently diagnosed cancer and third in mortality of all cancer deaths. Esophageal cancer accounted for 5,72,000 new cases and 5,09,000 deaths in 2018. Esophageal cancer lines are ranked seventh in terms of incidence and sixth in overall cancer-related death [1].

Currently, cancer treatment involves multiple approaches using targeted drug therapy, chemotherapy, radiotherapy, hormonal therapy, and surgery. Albeit, all the current therapieshave some problems like they fail to destroy tumor cells without any side-effects on healthy cells of the body. Radiotherapy does not differentiate between healthy cells and cancerous cells and causes extensive damage to healthy ones. Chemotherapy resistance is one of the prime problems when used for long-term treatment. Thus, mono-drug therapy is not a viable option to treat cancer cells. Many cancer types have a higher recurrence rate after chemotherapy. For example, breast cancer has a 30% recurrence rate, melanoma has an 87% recurrence rate in the metastatic state, and non-small cell lung cancer has a 27% recurrence rate. Chemotherapy also causes different kinds of toxicities. 5-fluorouracil, a widely used chemotherapeutic drug, is known to cause cardiotoxicity and myelosuppression. Doxorubicin is a commonly used anthracycline drug that causes cardiotoxicity and renal toxicity. Bleomycin is also known to cause pulmonary toxicity. Cyclophosphamide has been shown to have bladder toxicity and immunosuppression. Other unwanted effects of current anticancer drugs are anemia, GIT disturbance, inflammation, alopecia, immunosuppression, and heart and nerve disorders. Surgery in cancer is mainly used for the removal of the tumor and surrounding tissues if required. Although some complications are associated with cancer surgery like blood loss, wound complications like delayed healing and wound infection, other infections like pneumonia, unbearable pain, and blood clots.

Newer targets and treatments are required to tackle the disease, particularly in the GI tract cancer.

In this chapter, we will discuss the sphingolipid metabolic pathway and the role of its enzymes and metabolites in cancer. Further, we will discuss existing knowledge regarding the role of sphingolipid metabolism in GI tract cancer.

## Currently Available Therapies to Treat Gastrointestinal Cancer

Systemic chemotherapy treatment is one of the most common and widely used strategies to combat GI tract cancer [2]. The metastasis of GI tract tumors generally involves the overexpression of p21 proteins and mutated Ras proteins [3]. The most commonly used chemotherapeutic agents in GI tract cancers are alkylating agents mainly cyclophosphamide, melphalan, ifosfamide, and busulfan, antimetabolites with first preference to 5-Fluorouracil followed by gemcitabine, and methotrexate, antibiotics such as doxorubicin daunorubicin and epirubicin, platinum-based agents (cisplatin, carboplatin, oxaliplatin) and topoisomerase inhibitors (topotecan, irinotecan, etoposide, teniposide) [4]. Asirinotecan and docetaxel are not commonly used and are considered as a treatment only during drug-resistance scenarios. The most common challenges regarding these drugs are anorexia, diarrhea, rash, and skin problems. Platinum-based drugs are considered first-line therapy for advanced gastric cancer while treatment for advanced gastric cancer includes platinum, taxanes, anthracyclines, doxorubicin, fluoropyrimidines, and irinotecan. Neurotoxicity (central and peripheral) produced as a by-product of anti-cancer drugs can affect the body for many years even after the completion of chemotherapy and can affect functional ability and quality of life in cancer patients. Chemotherapy-induced peripheral neuropathy (CIPN) is another major problem caused by anti-cancer agents including angiogenesis inhibitors, vinca alkaloids, platinum-based agents, taxanes, and proteasome inhibitors. Lifelong CIPN is linked with a complication like insomnia, anxiety, and depression [5].

## Sphingolipid Metabolism

In the past 2 decades, research on the role of 'bioactive lipids' has extensively emerged. Before the last 2 decades, the role of lipids in the body is thought to be involved only in energy metabolism and cellular structure. In the 1950s, Hokin and Hokin identified that the amount of inositol phospholipids drastically increased in pancreatic cells that were treated with acetylcholine [6]. Only years later, the role of diacylglycerol (DAG) and inositol1,4,5-trisphosphate was identified in the regulation of protein kinase C (PKC) and calcium release, respectively [7]. Over many years, different bioactive lipids like eicosanoid [8], phospholipids, sphingolipids, phosphatidic acid, monoacylglycerols, anandamide, and platelet-activating factors (PAF) were identified in various inter and intramolecular signaling in cells.

In the last decade, a group of bioactive lipids known as 'sphingolipids' is identified and their role in metabolism is studied [9]. Sphingolipids are a type of lipids containing sphingoid bases and a set of aliphatic amino alcohols [10]. The first molecule identified as a part of sphingolipid metabolism was sphingosine, which exerts molecular signaling on kinases and genes. Sphingosine and its counterparts have roles in the cell cycle, apoptosis, maintaining cell structure, and endocytosis [11, 12]. Though sphingosine was identified as the first molecule, much of the research remained focused on ceramide and sphingosine-1-phosphate (S1P). Ceramide is converted into sphingosine by the ceramidase enzyme. Sphingosine is further converted into S1P by sphingosine kinase [13]. Ceramide and S1P mediate opposite cellar responses. Ceramide is involved in cellular stress responses and apoptosis while S1P is involved in cell survival, and cell migration [14 - 16]. The overview of sphingolipid metabolism is represented in Fig. (1).

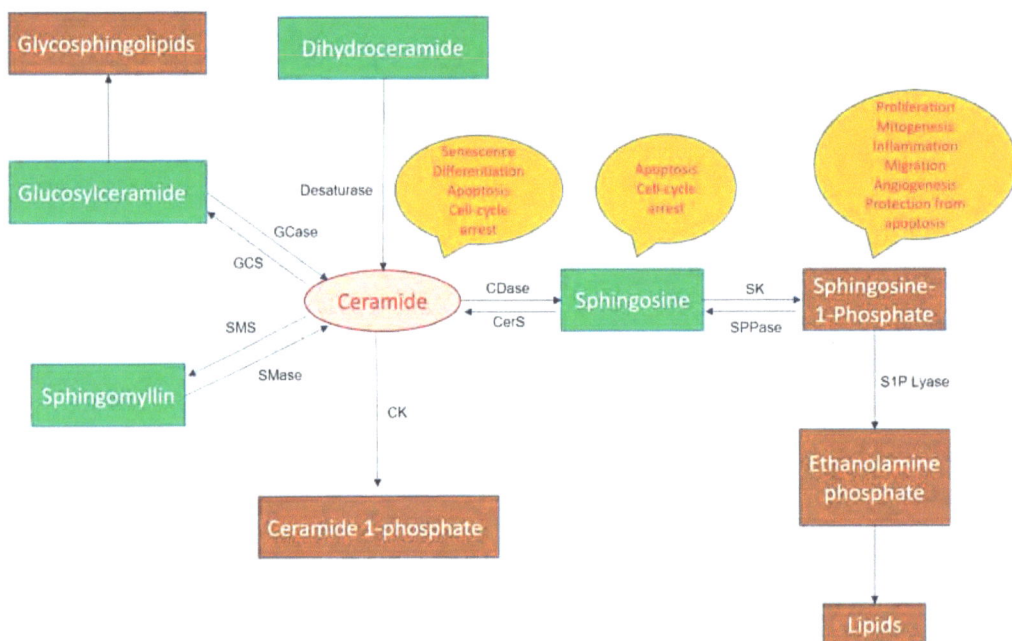

**Fig. (1).** Overview of Sphingolipid metabolism with the specific role of ceramide, sphingosine, and sphingosine-1-phosphate in cancer cells. CDase, ceramidase; CK, ceramide kinase; GCase, glucosyl ceramidase; GCS, glucosylceramide synthase; SK, sphingosine kinase; SMase, sphingomyelinase; SMS, sphingomyelin synthase; SPPase, sphingosine phosphate phosphatase.

The metabolic pathway of sphingolipids begins with the formation of 3-ket--dihydrosphingosine through the condensation of serine and palmitate by the serine palmitoyltransferase (SPT) enzyme [17, 18]. Reduction of 3-ket--dihydrosphingosine forms dihydrosphingosine, which is further acetylated to dihydroceramide by dihydroceramide synthase. The desaturation of dihydroceramide leads to the formation of ceramide [19]. Ceramide is known as a central player in sphingolipid metabolism and can be converted or broken down by different enzymes to exert different responses at the molecular level. Many molecular signaling pathways exhibit linear signaling involving molecules and receptors. However, sphingolipid signaling contains additional levels of molecules and enzymes, which form a complex and interconnected network. Moreover, many pathways in the synthesis of sphingolipids run parallel. As sphingolipids contain hydrophobic properties, the physiological process and synthesis of sphingolipids remain restricted to biological membranes [20]. Activation of sphingomyelinases (SMases) converts Sphingomyelin into ceramide as an immediate lipid product [21]. However, many pathways and molecules can arise from ceramide by activation of different enzymes

## Sphingolipid Enzymes

### Sphingosine Kinases

Sphingosine kinase (SPHKs) are critical enzyme, that maintains a balance between ceramide-induced apoptotic signaling and S1P-induced cell migration and survival signaling [22]. SPHKs are considered as degradation enzymes for sphingolipids, as theycarry out ceramide to S1P conversion, and then decimation of S1P by S1P lyase. Many studies have focused on the biosynthesis of S1P by SPHK due to the role of S1P in the survival of the cell as well as overexpression of proto-oncogenes genes by activating S1P-selective G-protein-coupled receptors and as secondary messengers [22].

Two isoforms of SPHK, SPHK1 and SPHK2 exert a little bit different stimuli for biological functions. Studies have shown that SPHK1 is involved in an anti-apoptotic role. Under normal conditions, SPHK1 activity maintains a level of ceramide to prevent unnecessary cell death [23]. Extracellular signal-regulated kinases 1/2 (ERK1/2) phosphorylate SPHK1, which is further transfered to the plasma membrane, through binding with calcium and integrin-binding protein 1 (CIB1) and carries out the conversion of sphingosine to S1P [24]. As the RAS pathway is overexpressed in cancer cells, the activation and migration of SPHK1 are thought to be involved in drug resistance mechanisms by decreasing ceramide levels and further activating survival mechanisms [25, 26]. Moreover, drug-resistant cell lines have shown high activity of SPHK1 which decreases ceramide levels and inhibits ceramide-induced apoptosis. Several studies have shown that inhibiting SPHK1 blocks the conversion of sphingosine to S1P thereby activating apoptosis through the accumulation of ceramide [27, 28]. Although having the same characteristics, SPHK2 has proved more difficult with different opinions and results regarding its role in angiogenesis [29, 30]. Even with conflicting results, SPHK2 provided positive outcomes in mammary cancer, acute lymphoblastic leukemia (ALL) [31], and myeloma [32].

## *Ceramidase*

Synthesis of sphingosine from ceramide is carried out by ceramidases. Ceramidases have different isoforms, which function based on their affinity towards acidic, neutral, or alkaline pH. A highly abundant form of ceramidase, acid ceramidase (AC) is thought to be present in acidic environments, such as lysosomes [33]. In several solid tumors, AC overexpression has been documented [34]. Some pre-clinical studies have demonstrated a positive effect of AC inhibitors on cancer cells by decreasing drug resistance. As of now, no drug is under investigation for blockade of AC. Only one drug, Tamoxifen has shown some level of AC inhibition, making it a potential candidate for adj chemotherapy [34 - 36].

## *Glucosylceramide Synthase*

Glucosylceramide synthase (GCS) is involved in the generation of glycosphingolipids by converting ceramide to glucosylceramide. As GCS is involved in the utilization of ceramide and decreases its concentration, research has been focused on targeting GCS [37 - 39]. Eliglustat, a GCS inhibitor has been approved to treat Gaucher's disease and lysosomal storage disorder suggests that the inhibition of GCS is possible in humans without serious side effects and could provide insight into studying a combination therapy of GCS inhibition and chemotherapy [40].

## *Ceramide Synthase*

Six different types of ceramide synthases (CerS) have been identified, each capable of generating different lengths of sphingolipids as well as converting sphingosine into ceramides as a part of the classical sphingolipid salvage pathway [41]. Several pre-clinical studies have shown that activation of CerS is important for chemotherapy to kill cancer. Although activation of CerS showed an attractive anti-cancer target, the regulation of CerS remains poorly understood [42 - 45].

## Importance of Ceramide

To understand how these sphingolipids transmit signals to exert their physiological and molecular effects, in-depth knowledge is required to elucidate its functions. There are two possible mechanistic pathways to understanding the nature of lipids: one is lipid-lipid interaction where sphingolipids interact with the membrane layer or other lipids and another is lipid-protein interaction where lipids impart functional changes in target proteins to exert further downstream signaling. At physiological levels, sphingolipids exert their effect at different affinity and concentration. For example, small amounts of S1P are capable of interaction with high affinity receptors which can sense S1P at very low levels. Lipids such as ceramide or DAG found at intermediate levels of 0.1 to 1.0% in membrane act on target with intermediary affinity. However, it is difficult to identify that highly abundant lipids like SM exert their effect on targets as their affinity must be on the lower side. For ceramide and S1P, research has been focused on identifying the target proteins [46]. Ceramide exerts its anti-tumor activity by activating catalytic subunits protein phosphatases 1 (PP1) and protein phosphatases 2A (PP2A) and inhibiting certain genes such as Akt49, and Bcr [46]. Disruption in sphingolipid metabolism and accumulation of ceramide within cell membranes also play an important role by activating apoptotic signaling through autophagy, mitophagy, and unfolded protein response. Furthermore, the accumulation of ceramide is capable of direct apoptosis by creating pores within the outer mitochondrial membrane and facilitates the release of cytochrome c, activation of mitochondria-derived activator of caspases, and apoptosis-inducing factors [47]. Based on the above discussion, one fact has been cleared that the accumulation of ceramide may be helpful during chemotherapy (Fig. **2**).

## Role of S1P in the Growth of Cancer and Metastasis

Conversion from ceramide to S1P is facilitated by SPHK1 and SPHK2 in the S1P receptor (S1PR) dependent and S1PR independent manner. Transduction of signals through S1PR-1-5 has different roles in cell proliferation, cell migration, tumorigenesis, and angiogenesis. Moreover, downstream signals generated from SPHK1 and SPHK2, independent of S1PR are found to be different. At the plasma membrane, activation of SPHK1 leads to the conversion of ceramide to S1P, and S1P further interacts with S1PR receptors, activating the pro-oncogenic signaling pathway [20]. Oestradiol was found to be involved in the activation of S1P *via* activating ATP-binding cassette sub-family C member 1 (ABCC1) and ATP-binding cassette sub-family G member 2 (ABCG2) activates S1PR signalling and downstream pathway, which leads to survival of breast cancer cells [48]. Protein spinster homolog 2 (SPNS2) was able to secrete S1P in endothelial cells and the absence of spns2 resulted in a significant decrease in the metastatic nature of lung carcinoma when different lung metastatic cell lines were injected in mice [49]. The study also found that increased infiltration of immune cells such as NK cells and T cells to the lungs increases the invasion of cancer cells and halts angiogenesis in Spns2$^{-/-}$ mice [50]. This evidence was supported by another study which found that metastasis was increased in lung carcinoma of Sphk1$^{+/+}$ control mice and attenuated in Sphk1$^{-/-}$ mice [51]. Master suppressor of metastasis breast cancer metastasis-suppressor 1 (BRMS1) suppressed by S1P-mediated activation of S1PR2 and attenuation of systemic S1P leads to reactivation of BRMS1 results in the inhibition of metastasis in bladder and melanoma cancer allografts [51]. In addition, high systemic levels of S1P in Sphk2$^{-/-}$ mice aggravate inflammatory markers in the intestine, resulting in colitis and colitis-associated cancer (CAC) through the activation of S1PR1-mediated nuclear factor-κB (NFκB) activation [52]. Pro-drug FTY720 effectively delays the development of CAC in mice by inhibiting S1PR1 signalling. Moreover, S1P isolated from osteoblast induces cell proliferation with drug resistance in bone-metastasis-derived prostate cancer cells [52, 53]. Thus, these result highlights the involvement of systemic S1P signalling in controlling cell proliferation, angiogenesis, and metastasis, by activating S1PR downstream pathway in cancer cells.

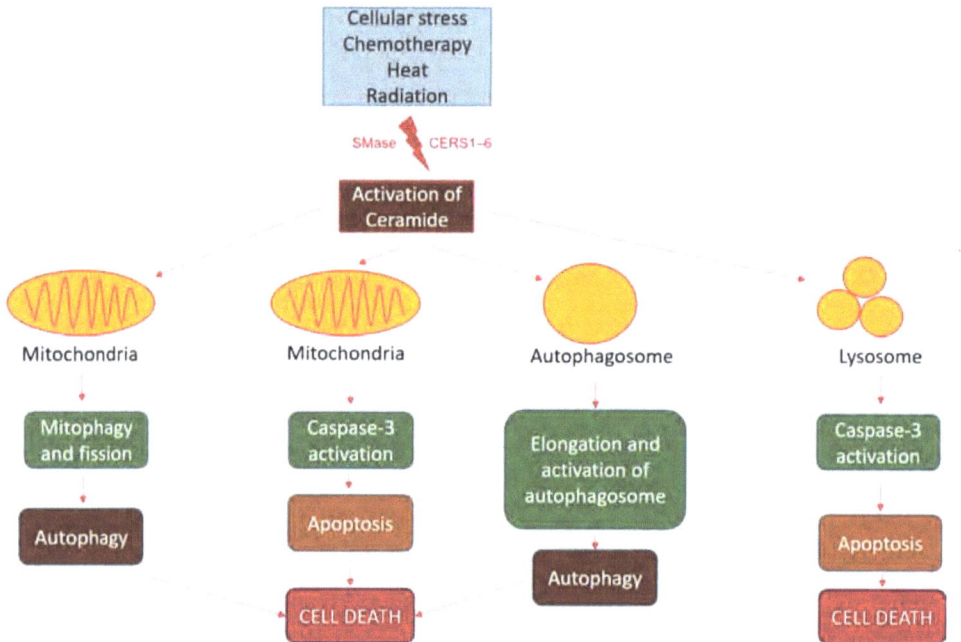

**Fig. (2).** Role of ceramide. Activation of ceramide *via* SMase and CERS1-6 leads to cell death *via* activating different pathways. Ceramide activation leads to fission and autophagy as well as activation of caspase-3 results in cell death *via* apoptosis. Activation of autophagosomes leads to elongation and subsequently activating autophagy in cells. Lysosomal-mediated activation of caspase leads to cell death.

## S1P Receptors

The role of S1PR1 was first recognised as a possible target to inhibit the STAT3 signaling pathway in B cell lymphomas [54]. Moreover, increased S1PR1 levels in T lymphocytic cells were strongly linked with the blockade of intercellular adhesion molecule 1 (ICAM1) and changes in cell-cell interaction and adhesion [55]. S1PR2 signaling in HeLa cells in a culture environment mediates AML proliferation and induces ERM proteins to increase mobility and metastasis [28]. The same results were obtained in tumor-mediated invasion in melanoma and bladder cancer in rodents [56]. Although systemic signaling of S1PR2 in bone marrow-derived and endothelial cells showed inhibition of tumor metastasis in rodent models [57]. Although controversial debate on the role of S1PR2 in cancer, targeting A1PR2 in the bladder, and melanoma cancer might be beneficial. S1PR3 signaling promotes aldehyde dehydrogenase (ALDH)-positive cancer stem cells through the activation of Notch signaling *via* stimulation of S1P [58]. Cancer stem cells were found to be overexpressing SPHK1 and induced tumor proliferation in xenograft tumor models. Knockdown of S1PR3 decreases tumor proliferation. Breast cancer cells derived from patients showed the presence of both SPHK, S1PR3, and ALDH1. However, no data is available regarding how S1PR3 signaling changes the characteristics of cancer cells. In a study, transforming growth factorβ (TGFβ)-mediated S1PR3 activation promoted lung cancer progression and metastasis inrodent models [59]. Increased expression of S1PR4 was found and thought to be associated with shortened survival in 140 ER-negative breast cancer patients [60]. Continuation of these studies found that S1P generated through SPHK2-mediated S1PR4 prevents S1PR2 translocation to induce the growth of ER-negative breast cancer cells [61]. However, the mechanism behind how S1PR4 regulates S1PR2 is still unknown. Overall, these studies indicate that targeting different types of S1P receptors in different types of cancer effectively alleviates cell proliferation, tumor growth, and angiogenesis through S1PR-dependent signaling.

S1P is also able to transduce signals without binding to the S1P receptor and activate different downstream pathways. For example, S1P generated through SPHK1 directly binds to TNF receptor-associated factor 2, which further phosphorylates IKK, translocates NF-κB, and activates further signaling cascade in HeLa cells [62]. However some studies have found that S1P was not required to mediate the activation of the NFκB pathway in macrophages [63]. Moreover, S1P generated through SPHK1 was found to act as a ligand for peroxisome proliferator-activated receptor γ (PPARγ) that governs angiogenesis in human endothelial cells, possibly by activating downstream signaling of PPARγ influenced genes [64]. S1P generated through SPHK2 was able to bind with HDAC1 and HDAC2 and inhibit them to prevent deacetylation of histone 3 in the MCF7 breast cancer cell line [65]. However, more data is required to justify whether S1P-SPHK2 mediated blockade of HDAC enzymes alters gene expression in every cancer cell in the body to promote or inhibit cell proliferation, tumor growth, and angiogenesis. In another study, SPHK2-generated S1P binds to prohibitin 2 (PHB2) in mitochondria to activate cytochrome c oxidase followed by mitochondrial respiration [66]. In addition, nuclear S1P derived from SPHK2 was able to interact with telomerase reverse transcriptase (TERT), thereby blocking telomere damage and senescence. SPHK2 inhibition demonstrated rapid loss of TERT, damage of telomeres, and fast senescence, leading to the inhibition of cell proliferation [67]. Thus, these results point out that SPHK1 and SPHK2 both are involved in the conversion of ceramidase to S1P through S1PR-dependent and non-dependent pathways, and the role of SPHK1 and SPHK2 is prominent in cancer initiation and progression.

## Presence of Sphingolipids in the Digestive System

Sphingolipids were found to be present in mucosal cells in the small and large intestines as well as in the liver and pancreatic parenchyma. The presence of sphingolipids is around 30-40% of all lipids present in the digestive tract [68]. Sphingolipids are double in amount in the colon compared to the small intestine and other digestive organs. The reason behind the high abundance of sphingolipids in colon mucosa is the high and rapid exfoliation and differentiation of mucosal cells in the upper digestive system. It is estimated that about 1.5 gm of sphingolipids are required for mucosal recovery [69]. In the colon lining, sphingolipids are abundantly present in the apical membrane and a trace amount is present in the basolateral membrane [70]. The mucosa of the small intestine and colon is highly abundant with ceramide, sphingomyelin, gangliosides, and glucosylceramide while stomach mucosa containing proton pumps are rich in sphingomyelin and gangliosides [71, 72]. Although the role of sphingolipids in the stomach remains controversial more studies are required to identify the protective role of sphingolipids in the stomach lining. Sphingolipids are either synthesized through the *de novo* pathway or delivered to mucosal cells through diet.

### Metabolism of Sphingolipids in the Gastrointestinal Tract

The *de novo* synthesis takes place in the liver, pancreas, and intestinal mucosa as cells of these organs have the enzyme required to catalyze the first reaction as discussed earlier in this chapter. After condensation of serine and palmitate, 3-ketosphinganine was quickly reduced to sphinganine. In the last step, dihydroceramide is converted into ceramide by different ceramide synthase isoforms. Almost all the isoforms of ceramide synthase are present in mucosal cells [73, 74]. Another pathway by which ceramide is synthesised is the hydrolysis of sphingomyelin. Three main isoforms of sphingomyelin phosphodiesterase were isolated from mucosal cells. Almost all the enzymes required to carry sphingolipids metabolism were identified in the gastrointestinal tract. The activity of SPT was found to be higher in the liver, followed by the pancreas and small intestine [75]. Mucosal cells of the small intestine showed the presence of alkaline and neutral SMase. Another study also proved the presence of alkaline SMase in the liver, pancreas bile salts, and pancreatic juice [76]. Out of three isoforms of ceramidases, alkaline ceramidase was found to be highly expressed in the intestinal mucosa which can catalyze the reaction in the alkaline environment of gut mucosa [77]. As sphingomyelinases and ceramides are present on the outer membrane of cells, their active sites are capable of carrying out catalytic reactions inside the cell and in the lumen of the gut [78]. Ceramide in the gut was also hydrolyzed through the reaction with pancreatic juice although BSSL knockout mice did not show a decrease in ceramide digestion and concluded that ceramidase was the prime enzyme in the hydrolysis of ceramides [79]. Certain drugs also affect the expression of these enzymes, for example, ursodeoxycholic acid, anti-inflammatory drugs, and psyllium increase the activity of alkaline sphingomyelinase and the concentration of ceramide in guts. The high-fat diet also decreases the activity of alkaline sphingomyelinase [77]. The expression of SPHK1 and SPHK2 has been found in the small intestine and colon mucosal cells. Despite the presence of sphingosine kinase, the amount of S1P was found very low maybe because of its quick degradation [80, 81].

## *Sphingolipids and Colorectal Tumorigenesis*

As previously discussed, sphingolipid metabolism is highly involved in the regulation of cell differentiation, cell proliferation, angiogenesis, and metastasis of different cancer cells. It is well established that ceramide and its counterpart sphingosine have apoptotic and anti-proliferative actions and their low concentration may increase the proliferation of cancer cells. Degradation of ceramide to S1P is mediated by catalytic enzymes SPHK1 and SPHK2 [82]. So targeting SPHKs may increase the concentration of ceramide as S1P also possesses cell survival and cell proliferation characteristics. Decreased levels of ceramide have been found in the liver, breast, colon, and ovarian cancer, indicating the overexpression of SPHKs and S1P in cells [82]. Moreover, ceramide levels decrease in cancer cells by glycosylation of ceramide to glycosylceramide, which causes drug resistance in cancer tissues [83]. The possible role of sphingolipids in colorectal cancer was first proposed by Dudeja *et al.*, in 1,2-dimethylhydrazine-induced colon cancer [84]. The result showed a high amount of SM levels in colon tissues. Further study showed that dietary supplements containing SM maintain almost constant levels of ceramide in colonic cells and prevent the formation of ulcers and crypt by 70% [85]. Another clinical study showed that levels of ceramide and SM decrease in colon cancer patients compared to healthy humans. The activity of alkaline SMase was found to be decreased in human colitis by 25%, colorectal cancer by 75%, and adenomatous polyposis by 90% [86]. Furthermore, a trace amount of alkaline

SMase was present in the feces samples of colorectal cancer patients as compared to healthy humans. A decrease in SMase activity results in the depletion of ceramide in colorectal cancer. Moreover, alkaline SMase was found to be involved in the inactivation of PAF which was found to be involved in cancer progression and inflammation, which concluded that lower SMase activity may increase the PAF activity in colon cancer progression [87]. S1P is another important sphingolipid involved in the progression of cancer. As discussed earlier regarding the nature of S1P in tumorigenesis, S1P promotes angiogenesis *via* activating platelet-derived growth factor and vascular endothelial growth factor [88]. S1P can be considered a carcinogenic factor since the overexpression of S1P is associated with poor survival in cancer patients of glioblastoma. The same mechanism may be working in colon cancer [89]. The high amount of S1P was identified in both pre-clinical and clinical studies of colon cancer due to the upregulation of SPHK enzymes. Another study also observed the upregulation of SPHK in human colon, breast, melanoma, and lung tumor cells [90]. Additionally, specific S1P inhibitors were able to decrease the cellular growth, proliferation and metastasis in different cancer cell lines including colon cancer [91]. In colon cancer cells, S1P lyase and S1P phosphatase responsible for the degradation of S1P were downregulated and increased the concentration of S1P in cells. Another study supports the fact that an increase in the expression of S1P lyase in colon cancer was able to induce apoptosis in cells, confirming the proliferative role of S1P in cancer cells. In the adenomatous polyposis SPHK$^{-/-}$ mice model, the concentration of S1P decreases which results in decreased cell proliferation confirming the role of SPHK in cancer cell proliferation [91].

**Sphingolipids and Intestinal Inflammation**

Sphingolipids are present at the outer membrane of gastric mucosa to protect the outer layer from bile salts, gastric juice, and different enzymes. Changes in the metabolism of sphingolipids may give rise to inflammatory diseases. In the rodent model, the inhibition of the *de novo* synthesis of sphingolipids leads to barrier dysfunction and initiation of inflammation [92]. In another study, sphingomyelinase increases inflammation and damages the intestinal barrier by a decrease in SM levels [93]. Ceramide-1-phosphate (C1P) is known to have proliferative properties. Increased C1P levels in the mucosal line mediate the overexpression of COX2 mainly PGE2, which plays an important role in colitis-associated cancer. S1P also stimulates the COX2 expression and produces proinflammatory markers [94]. Interestingly, the administration of sphingosine kinase inhibitors decreases levels of S1P and improves the colitis in the mice model [14].

## Sphingolipids in Liver Cancer

The involvement of sphingolipids in liver cancer remains controversial. Liver cancer cells showed similar properties to colon cancer cells regarding sphingolipid metabolism and low levels of ceramide were observed. Low levels of ceramide were a result of decreased activity of alkaline sphingomyelinase. Low levels of all three types of SMases were found in liver tissue samples obtained from patients with liver cancer development [95]. Moreover, in liver cancer cells, all the isoforms of SMases were found to be inactive. Another study established that the inhibition of ceramide synthesis in rat models developed cirrhosis and 66% of them developed hepatocellular carcinoma [96]. No other data is available to discuss the role of sphingolipid metabolism in liver cancer.

## CONCLUSION

Even though a marked decline in GI tract cancer patients in recent years, treatment of gastrointestinal tract cancer remains a challenge. Standard chemotherapy has its disadvantages and limitations to treat the disease. Research on different pathways influencing the proliferation and anti-apoptotic signals discovered in the last decade gave meaningful insight into the newer target approaches. The sphingolipid metabolism pathway is largely explored in recent years and the role of their metabolites is explored in the context of cancer signaling. The role of ceramide, S1P, and SPHK has been found promising and few drugs were assessed in the pre-clinical and clinical setup. Although no new drugs were present in the market targeting specific sphingolipid metabolites to treat GI tract cancer.

In conclusion, SPHK has been found to be a promising target to treat GI tract cancer as inhibiting SPHK showed promising results *in vivo* scenarios, which are devoid of side effects that are anticipated in case of conventional chemotherapy.

## REFERENCES

[1]     Bray F, Ferlay J, Soerjomataram I, Siegel RL, Torre LA, Jemal A. Global cancer statistics 2018: GLOBOCAN estimates of incidence and mortality worldwide for 36 cancers in 185 countries. CA Cancer J Clin 2018; 68(6): 394-424.
        [http://dx.doi.org/10.3322/caac.21492] [PMID: 30207593]

[2]     Kim HJ, Eun JY, Jeon YW, *et al.* Efficacy and safety of oxaliplatin, 5-Fluorouracil, and folinic Acid combination chemotherapy as first-line treatment in metastatic or recurrent gastric cancer. Cancer Res Treat 2011; 43(3): 154-9.
        [http://dx.doi.org/10.4143/crt.2011.43.3.154] [PMID: 22022292]

[3]     Wang M, Hong Y, Feng Q, *et al.* Recombinant adenovirus KGHV500 and CIK cells codeliver anti-p21-ras scfv for the treatment of gastric cancer with wild-type ras overexpression. Mol Ther Oncolytics 2018; 11: 90-101.
        [http://dx.doi.org/10.1016/j.omto.2018.10.003] [PMID: 30534583]

[4]     Escalante J, McQuade RM, Stojanovska V, Nurgali K. Impact of chemotherapy on gastrointestinal functions and the enteric nervous system. Maturitas 2017; 105: 23-9.
[http://dx.doi.org/10.1016/j.maturitas.2017.04.021] [PMID: 28545907]

[5]     Nurgali K, Jagoe RT, Abalo R. Editorial: Adverse effects of cancer chemotherapy: anything new to improve tolerance and reduce sequelae? Front Pharmacol 2018; 9: 245.
[http://dx.doi.org/10.3389/fphar.2018.00245] [PMID: 29623040]

[6]     Hokin MR, Hokin LE. Enzyme secretion and the incorporation of P32 into phospholipides of pancreas slices. J Biol Chem 1953; 203(2): 967-77.
[http://dx.doi.org/10.1016/S0021-9258(19)52367-5] [PMID: 13084667]

[7]     Nishizuka Y. Intracellular signaling by hydrolysis of phospholipids and activation of protein kinase C. Science 1992; 258(5082): 607-14.
[http://dx.doi.org/10.1126/science.1411571] [PMID: 1411571]

[8]     Serhan CN, Savill J. Resolution of inflammation: the beginning programs the end. Nat Immunol 2005; 6(12): 1191-7.
[http://dx.doi.org/10.1038/ni1276] [PMID: 16369558]

[9]     Smith ER, Merrill AH Jr, Obeid LM, Hannun YA. Effects of sphingosine and other sphingolipids on protein kinase C. Methods Enzymol 2000; 312: 361-73.
[http://dx.doi.org/10.1016/S0076-6879(00)12921-0] [PMID: 11070884]

[10]    Merrill AH Jr. Sphingolipid and glycosphingolipid metabolic pathways in the era of sphingolipidomics. Chem Rev 2011; 111(10): 6387-422.
[http://dx.doi.org/10.1021/cr2002917] [PMID: 21942574]

[11]    Obeid LM, Linardic CM, Karolak LA, Hannun YA. Programmed cell death induced by ceramide. Science 1993; 259(5102): 1769-71.
[http://dx.doi.org/10.1126/science.8456305] [PMID: 8456305]

[12]    Venable ME, Lee JY, Smyth MJ, Bielawska A, Obeid LM. Role of ceramide in cellular senescence. J Biol Chem 1995; 270(51): 30701-8.
[http://dx.doi.org/10.1074/jbc.270.51.30701] [PMID: 8530509]

[13]    Hla T. Physiological and pathological actions of sphingosine 1-phosphate. Semin Cell Dev Biol 2004; 15(5): 513-20.
[http://dx.doi.org/10.1016/j.semcdb.2004.05.002] [PMID: 15271296]

[14]    Chalfant CE, Spiegel S. Sphingosine 1-phosphate and ceramide 1-phosphate: expanding roles in cell signaling. J Cell Sci 2005; 118(20): 4605-12.
[http://dx.doi.org/10.1242/jcs.02637] [PMID: 16219683]

[15]    Mitsutake S, Kim TJ, Inagaki Y, Kato M, Yamashita T, Igarashi Y. Ceramide kinase is a mediator of calcium-dependent degranulation in mast cells. J Biol Chem 2004; 279(17): 17570-7.
[http://dx.doi.org/10.1074/jbc.M312885200] [PMID: 14769792]

[16]    Hinkovska-Galcheva V, Boxer LA, Kindzelskii A, *et al.* Ceramide 1-phosphate, a mediator of phagocytosis. J Biol Chem 2005; 280(28): 26612-21.
[http://dx.doi.org/10.1074/jbc.M501359200] [PMID: 15899891]

[17]    Hannun YA, Obeid LM. The Ceramide-centric universe of lipid-mediated cell regulation: stress encounters of the lipid kind. J Biol Chem 2002; 277(29): 25847-50.
[http://dx.doi.org/10.1074/jbc.R200008200] [PMID: 12011103]

[18]    Linn SC, Kim HS, Keane EM, Andras LM, Wang E, Merrill AH Jr. Regulation of *de novo* sphingolipid biosynthesis and the toxic consequences of its disruption. Biochem Soc Trans 2001; 29(6): 831-5.
[http://dx.doi.org/10.1042/bst0290831] [PMID: 11709083]

[19]    Causeret C, Geeraert L, Van der Hoeven G, Mannaerts GP, Van Veldhoven PP. Further

characterization of rat dihydroceramide desaturase: Tissue distribution, subcellular localization, and substrate specificity. Lipids 2000; 35(10): 1117-25.
[http://dx.doi.org/10.1007/s11745-000-0627-6] [PMID: 11104018]

[20]    Hannun YA, Obeid LM. Principles of bioactive lipid signalling: lessons from sphingolipids. Nat Rev Mol Cell Biol 2008; 9(2): 139-50.
[http://dx.doi.org/10.1038/nrm2329] [PMID: 18216770]

[21]    Marchesini N, Hannun YA. Acid and neutral sphingomyelinases: roles and mechanisms of regulation. Biochem Cell Biol 2004; 82(1): 27-44.
[http://dx.doi.org/10.1139/o03-091] [PMID: 15052326]

[22]    Pitson SM. Regulation of sphingosine kinase and sphingolipid signaling. Trends Biochem Sci 2011; 36(2): 97-107.
[http://dx.doi.org/10.1016/j.tibs.2010.08.001] [PMID: 20870412]

[23]    Pitson SM, Xia P, Leclercq TM, *et al.* Phosphorylation-dependent translocation of sphingosine kinase to the plasma membrane drives its oncogenic signalling. J Exp Med 2005; 201(1): 49-54.
[http://dx.doi.org/10.1084/jem.20040559] [PMID: 15623571]

[24]    Zhu W, Jarman KE, Lokman NA, *et al.* CIB2 negatively regulates oncogenic signaling in ovarian cancer *via* sphingosine kinase 1. Cancer Res 2017; 77(18): 4823-34.
[http://dx.doi.org/10.1158/0008-5472.CAN-17-0025] [PMID: 28729416]

[25]    Baran Y, Salas A, Senkal CE, *et al.* Alterations of ceramide/sphingosine 1-phosphate rheostat involved in the regulation of resistance to imatinib-induced apoptosis in K562 human chronic myeloid leukemia cells. J Biol Chem 2007; 282(15): 10922-34.
[http://dx.doi.org/10.1074/jbc.M610157200] [PMID: 17303574]

[26]    Bonhoure E, Pchejetski D, Aouali N, *et al.* Overcoming MDR-associated chemoresistance in HL-60 acute myeloid leukemia cells by targeting shingosine kinase-1. Leukemia 2006; 20(1): 95-102.
[http://dx.doi.org/10.1038/sj.leu.2404023] [PMID: 16281067]

[27]    Bonhoure E, Lauret A, Barnes DJ, *et al.* Sphingosine kinase-1 is a downstream regulator of imatinib-induced apoptosis in chronic myeloid leukemia cells. Leukemia 2008; 22(5): 971-9.
[http://dx.doi.org/10.1038/leu.2008.95] [PMID: 18401414]

[28]    Powell JA, Lewis AC, Zhu W, *et al.* Targeting sphingosine kinase 1 induces MCL1-dependent cell death in acute myeloid leukemia. Blood 2017; 129(6): 771-82.
[http://dx.doi.org/10.1182/blood-2016-06-720433] [PMID: 27956387]

[29]    Neubauer HA, Pham DH, Zebol JR, *et al.* An oncogenic role for sphingosine kinase 2. Oncotarget 2016; 7(40): 64886-99.
[http://dx.doi.org/10.18632/oncotarget.11714] [PMID: 27588496]

[30]    Neubauer HA, Pitson SM. Roles, regulation and inhibitors of sphingosine kinase 2. FEBS J 2013; 280(21): 5317-36.
[http://dx.doi.org/10.1111/febs.12314] [PMID: 23638983]

[31]    Wallington-Beddoe CT, Powell JA, Tong D, Pitson SM, Bradstock KF, Bendall LJ. Sphingosine kinase 2 promotes acute lymphoblastic leukemia by enhancing MYC expression. Cancer Res 2014; 74(10): 2803-15.
[http://dx.doi.org/10.1158/0008-5472.CAN-13-2732] [PMID: 24686171]

[32]    Kummetha Venkata J, An N, Stuart R, *et al.* Inhibition of sphingosine kinase 2 downregulates the expression of c-Myc and Mcl-1 and induces apoptosis in multiple myeloma. Blood 2014; 124(12): 1915-25.
[http://dx.doi.org/10.1182/blood-2014-03-559385] [PMID: 25122609]

[33]    Mao C, Obeid LM. Ceramidases: regulators of cellular responses mediated by ceramide, sphingosine, and sphingosine-1-phosphate. Biochim Biophys Acta Mol Cell Biol Lipids 2008; 1781(9): 424-34.
[http://dx.doi.org/10.1016/j.bbalip.2008.06.002] [PMID: 18619555]

[34]    Coant N, Sakamoto W, Mao C, Hannun YA. Ceramidases, roles in sphingolipid metabolism and in health and disease. Adv Biol Regul 2017; 63: 122-31.
[http://dx.doi.org/10.1016/j.jbior.2016.10.002] [PMID: 27771292]

[35]    Bedia C, Casas J, Andrieu-Abadie N, Fabriàs G, Levade T. Acid ceramidase expression modulates the sensitivity of A375 melanoma cells to dacarbazine. J Biol Chem 2011; 286(32): 28200-9.
[http://dx.doi.org/10.1074/jbc.M110.216382] [PMID: 21700700]

[36]    Morad SAF, Cabot MC. Tamoxifen regulation of sphingolipid metabolism—Therapeutic implications. Biochim Biophys Acta Mol Cell Biol Lipids 2015; 1851(9): 1134-45.
[http://dx.doi.org/10.1016/j.bbalip.2015.05.001] [PMID: 25964209]

[37]    Grazide S, Terrisse AD, Lerouge S, Laurent G, Jaffrézou JP. Cytoprotective effect of glucosylceramide synthase inhibition against daunorubicin-induced apoptosis in human leukemic cell lines. J Biol Chem 2004; 279(18): 18256-61.
[http://dx.doi.org/10.1074/jbc.M314105200] [PMID: 14766899]

[38]    Gouazé V, Yu JY, Bleicher RJ, *et al.* Overexpression of glucosylceramide synthase and P-glycoprotein in cancer cells selected for resistance to natural product chemotherapy. Mol Cancer Ther 2004; 3(5): 633-40.
[http://dx.doi.org/10.1158/1535-7163.633.3.5] [PMID: 15141021]

[39]    Baran Y, Bielawski J, Gunduz U, Ogretmen B. Targeting glucosylceramide synthase sensitizes imatinib-resistant chronic myeloid leukemia cells *via* endogenous ceramide accumulation. J Cancer Res Clin Oncol 2011; 137(10): 1535-44.
[http://dx.doi.org/10.1007/s00432-011-1016-y] [PMID: 21833718]

[40]    Cox TM, Drelichman G, Cravo R, *et al.* Eliglustat maintains long-term clinical stability in patients with Gaucher disease type 1 stabilized on enzyme therapy. Blood 2017; 129(17): 2375-83.
[http://dx.doi.org/10.1182/blood-2016-12-758409] [PMID: 28167660]

[41]    Levy M, Futerman AH. Mammalian ceramide synthases. IUBMB Life 2010; 62(5): 347-56.
[http://dx.doi.org/10.1002/iub.319] [PMID: 20222015]

[42]    Senkal CE, Ponnusamy S, Rossi MJ, *et al.* Role of human longevity assurance gene 1 and C18-ceramide in chemotherapy-induced cell death in human head and neck squamous cell carcinomas. Mol Cancer Ther 2007; 6(2): 712-22.
[http://dx.doi.org/10.1158/1535-7163.MCT-06-0558] [PMID: 17308067]

[43]    White-Gilbertson S, Mullen T, Senkal C, *et al.* Ceramide synthase 6 modulates TRAIL sensitivity and nuclear translocation of active caspase-3 in colon cancer cells. Oncogene 2009; 28(8): 1132-41.
[http://dx.doi.org/10.1038/onc.2008.468] [PMID: 19137010]

[44]    Panjarian S, Kozhaya L, Arayssi S, *et al. De novo* N-palmitoylsphingosine synthesis is the major biochemical mechanism of ceramide accumulation following p53 up-regulation. Prostaglandins Other Lipid Mediat 2008; 86(1-4): 41-8.
[http://dx.doi.org/10.1016/j.prostaglandins.2008.02.004] [PMID: 18400537]

[45]    Dany M, Gencer S, Nganga R, *et al.* Targeting FLT3-ITD signaling mediates ceramide-dependent mitophagy and attenuates drug resistance in AML. Blood 2016; 128(15): 1944-58.
[http://dx.doi.org/10.1182/blood-2016-04-708750] [PMID: 27540013]

[46]    Chalfant CE, Szulc Z, Roddy P, Bielawska A, Hannun YA. The structural requirements for ceramide activation of serine-threonine protein phosphatases. J Lipid Res 2004; 45(3): 496-506.
[http://dx.doi.org/10.1194/jlr.M300347-JLR200] [PMID: 14657198]

[47]    Heinrich M, Neumeyer J, Jakob M, *et al.* Cathepsin D links TNF-induced acid sphingomyelinase to Bid-mediated caspase-9 and -3 activation. Cell Death Differ 2004; 11(5): 550-63.
[http://dx.doi.org/10.1038/sj.cdd.4401382] [PMID: 14739942]

[48]    Takabe K, Kim RH, Allegood JC, *et al.* Estradiol induces export of sphingosine 1-phosphate from breast cancer cells *via* ABCC1 and ABCG2. J Biol Chem 2010; 285(14): 10477-86.

[http://dx.doi.org/10.1074/jbc.M109.064162] [PMID: 20110355]

[49]   Hisano Y, Kobayashi N, Yamaguchi A, Nishi T. Mouse SPNS2 functions as a sphingosine--
       -phosphate transporter in vascular endothelial cells. PLoS One 2012; 7(6): e38941.
       [http://dx.doi.org/10.1371/journal.pone.0038941] [PMID: 22723910]

[50]   van der Weyden L, Arends MJ, Campbell AD, *et al.* Genome-wide *in vivo* screen identifies novel host
       regulators of metastatic colonization. Nature 2017; 541(7636): 233-6.
       [http://dx.doi.org/10.1038/nature20792] [PMID: 28052056]

[51]   Ponnusamy S, Selvam SP, Mehrotra S, *et al.* Communication between host organism and cancer cells
       is transduced by systemic sphingosine kinase 1/sphingosine 1-phosphate signalling to regulate tumour
       metastasis. EMBO Mol Med 2012; 4(8): 761-75.
       [http://dx.doi.org/10.1002/emmm.201200244] [PMID: 22707406]

[52]   Liang J, Nagahashi M, Kim EY, *et al.* Sphingosine-1-phosphate links persistent STAT3 activation,
       chronic intestinal inflammation, and development of colitis-associated cancer. Cancer Cell 2013;
       23(1): 107-20.
       [http://dx.doi.org/10.1016/j.ccr.2012.11.013] [PMID: 23273921]

[53]   Brizuela L, Martin C, Jeannot P, *et al.* Osteoblast-derived sphingosine 1-phosphate to induce
       proliferation and confer resistance to therapeutics to bone metastasis-derived prostate cancer cells. Mol
       Oncol 2014; 8(7): 1181-95.
       [http://dx.doi.org/10.1016/j.molonc.2014.04.001] [PMID: 24768038]

[54]   Liu Y, Deng J, Wang L, *et al.* S1PR1 is an effective target to block STAT3 signaling in activated B
       cell–like diffuse large B-cell lymphoma. Blood 2012; 120(7): 1458-65.
       [http://dx.doi.org/10.1182/blood-2011-12-399030] [PMID: 22745305]

[55]   Feng H, Stachura DL, White RM, *et al.* T-lymphoblastic lymphoma cells express high levels of BCL2,
       S1P1, and ICAM1, leading to a blockade of tumor cell intravasation. Cancer Cell 2010; 18(4): 353-66.
       [http://dx.doi.org/10.1016/j.ccr.2010.09.009] [PMID: 20951945]

[56]   Adada MM, Canals D, Jeong N, *et al.* Intracellular sphingosine kinase 2-derived sphingosine--
       -phosphate mediates epidermal growth factor-induced ezrin-radixin-moesin phosphorylation and
       cancer cell invasion. FASEB J 2015; 29(11): 4654-69.
       [http://dx.doi.org/10.1096/fj.15-274340] [PMID: 26209696]

[57]   Du W, Takuwa N, Yoshioka K, *et al.* S1P(2), the G protein-coupled receptor for sphingosine--
       -phosphate, negatively regulates tumor angiogenesis and tumor growth *in vivo* in mice. Cancer Res
       2010; 70(2): 772-81.
       [http://dx.doi.org/10.1158/0008-5472.CAN-09-2722] [PMID: 20068174]

[58]   Hirata N, Yamada S, Shoda T, Kurihara M, Sekino Y, Kanda Y. Sphingosine-1-phosphate promotes
       expansion of cancer stem cells *via* S1PR3 by a ligand-independent Notch activation. Nat Commun
       2014; 5(1): 4806.
       [http://dx.doi.org/10.1038/ncomms5806] [PMID: 25254944]

[59]   Zhao J, Liu J, Lee JF, *et al.* TGF-β/SMAD3 pathway stimulates sphingosine-1 phosphate receptor 3
       expression implication of sphingosine-1 phosphate receptor 3 in lung adenocarcinoma progression. J
       Biol Chem 2016; 291(53): 27343-53.
       [http://dx.doi.org/10.1074/jbc.M116.740084] [PMID: 27856637]

[60]   Ohotski J, Long JS, Orange C, *et al.* Expression of sphingosine 1-phosphate receptor 4 and
       sphingosine kinase 1 is associated with outcome in oestrogen receptor-negative breast cancer. Br J
       Cancer 2012; 106(8): 1453-9.
       [http://dx.doi.org/10.1038/bjc.2012.98] [PMID: 22460268]

[61]   Ohotski J, Rosen H, Bittman R, Pyne S, Pyne NJ. Sphingosine kinase 2 prevents the nuclear
       translocation of sphingosine 1-phosphate receptor-2 and tyrosine 416 phosphorylated c-Src and
       increases estrogen receptor negative MDA-MB-231 breast cancer cell growth: The role of sphingosine
       1-phosphate receptor-4. Cell Signal 2014; 26(5): 1040-7.

[http://dx.doi.org/10.1016/j.cellsig.2014.01.023] [PMID: 24486401]

[62]   Alvarez SE, Harikumar KB, Hait NC, *et al.* Sphingosine-1-phosphate is a missing cofactor for the E3 ubiquitin ligase TRAF2. Nature 2010; 465(7301): 1084-8.
[http://dx.doi.org/10.1038/nature09128] [PMID: 20577214]

[63]   Xiong Y, Lee HJ, Mariko B, *et al.* Sphingosine kinases are not required for inflammatory responses in macrophages. J Biol Chem 2013; 288(45): 32563-73.
[http://dx.doi.org/10.1074/jbc.M113.483750] [PMID: 24081141]

[64]   Parham KA, Zebol JR, Tooley KL, *et al.* Sphingosine 1-phosphate is a ligand for peroxisome proliferator-activated receptor-γ that regulates neoangiogenesis. FASEB J 2015; 29(9): 3638-53.
[http://dx.doi.org/10.1096/fj.14-261289] [PMID: 25985799]

[65]   Hait NC, Allegood J, Maceyka M, *et al.* Regulation of histone acetylation in the nucleus by sphingosine-1-phosphate. Science 2009; 325(5945): 1254-7.
[http://dx.doi.org/10.1126/science.1176709] [PMID: 19729656]

[66]   Strub GM, Paillard M, Liang J, *et al.* Sphingosine-1-phosphate produced by sphingosine kinase 2 in mitochondria interacts with prohibitin 2 to regulate complex IV assembly and respiration. FASEB J 2011; 25(2): 600-12.
[http://dx.doi.org/10.1096/fj.10-167502] [PMID: 20959514]

[67]   Panneer Selvam S, De Palma RM, Oaks JJ, *et al.* Binding of the sphingolipid S1P to hTERT stabilizes telomerase at the nuclear periphery by allosterically mimicking protein phosphorylation. Sci Signal 2015; 8(381): ra58.
[http://dx.doi.org/10.1126/scisignal.aaa4998] [PMID: 26082434]

[68]   Duan R, Nilsson A. Metabolism of sphingolipids in the gut and its relation to inflammation and cancer development. Prog Lipid Res 2009; 48(1): 62-72.
[http://dx.doi.org/10.1016/j.plipres.2008.04.003] [PMID: 19027789]

[69]   Nilsson Å, Duan RD. Absorption and lipoprotein transport of sphingomyelin. J Lipid Res 2006; 47(1): 154-71.
[http://dx.doi.org/10.1194/jlr.M500357-JLR200] [PMID: 16251722]

[70]   Michael Danielsen E, Hansen GH. Lipid raft organization and function in brush borders of epithelial cells (Review). Mol Membr Biol 2006; 23(1): 71-9.
[http://dx.doi.org/10.1080/09687860500445604] [PMID: 16611582]

[71]   Olaisson H, Mårdh S, Arvidson G. Phospholipid organization in H,K-ATPase-containing membranes from pig gastric mucosa. J Biol Chem 1985; 260(20): 11262-7.
[http://dx.doi.org/10.1016/S0021-9258(17)39175-5] [PMID: 2993306]

[72]   Breimer ME. Distribution of molecular species of sphingomyelins in different parts of bovine digestive tract. J Lipid Res 1975; 16(3): 189-94.
[http://dx.doi.org/10.1016/S0022-2275(20)36725-0] [PMID: 1168686]

[73]   Hanada K. Serine palmitoyltransferase, a key enzyme of sphingolipid metabolism. Biochim Biophys Acta Mol Cell Biol Lipids 2003; 1632(1-3): 16-30.
[http://dx.doi.org/10.1016/S1388-1981(03)00059-3] [PMID: 12782147]

[74]   Futerman AH, Riezman H. The ins and outs of sphingolipid synthesis. Trends Cell Biol 2005; 15(6): 312-8.
[http://dx.doi.org/10.1016/j.tcb.2005.04.006] [PMID: 15953549]

[75]   Merrill AH Jr, Nixon DW, Williams RD. Activities of serine palmitoyltransferase (3-ketosphinganine synthase) in microsomes from different rat tissues. J Lipid Res 1985; 26(5): 617-22.
[http://dx.doi.org/10.1016/S0022-2275(20)34349-2] [PMID: 4020300]

[76]   Duan R. Alkaline sphingomyelinase: An old enzyme with novel implications. Biochim Biophys Acta Mol Cell Biol Lipids 2006; 1761(3): 281-91.
[http://dx.doi.org/10.1016/j.bbalip.2006.03.007] [PMID: 16631405]

[77]     Duan RD, Cheng Y, Hansen G, *et al.* Purification, localization, and expression of human intestinal alkaline sphingomyelinase. J Lipid Res 2003; 44(6): 1241-50.
[http://dx.doi.org/10.1194/jlr.M300037-JLR200] [PMID: 12671034]

[78]     Duan RD, Bergman T, Xu N, *et al.* Identification of human intestinal alkaline sphingomyelinase as a novel ecto-enzyme related to the nucleotide phosphodiesterase family. J Biol Chem 2003; 278(40): 38528-36.
[http://dx.doi.org/10.1074/jbc.M305437200] [PMID: 12885774]

[79]     Kono M, Dreier JL, Ellis JM, *et al.* Neutral ceramidase encoded by the Asah2 gene is essential for the intestinal degradation of sphingolipids. J Biol Chem 2006; 281(11): 7324-31.
[http://dx.doi.org/10.1074/jbc.M508382200] [PMID: 16380386]

[80]     Fukuda Y, Kihara A, Igarashi Y. Distribution of sphingosine kinase activity in mouse tissues: contribution of SPHK1. Biochem Biophys Res Commun 2003; 309(1): 155-60.
[http://dx.doi.org/10.1016/S0006-291X(03)01551-1] [PMID: 12943676]

[81]     Sugiura M, Kono K, Liu H, *et al.* Ceramide kinase, a novel lipid kinase. Molecular cloning and functional characterization. J Biol Chem 2002; 277(26): 23294-300.
[http://dx.doi.org/10.1074/jbc.M201535200] [PMID: 11956206]

[82]     Ogretmen B, Hannun YA. Biologically active sphingolipids in cancer pathogenesis and treatment. Nat Rev Cancer 2004; 4(8): 604-16.
[http://dx.doi.org/10.1038/nrc1411] [PMID: 15286740]

[83]     Liu YY, Han TY, Giuliano A, Cabot MC. Ceramide glycosylation potentiates cellular multidrug resistance. FASEB J 2001; 15(3): 719-30.
[http://dx.doi.org/10.1096/fj.00-0223com] [PMID: 11259390]

[84]     Dudeja PK, Dahiya R, Brasitus TA. The role of sphingomyelin synthetase and sphingomyelinase in 1,2-dimethylhydrazine-induced lipid alterations of rat colonic plasma membranes. Biochim Biophys Acta Biomembr 1986; 863(2): 309-12.
[http://dx.doi.org/10.1016/0005-2736(86)90272-5] [PMID: 3024722]

[85]     Dillehay DL, Webb SK, Schmelz EM, Merrill AH Jr. Dietary sphingomyelin inhibits 1,2-dimethylhydrazine-induced colon cancer in CF1 mice. J Nutr 1994; 124(5): 615-20.
[http://dx.doi.org/10.1093/jn/124.5.615] [PMID: 8169652]

[86]     Di Marzio L, Di Leo A, Cinque B, *et al.* Detection of alkaline sphingomyelinase activity in human stool: proposed role as a new diagnostic and prognostic marker of colorectal cancer. Cancer Epidemiol Biomarkers Prev 2005; 14(4): 856-62.
[http://dx.doi.org/10.1158/1055-9965.EPI-04-0434] [PMID: 15824156]

[87]     Shida D, Kitayama J, Yamaguchi H, *et al.* Lysophosphatidic acid (LPA) enhances the metastatic potential of human colon carcinoma DLD1 cells through LPA1. Cancer Res 2003; 63(7): 1706-11.
[PMID: 12670925]

[88]     Zalatan JG, Fenn TD, Brunger AT, Herschlag D. Structural and functional comparisons of nucleotide pyrophosphatase/phosphodiesterase and alkaline phosphatase: implications for mechanism and evolution. Biochemistry 2006; 45(32): 9788-803.
[http://dx.doi.org/10.1021/bi060847t] [PMID: 16893180]

[89]     Van Brocklyn JR, Jackson CA, Pearl DK, Kotur MS, Snyder PJ, Prior TW. Sphingosine kinase-1 expression correlates with poor survival of patients with glioblastoma multiforme: roles of sphingosine kinase isoforms in growth of glioblastoma cell lines. J Neuropathol Exp Neurol 2005; 64(8): 695-705.
[http://dx.doi.org/10.1097/01.jnen.0000175329.59092.2c] [PMID: 16106218]

[90]     Müller R, Berliner C, Leptin J, *et al.* Expression of sphingosine-1-phosphate receptors and lysophosphatidic acid receptors on cultured and xenografted human colon, breast, melanoma, and lung tumor cells. Tumour Biol 2010; 31(4): 341-9.
[http://dx.doi.org/10.1007/s13277-010-0043-7] [PMID: 20480410]

[91]    Kohno M, Momoi M, Oo ML, *et al.* Intracellular role for sphingosine kinase 1 in intestinal adenoma cell proliferation. Mol Cell Biol 2006; 26(19): 7211-23.
[http://dx.doi.org/10.1128/MCB.02341-05] [PMID: 16980623]

[92]    Bouhet S, Hourcade E, Loiseau N, *et al.* The mycotoxin fumonisin B1 alters the proliferation and the barrier function of porcine intestinal epithelial cells. Toxicol Sci 2003; 77(1): 165-71.
[http://dx.doi.org/10.1093/toxsci/kfh006] [PMID: 14600282]

[93]    Bock J, Liebisch G, Schweimer J, Schmitz G, Rogler G. Exogenous sphingomyelinase causes impaired intestinal epithelial barrier function. World J Gastroenterol 2007; 13(39): 5217-25.
[http://dx.doi.org/10.3748/wjg.v13.i39.5217] [PMID: 17876892]

[94]    Subramanian P, Stahelin RV, Szulc Z, Bielawska A, Cho W, Chalfant CE. Ceramide 1-phosphate acts as a positive allosteric activator of group IVA cytosolic phospholipase A2 alpha and enhances the interaction of the enzyme with phosphatidylcholine. J Biol Chem 2005; 280(18): 17601-7.
[http://dx.doi.org/10.1074/jbc.M414173200] [PMID: 15743759]

[95]    Cheng Y, Wu J, Hertervig E, *et al.* Identification of aberrant forms of alkaline sphingomyelinase (NPP7) associated with human liver tumorigenesis. Br J Cancer 2007; 97(10): 1441-8.
[http://dx.doi.org/10.1038/sj.bjc.6604013] [PMID: 17923876]

[96]    Gelderblom WCA, Kriek NPJ, Marasas WFO, Thiel PG. Toxicity and carcinogenicity of the *Fusanum monilzforine* metabolite, fumonisin B $_1$, in rats. Carcinogenesis 1991; 12(7): 1247-51.
[http://dx.doi.org/10.1093/carcin/12.7.1247] [PMID: 1649015]

# CHAPTER 7

# Hippo Signaling and its Regulation in Liver Cancer

**Naveen Kumar Perumal[1], Vasudevan Sekar[2], Annapoorna Bangalore Ramachandra[2,3], Nivya Vijayan[2,3], Vani Vijay[2,3], Venkat Prashanth[2,3]** and **Madan Kumar Perumal[2,3,*]**

[1] *Department of Bio-Medical Sciences, School of Biosciences and Technology, Vellore Institute of Technology, Vellore-632014, Tamil Nadu, India*

[2] *Department of Biochemistry, CSIR-Central Food Technological Research Institute, Mysore-570020, Karnataka, India*

[3] *Academy of Scientific and Innovative Research (AcSIR), Ghaziabad-201002, India*

**Abstract:** Globally, liver cancer is a severe health problem, which affects both men and women. A large number of scientific studies have suggested dysregulation of signaling cascades as a major characteristic feature in cancer. Hippo is one of the key pathways, which is dysregulated in several human cancers including liver cancer. Therefore, targeting such dysregulated signaling pathways with small molecules and phytochemicals offers significance for liver cancer therapeutics. Numerous phytochemicals were tested for their effect against the dysregulated hippo pathway. This chapter will focus on the phytochemicals that were reported in regulating the hippo pathway in experimental liver cancer.

**Keywords:** Anti-cancer, Dysregulated signaling, Hippo pathway, Liver cancer, Phytochemicals, Small molecules.

## INTRODUCTION

Coordination of fundamental biological processes such as proliferation, differentiation, and cell death is important for development, tissue homeostasis, and tumorigenesis [1, 2]. During the development process, cell number is increased to enhance organ size. During wound healing and organ regeneration, cell division and differentiation of tissue-specific progenitor cells are upregulated to compensate for the lost cells [3]. However, the coordination and integration of cellular proliferation, cell death, and cell differentiation are poorly understood. In very recent years, hippo signaling has been shown to possess coordination of the

---
* **Corresponding author Madan Kumar Perumal:** Department of Biochemistry, CSIR-Central Food Technological Research Institute, Mysore-570020, Karnataka, India and Academy of Scientific and Innovative Research (AcSIR), Ghaziabad-201002, India; E-mail: madanperumal@cftri.res.in

**Ashok Kumar Pandurangan (Ed.)**

cellular processes, including the inhibition of cell proliferation, promotion of cell death, and cellular differentiation [3 - 5].

## Hippo Pathway

The hippo pathway was first identified by genetic mosaic screens for tumor suppressor genes in Drosophila. The major hippo components include hippo (hpo), warts (wts) and yorkie (Yki) [6]. Hpo interacts directly with Sav (WW domain-containing protein) and promotes Sav and Wts phosphorylation [7]. The Mats protein interacts with Wts as an activating subunit [8, 9]. Mats is also phosphorylated by Hpo, resulting in increased interaction with Wts, and forms the core components of the Drosophila hippo pathway. On attenuation of hippo signaling, Yki phosphorylation is reduced, leading to its nuclear localization, binding to the sequence-specific DNA-binding protein scalloped (Sd), and regulation of target genes promoting proliferation and survival [10, 11].

## The Mammalian Hippo Pathway

In mammals, Msts, Lats, YAP, and TAZ are human homologues of the Drosophila Hpo, Wts, and Yki respectively [11, 12]. Mst1/2 belongs to the STE20 family protein kinases and phosphorylate Sav1, Lats1/2, and Mob1 [7, 13 - 15]. The kinase activity of Mst1/2 is enhanced through interaction with Sav1, which is mediated by SARAH (Sav/Rassf/Hpo) domains present in both Mst1/2 and Sav1 [14]. Mst1/2 directly phosphorylates Lats1/2 at the hydrophobic motif (Lats1 T1079 and Lats2 T1041), and this phosphorylation is required for Lats1/2 activation [13]. Mob1, when phosphorylated by Mst1/2, binds to the auto-inhibitory motif in Lats1/2, which in turn leads to the phosphorylation of the Lats activation loop (Lats1 S909 and Lats2 S872) and thereby increases the Lats1/2 kinase activity [13, 15]. Also, the protein levels of Lats1/2 kinases are controlled by Itch E3 ubiquitin ligase-mediated degradation [16].

Lats1/2 directly interacts and phosphorylates YAP/TAZ [6, 17, 18]. The phosphorylated YAP (Ser127) is sequestered in the cytoplasm *via* a 14-3-3 interaction [19]. In contrast, when upstream kinases are inactive, YAP/TAZ will be hypophosphorylated and translocated into the nucleus [6, 18 - 21]. Phospho-rylation of YAP (S381) and TAZ (S311) by Lats1/2 primes subsequent phosphorylation events by casein kinase 1; this sequential phosphorylation results in the recruitment of b-transducin repeat-containing proteins (b-TRCP) and consequently leads to the degradation of YAP/TAZ (Scheme **1**) [22, 23]. Hypophosphorylated YAP/TAZ in the nucleus binds to TEAD1-4 to regulate key genes [10, 11, 24 - 26]. Besides TEADs, YAP/TAZ may also interact with other transcription factors, such as Smad1 [27], smad2/3 [28], Smad7 [29], RUNX1/2 [30], p63/p73 [31], and ErbB4 [32].

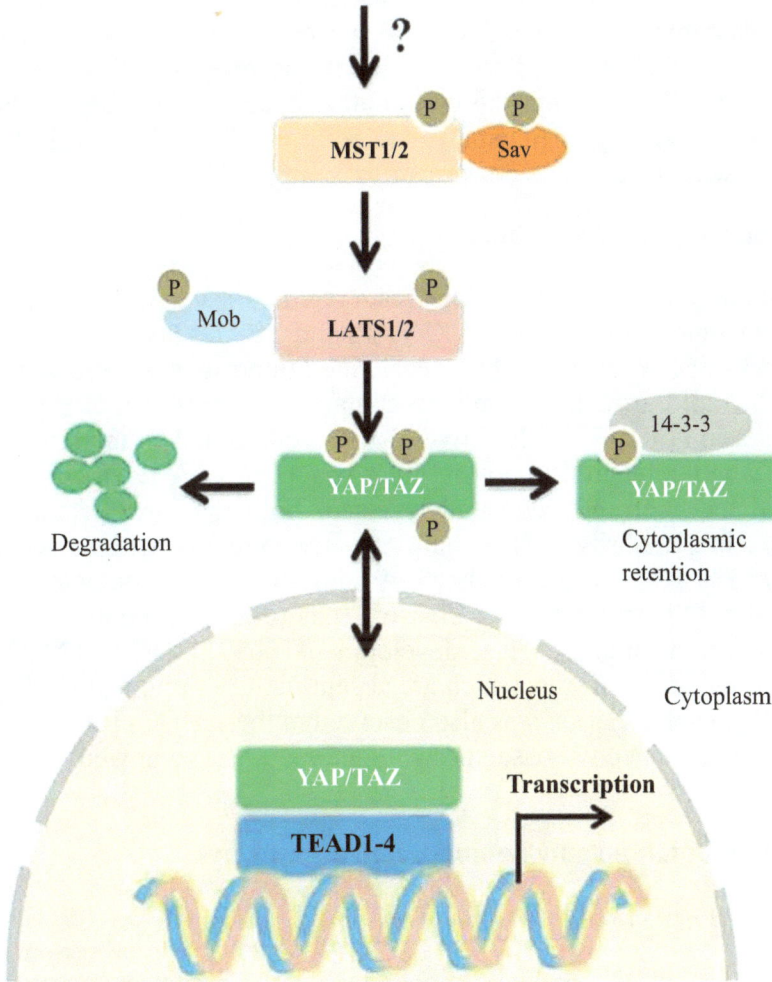

**Scheme (1).** Central components of mammalian hippo pathway.

## Hippo Pathway in Cancer

Mutations of Sav1 and Mob1 have been observed in a human renal carcinoma cell line [33] and colorectal cancer [34]. Downregulation of Lats1/2 has been reported in human cancer including ovarian, breast, retinoblastomas, and acute lymphoblastic leukemia [35 - 37]. In some cases, attenuated Lats1/2 expression with promoter hypermethylation has also been reported [38, 39]. Differential expression of Mst1/2 has been observed in human colorectal and soft tissue sarcomas [40, 41]. The germline Mst1$^{-/-}$ Mst2$^{+/-}$ mice mainly developed hepatocellular carcinoma (HCC) due to Mst2 loss of heterozygosity [42].

Overexpression of YAP is observed in several human cancers including liver, breast, colon, ovarian, lung, prostate intracranial ependymomas, oral, and medulloblastomas [43 - 49]. YAP is also reported to have pro-apoptotic activity by coactivation of p73 [31, 50, 51] and was proposed to be a breast tumor suppressor [52]. This might be cell context-specific and needs to be supported further by *in vivo* genetic study. In addition, TAZ has been shown to be overexpressed in ~20% of breast cancer samples [46].

## Hippo Pathway in Liver Cancer

The hippo core components and upstream regulators are chiefly involved in tumor suppressor function, whereas TAZ, YAP, and TEADs are involved in oncogenic events [53 - 55]. YAP and cIAP1 accelerated tumorigenesis and were required to sustain the rapid growth of amplicon-containing tumors [56, 57]. Studies showed overexpression of YAP in HCC liver tissues determined by immunohistochemical staining when compared to normal liver tissues [58]. A research group in China identified the aberrantly elevated levels of both the YAP protein and mRNA transcripts in a majority of HCC tumor tissues compared with adjacent non-tumor tissue by 62% to 9%, respectively [6, 49]. Furthermore, recent work demonstrated combined deficiency of Mst1/2 kinases leads to loss of the inactivation of YAP phosphorylation leading to HCC development [6, 59]. Mst1 and Mst2 are cleaved to shorter and active forms, which are absent in 30% of human HCC. In addition, low YAP phosphorylation was also observed in these HCCs [60]. Upregulation of nuclear YAP, connective tissue growth factor, and survivin were observed in oval cells [61, 62].

## Association of Hippo and Tumor-Related Pathways

### *Hippo and Wnt Pathway*

The influence of Wnt pathway molecules on the hippo pathway is reported to regulate mouse heart development (Scheme **2**) [63 - 66]. A cardiac muscle-specific conditional knockout of Sav, or Lats2, or conditional double knockout of Mst1 and Mst2 showed increased nuclear YAP activity and caused cardiomyocyte proliferation. YAP is recruited to TCF/LEF binding sites together with β-catenin, revealing that YAP participates *via* its nuclear functions in Wnt signaling [65]. Inhibition of Wnt signaling is due to alterations in DVL phosphorylation. TAZ binds to DVL proteins, thereby inhibiting DVL phosphorylation by casein kinase 1-delta and epsilon kinases (CK1d/e), thus promoting β-catenin degradation.

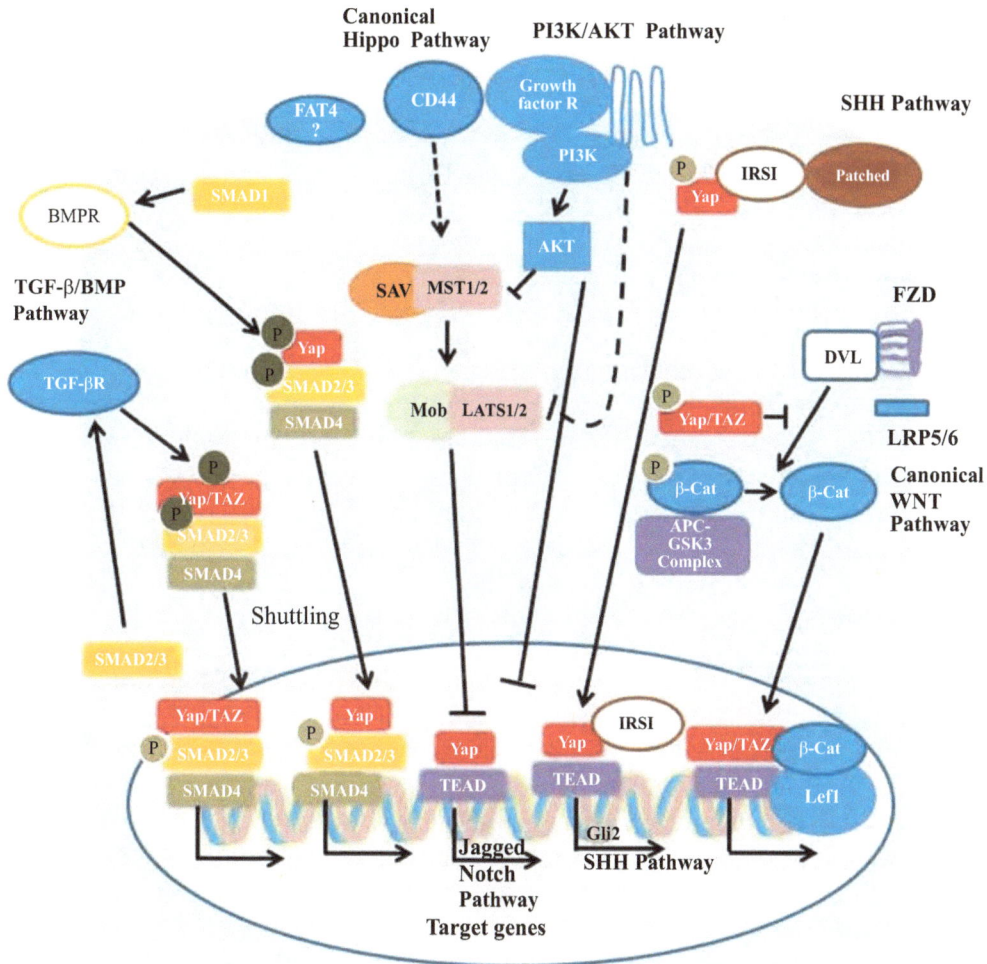

**Scheme (2).** Association of hippo and tumor-related pathways.

## Hippo and TGF-β Pathway

The TGF-β superfamily of proteins is a group of secreted morphogens that signal *via* binding to serine threonine kinase receptors, which phosphorylate the receptor-regulated Smad (R-Smad) proteins. Phosphorylated R-Smads bind to the Smad4, and subsequently accumulate in the nucleus to regulate gene transcription [67 - 69]. Hippo and TGF-β signaling are connected when YAP/TAZ binds to phosphorylated R-SMADs (Scheme **2**). The activity of SMAD nuclear is enhanced by nuclear YAP/TAZ whereas nuclear accumulation of SMAD is restricted by cytoplasmic YAP/TAZ. TGF-β activation induced by low cell density depends on nuclear YAP/TAZ, while YAP/TAZ-induced stem cell self-renewal depends on nuclear SMADs [28, 70]. Overall, hippo signaling directs the opposing roles of the TGF-β in different stages of cancer. Normally polarized epithelial cells possess cytoplasmic YAP/TAZ, which restricts TGF-β induced SMAD activity. Also, cells that exhibit impaired cell polarity show elevated nuclear YAP/TAZ, increased nuclear SMADs, and enhanced sensitivity to the TGF-β ligand [70].

## Hippo and other Pathways

The other hippo network tumor-regulated pathways, include the SHH pathway, AKT signaling, and Notch signaling (Scheme **2**). The activation of the SHH pathway leads to YAP stabilization and nuclear accumulation [46]. Also, the expressions of TEAD1 and IRS1 are modulated by SHH. In YAP overexpressed mice, neuronal differentiation defect in primary cortical progenitors was observed which was caused due to hyperactivation of SHH signaling. In human medulloblastomas, there was increased YAP1 expression with aberrant SHH signaling which suggested YAP as a therapeutic target for medulloblastoma recurrence [46].

A study by Jang *et al.* (2007) demonstrated the anti-apoptotic function of AKT where AKT inhibited apoptosis by phosphorylating Mst1/2 [71]. Reciprocal regulation also exists where Mst1/2 overexpression in prostate cancer cells inhibits AKT activity. However, AKT-mediated YAP (Ser127) phosphorylation promotes YAP localization in the cytoplasm and attenuation of p73-mediated apoptosis [72]. Jagged-1 is a YAP target in hepatocytes, and hippo pathway activation in these cells inhibits their proliferation and survival. Conversely, the overexpression of constitutively active YAP upregulates Jagged-1 and increases hepatocyte proliferation. Jagged-1 induction is required for YAP binding to TEAD-4 after Mst stimulation [73].

## Role of Hippo Signaling in Liver Cancer Development

Liver cancer, especially HCC is one of the deadliest cancers occurring worldwide. The hippo pathway is a critical pathway required for regulating organ size, tissue growth, regeneration, and tumorigenesis [74]. In normal cells, the hippo signaling module is activated to regulate the organ size by limiting cell proliferation. On the other hand, the abnormal activation of YAP/TAZ and downstream effectors has been implicated in HCC (Scheme **3**). Thus the key function of hippo signaling is to inhibit YAP and its paralog, TAZ for controlling cell proliferation and differentiation [75]. The Mst1/2 is a set of core kinases acting upstream of the hippo pathway. Mst1/2 knockdown in mouse livers resulted in the development of liver tumors. Inactivation of Mst1/2 in the liver is associated with the rapid loss of

YAP phosphorylation, increased YAP nuclear localization and protein expression, resistance to Fas-induced apoptosis, and subsequent development of HCC [42]. Perumal *et al.* (2017) in their study reported morin (a bioflavonoid) activated hippo signaling by inhibiting YAP nuclear translocation by concomitant reduction of MST1/2, Lats1/2 in cultured LX-2 cells and DEN-induced rats and thereby regulated TGF-β/Smad pathway, which is an important pathway resulting in liver fibrosis [76]. Nailing Zhang *et al.* (2010) showed genetic disruption of NF2, WW45, and Mst1/2 upstream effectors of the hippo pathway, resulting in liver tumorigenesis in *Mst1$^{Δ/Δ}$;Mst2$^{c/Δ}$;CAGGCre-ER* mice [77, 78].

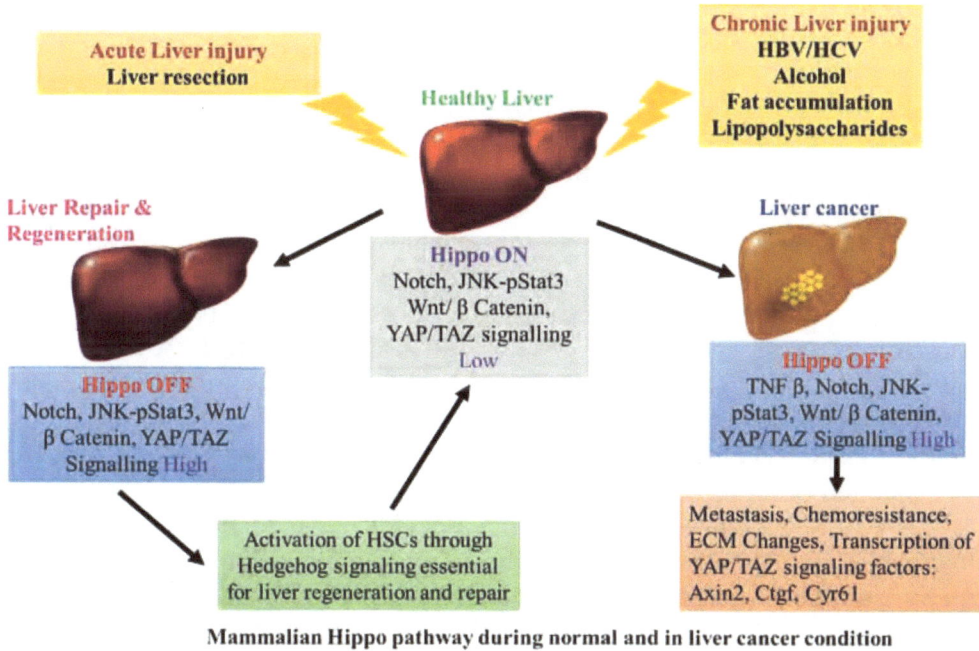

Mammalian Hippo pathway during normal and in liver cancer condition

**Scheme (3). Hippo signaling in liver cancer.** The hippo pathway is activated under normal physiological conditions to regulate YAP functions and maintain liver homeostasis. Following liver injury, the hippo pathway is immediately repressed, allowing activation of its interactors (Notch, Wnt, TGF-β, and KNK-pSTAT3 pathways) and recruitment of YAP/TAZ to the nucleus. Mechanosensing and nutrient-sensing systems will turn the hippo pathway back on once the liver achieves its hepatostat, and YAP will be inactivated *via* cytoplasmic retention or degradation. The hippo pathway is dysregulated in liver tumors, resulting in hyperactivation of YAP/TAZ.

Upstream effectors of the hippo pathway and many other proteins act in concert to regulate YAP activity mainly *via* phosphorylation of Ser 127/S381 resulting in its binding to 14-3-3, its inactivation and subsequent cytoplasmic retention. It was demonstrated that LATS phosphorylation of YAP at a site other than S127 catalyzed YAP ubiquitination by recruiting the SCFb-TRCP E3 ubiquitin ligase [79]. GABP, a heteromeric transcription factor of the Ets family activates YAP expression by specifically binding to multiple Ets binding sequences (GGAAG) of the YAP promoter and YAP acts as a downstream effector of GABP for cell proliferation and survival. The depletion of GABP downregulates YAP, resulting in a G1/S cell-cycle block and increased cell death [80].

## Role of Key Proteins in Regulating Hippo Pathway

Multiple proteins come into play, which either directly or indirectly act on the candidate upstream regulators of the hippo signaling cascade. c-Src (non-receptor tyrosine kinase) is a proto-oncogene essential for tumor growth and metastasis. c-Src gene activation is seen during the early stages of HCC. Jing Yang and colleagues reported that c-Src impeded YAP translocation from the nucleus to the cytoplasm and promoted YAP transcriptional activity [81]. Survivin is an anti-apoptotic protein belonging to the inhibitor of apoptosis protein (IAP) family. The expression levels of survivin are high in HCC cells. It has been found that the knockout of the survivin gene in PLC/PRF/5 significantly enhanced the cell-killing effect of platinum-based chemotherapy drugs toward HCC cells [82, 83]. Sirtuin1 (SIRT1), a deacetylase, is responsible for YAP deacetylation. It was reported that SIRT1 deacetylates YAP and thus enhances YAP/TEAD4 association and transcriptional activity in HCC cells, leading to cell growth and tumor formation [84]. Angiomotin family of proteins (AMOT, AMOTL1, and AMOTL2) act as negative regulators of YAP/TAZ. It was demonstrated that AMOT proteins act as adaptor proteins to promote Mst2 activation of LATS2, thereby phosphorylating YAP/TAZ leading to their cytoplasmic retention [85]. Upon deletion of all three angiomotins, it was shown to reduce the association of LATS1 with SAV1-Mst1 and decrease Mst1/2-mediated LATS1/2-HM phosphorylation. AMOTs along with MOB1 also promote autophosphorylation of LATS1/2 on the activation loop motif independent of HM phosphorylation [86]. In addition, miR-375 has also been shown to suppress the endogenous YAP protein level and inhibit the proliferation and invasion of HCC cells. In addition, small noncoding RNAs, and microRNAs (miRNAs) play a critical role in apoptosis and development of cancer including liver cancer. miR-375 has been shown to modulate Hippo signaling in the liver by suppressing endogenous YAP and inhibiting the proliferation of HCC cells [87]. Li *et al.* have demonstrated that MEK1 is required for maintaining the expression and function of YAP, which was proven in cells inactivated with MEK1/YAP knockdown which inhibited cell proliferation and maintenance of transformative phenotype was seen in both cases. Furthermore, it was shown that reduced phosphorylation of MEK1 by potent inhibitors reduced YAP expression [88].

## Role of Mst1 in Liver Cancer

Mst 1/2, a 54-60 KDa GC kinase, act as a tumor suppressor gene and are the upstream regulators of the Hippo pathway [89, 90]. Mst1 also known as serine threonine kinase 4 (STK4), belongs to the STE20 family of proteins, which plays a crucial role in regulating cell morphology, apoptosis, oncogenesis, and organ growth by inducing mitogen-activated protein kinase. Mst1 is a pro-apoptotic kinase that complexes with Mst2, a mutant or loss of Mst1 induces the hyperproliferation and suppresses the developmental apoptosis leading to tumorigenesis [91]. The activation of Mst1 *via* Akt involves inhibitory phosphorylation on Thr387 cell proliferation and evasion of apoptosis, under stressed conditions, Mst1 becomes autophosphorylated [71].

In normal physiology, Mst1 which maintains the quiescence of the hepatocytes, induces apoptosis. Mst1 suppresses the HCC development through the inactivation of the YAP. Approximately 30% of the human HCC shows overexpression of Mst1, leading to YAP phosphorylation and inhibition of developmental apoptosis. Mst1/2 knockout animals exhibit at the age of 7 months that in Mst1 null animals began to show signs of illness, including lethargy and the presence of a palpable abdominal mass. Histopathological assessment of Mst1/2 mutant animal liver showed highly aggressive HCC development [42]. In most of the HCC cells, the mutant Mst1 or the loss of the gene induced aberrant cell proliferation and protected against FAS-induced apoptosis [11].

## Effects of Targeting Mst1 Protein During Liver Carcinogenesis

The hippo pathway dynamically regulates the cellular physiology of the liver [92]. Mst1/2 are the central components of the hippo pathway and these kinases mediate the phosphorylation of YAP leading to rapid cell proliferation [91]. Thus, the pharmacological modulation of Mst1/2 kinase will be the ideal target candidate for liver cancer. Emerging reports show that food bioactives are gaining interest for use as therapeutic agents targeting the Mst1/2 for liver cancer. Morin, bioflavonoid-induced apoptosis of HCC cells through regulating the Wnt and NF-κB signaling by the activation of Mst1 *via* cleavage and phosphorylation [76, 93]. Berberine is an alkaloid that activates Mst1 by the phosphorylation of the active site and leads to the inhibition of PI3K/AKT cell survival and signaling cascade-induced mitochondrial-mediated apoptosis in HCC (Scheme **4**) [94].

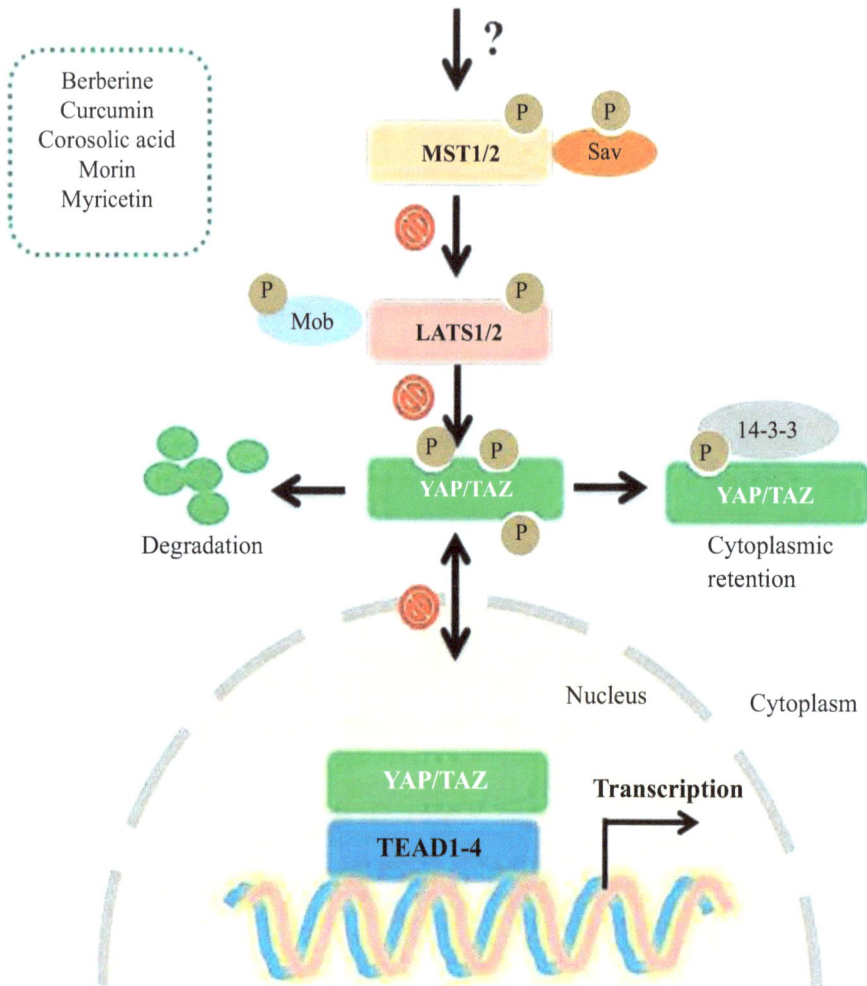

**Scheme (4).** Effect of food bioactives on the dysregulated hippo pathway during liver cancer.

## Role of YAP in Liver Cancer

Hippo signaling plays a key role in inhibiting its downstream transcriptional co-activator, YAP [95, 96]. YAP is a mammalian ortholog of Drosophila Yki [97]. Increased YAP expression has been observed in rat and human HCC cells. Studies have shown that 60% of human HCC showed increased YAP/TAZ activity indicating the role of YAP/TAZ in liver cancer progression. Therefore, the regulation of YAP expression is critical in maintaining liver homeostasis [98]. In mouse or human HCC cells, transcription factors like GABP, c-Jun, β-catenin/TCF4 complex, and CREB are known to directly bind to the YAP promoter and initiate gene transcription [99 - 101]. Hepatitis B virus (HBV) is a major risk factor for HCC where the protein HBV X is known to bind to the YAP promoter in a CREB-dependent manner and activate the transcription of the YAP gene [99]. miR-375 and miR-590-5p suppressed HCC cell proliferation and invasion by downregulating YAP expression [102, 103]. YAP is also regulated through various post-translational modifications like phosphorylation, acetylation, methylation, and O-glycosylation [104, 105].

YAP/TAZ pathway plays an important role in different facets of carcinogenesis including cell proliferation, metastasis, and cancer stemness. The upregulation of YAP/TAZ leads to chemoresistance, metastasis, and relapse of cancer. Activated YAP/TAZ also leads to increased cell survival through the repression of apoptosis-inducing factors such as CTGF, and CCN1 and through the upregulation of pro-survival factors such as BCL2 family proteins, BIRC2, BIRC5, and MCL [106]. Increased YAP activity also activates survivin leading to liver carcinogenesis. Altered YAP expression can also lead to liver cell polyploidy, aneuploidy, and chromosomal instability [107]. Metabolic reprogramming by increased YAP expression leads to liver tumorigenesis via an increase in glycolysis, glutaminolysis, and fatty acid oxidation [104, 108, 109]. YAP/TAZ activation also results in the infiltration of inflammatory cells and increased production of pro-inflammatory cytokines in the liver [110]. The crosstalk between YAP/TAZ and other oncogenic signaling promotes tumor progression. Studies have shown that increased YAP activity reduced cell senescence while YAP silencing inhibited cell proliferation and induced premature senescence. The frequency of YAP/TAZ activation was found to be the highest in liver cancer [111]. In a study conducted with 177 HCC patients, an increased expression of YAP was associated with poor tumor cell differentiation and increased serum AFP levels. YAP is also associated with drug resistance in HCC patients. Studies have shown that the increased expression of YAP in HCC cells leads to doxorubicin-induced apoptosis. This effect was reversed upon the suppression of YAP activity using the RNA interference mechanism [112].

The activation of Hepatic stellate cells (HSCs) occurs during the progression from liver fibrosis to cirrhosis, further promoting the proliferation and survival of HCC cells. A complex relationship exists between YAP and HSC activation. Increased YAP activity leads to the release of TGF-β from HCC cells, which in turn regulates the HSCs function. Activated HSCs further activate the ECM proteins. Increased ECM proteins activate the translocation of YAP from the cytoplasm to the nucleus in HCC cells leading to HCC proliferation and transformation [113].

## Effect of Targeting Yap Protein During Liver Carcinogenesis

A study by Perumal *et al.* (2017) reported that morin treatment impeded nuclear translocation of YAP thereby promoting apoptosis through the downregulation of Wnt/β-catenin and NF-KB signaling in HepG2 cells overexpressing Mst1. The study also revealed activation of Mst1 by caspase-3-dependent cleavage upon treatment of Mst-1 overexpressing HepG2 cells with morin. Apoptosis was confirmed using Annexin-V/PI staining of morin-treated F-Mst1 overexpressing cells. Morin treatment also elevated the levels of Mst1 and Lats1 and reduced YAP protein expression (Scheme **4**) [114]. Myricetin, a flavonoid abundantly present in fruits and vegetables is reported for anti-cancer properties against various cancers such as ovarian, liver, breast, gastric, skin, and placental carcinomas. Minjing Li *et al.* (2019) showed that myricetin treatment inhibited cell proliferation and potentiated apoptosis in HCC cells. Myricetin treatment also downregulated YAP expression through proteasomal degradation of YAP and reduced expression of its target genes like c-myc, survivin, and CYR61 in HepG2 and Huh-7 cells. The study also demonstrated the sensitization of cisplatin and sorafenib-resistant HCC upon myricetin treatment through YAP inhibition [115].

Curcumin, a chemical compound isolated from the Rhizome of plant species Zingiberaceae and Araceae has been reported to suppress tumor progression in different cancer types. A study by Lihua Wang *et al.* demonstrated WZ35, a derivative of curcumin, to exhibit tumor suppressive effects in experimental HCC. WZ35 significantly suppressed autophagy in HCC cells - HCCLM3 in a YAP-dependent manner [116]. Corosolic acid, a pentacyclic triterpenoid is a Chinese herbal monomer extracted from Valerians. Congcong Zang *et al.* showed that corosolic acid inhibited the YAP expression and proliferation of HCC cells (Scheme **4**) [117]. They showed that under high glucose conditions, corosolic acid inhibited YAP expression and O-GlcNAcylation through CDK19 inhibition [118].

## Role of LATS 1/2 in Liver Cancer

The imminent protein family LATS encompassing LATS1 and LATS2 has been instrumental in the maintenance of cellular homeostasis in the mammalian systems. LATS1 and LATS2 represent a distinctive signaling family within the cell owing to their high degree of homology and significant functional overlap. Both LATS1 and LATS2 perform more specific roles in the modulation of cell cycle checkpoints, induction of apoptosis, and inhibition of cell migration [119]. In addition to the latter, they are key signaling molecules that function as Ser/Thr kinases with diverse regulatory mechanisms such as transcriptional regulation and genetic stability [120].

Albeit, essentially known as a crucial player in the Hippo-LATS pathway, research suggests that LATS1 and LATS2 have broader functional capabilities. On the other hand, the loss of either of these genes will lead to malevolent phenotypes. So, it is critical to recognize the functioning of LATS1 and LATS2 in order to understand tumorigenesis. These tumor suppressors operate both as individual proteins and as a collective, showcasing their distinct potential redundant roles [121]. The LATS1 and LATS2 kinases have caused quite a stir in recent years. They are gaining popularity due to their diverse biological activities in genome integrity, cell cycle regulation, differentiation, and organism fitness. Their deregulation also has significant and diverse pathological consequences. Moreover, LATS kinases play a vital role in cancer prevention and cell motility [22, 122 - 124].   -

Aside from the traditional Hippo-YAP axis, the network also seems to include novel kinases such as NDR1/2 (STK38/STK38L), MAP4Ks, and CK1. MAP4Ks that are activated may also phosphorylate LATS1/2 and NDR1/2. While LATS phosphorylates YAP on five serine residues: S61, S109, S127, S164, and S381, NDR phosphorylates YAP directly on S127, preventing it from entering the nucleus [125]. Aside from phosphorylation status, the Hippo pathway is influenced by cell architecture and mechanical signals. YAP interacts with tight junction proteins, which seems to restrict target gene expression although YAP activation is an early event in the development of HCC, mutations in the hippo pathway are uncommon in human tumors [126].

## Effects of Targeting LATS1 and LATS2 Protein During Liver Carcinogenesis

The bioflavonoid, morin's anti-cancer action is mediated by the induction of Mst1/Hippo signaling in liver cancer cells, according to a study performed by Perumal N (2017). Morin triggered Mst1 *via* cleavage and phosphorylation, thereby stimulating LATS 1/2, promoting hippo signaling in HepG2 cells. Subsequently, substantial reductions in YAP and TAZ levels are revealed, restricting cell growth and amplifying HepG2 cell death [93]. Curcumin, a significant part of turmeric, decreased TAZ and YAP expressions and had anti-cancer activity in HCC cell lines (HepG2 and HLF, which exhibited high TAZ expression), as shown in a study by Hiromitsu Hayashi (2015). TAZ/YAP co-inhibition seemed to be a potential therapeutic method for treating HCC. By shifting the predominant coactivator, TAZ and YAP, downstream components of Hippo signaling enhance cell proliferation, chemoresistance, and tumorigenicity amid cancer progression [127].

According to Hui Liu (2021), ethanol extract from Chinese poplar propolis was observed to activate LATS 2 and, as a consequence, inhibit the levels of YAP, TAZ, and their target protein TEAD1. Hippo/YAP signaling pathways are important for HCC proliferation. Poplar propolis extract suppresses the loop between the Hippo/YAP and PI3K/AKT pathways. Moreover, it imposes good anti-proliferation and pro-apoptosis effects in HepG2 cells. Future research could develop this extract as a therapeutic agent for HCC [128].

Myricetin possesses therapeutic potential against ovarian cancer, breast cancer, stomach cancer, skin cancer, and placental choriocarcinoma, among other cancers. Myricetin, for example, has been found to cause cell-cycle arrest, inhibit proliferation, and fatality by targeting the cyclin B/Cdc2 complex, Akt/p70S6K/Bad signaling, mitochondrial apoptotic cascades, and oxidants. Minjing Li (2019) observed that Myricetin inhibited proliferation and activated apoptosis in HepG2 and Huh-7 cells, by restricting the phosphorylation of YAP. Myricetin has also been found to suppress the YAP expression by inducing the LATS1/2 kinase. Myricetin-induced phosphorylation and degradation of YAP were attenuated while LATS1/2 expression was knocked down employing shRNA [115].

Yen-Lin Chen (2020) showed that 4-acetylantrocamol LT3 (4AALT3), a novel ubiquinone from the mycelium of *Antrodia cinnamomea* (Polyporaceae), exhibits anti-cancer activities. *Antrodia cinnamomea*has long been used in Taiwan to treat liver ailments. According to pharmacological studies, *Antrodia cinnamomea* and its bioactives exhibited anti-cancer effects. The subsequent results showed that 4AALT3 inhibited the nuclear localization of YAP/TAZ and the expression of its target genes, revealing that 4AALT3 plays a role in the YAP-driven signaling network that can be either by direct or through hippo pathway key factors like Mst1/2 and LATS1/2 [129].

## CONCLUSION

Liver cancer is a pathological condition, which affects both men and women worldwide. Numerous studies conducted to understand the mechanisms involved in liver tumor progression have revealed the hippo pathway as the key signaling pathway undergoing activation in humans. Therefore, targeting this exacerbated hippo signaling, which could be one effective strategy to treat human liver cancer. Sorafenib, Lenvatinib, and Cabozantinib are FDA-approved chemodrugs for the treatment of advanced HCC. Although these drugs mediate anti-cancer effects, the main concern is their side effects. A large number of studies showed the hepatoprotective effects of plant phytochemicals including liver cancer. This chapter focused on elucidating the hippo pathway regulation in liver cancer and the anti-cancer effects of phytochemicals targeting hippo components exerting their anti-cancer effect. Despite the enormous availability of pre-clinical data showing the anti-cancer effects of these phytochemicals, clinical trials are still challenging.

## REFERENCES

[1]     Pellettieri J, Alvarado AS. Cell turnover and adult tissue homeostasis: from humans to planarians. Annu Rev Genet 2007; 41(1): 83-105.
[http://dx.doi.org/10.1146/annurev.genet.41.110306.130244] [PMID: 18076325]

[2]     Galliot B, Ghila L. Cell plasticity in homeostasis and regeneration. Mol Reprod Dev 2010; 77(10): 837-55.
[http://dx.doi.org/10.1002/mrd.21206] [PMID: 20602493]

[3]     Yu FX, Guan KL. The Hippo pathway: regulators and regulations. Genes Dev 2013; 27(4): 355-71.
[http://dx.doi.org/10.1101/gad.210773.112] [PMID: 23431053]

[4]     Edgar BA. From cell structure to transcription: Hippo forges a new path. Cell 2006; 124(2): 267-73.
[http://dx.doi.org/10.1016/j.cell.2006.01.005] [PMID: 16439203]

[5]     Harvey K, Tapon N. The Salvador–Warts–Hippo pathway — an emerging tumour-suppressor network. Nat Rev Cancer 2007; 7(3): 182-91.
[http://dx.doi.org/10.1038/nrc2070] [PMID: 17318211]

[6]     Dong J, Feldmann G, Huang J, *et al.* Elucidation of a universal size-control mechanism in Drosophila and mammals. Cell 2007; 130(6): 1120-33.
[http://dx.doi.org/10.1016/j.cell.2007.07.019] [PMID: 17889654]

[7]     Wu S, Huang J, Dong J, Pan D. hippo encodes a Ste-20 family protein kinase that restricts cell proliferation and promotes apoptosis in conjunction with salvador and warts. Cell 2003; 114(4): 445-56.
[http://dx.doi.org/10.1016/S0092-8674(03)00549-X] [PMID: 12941273]

[8]     Lai ZC, Wei X, Shimizu T, *et al.* Control of cell proliferation and apoptosis by mob as tumor suppressor, mats. Cell 2005; 120(5): 675-85.
[http://dx.doi.org/10.1016/j.cell.2004.12.036] [PMID: 15766530]

[9]     Wei X, Shimizu T, Lai ZC. Mob as tumor suppressor is activated by Hippo kinase for growth inhibition in Drosophila. EMBO J 2007; 26(7): 1772-81.
[http://dx.doi.org/10.1038/sj.emboj.7601630] [PMID: 17347649]

[10]    Zhang L, Ren F, Zhang Q, Chen Y, Wang B, Jiang J. The TEAD/TEF family of transcription factor Scalloped mediates Hippo signaling in organ size control. Dev Cell 2008; 14(3): 377-87.
[http://dx.doi.org/10.1016/j.devcel.2008.01.006] [PMID: 18258485]

[11]    Zhao B, Lei QY, Guan KL. The Hippo–YAP pathway: new connections between regulation of organ size and cancer. Curr Opin Cell Biol 2008; 20(6): 638-46.
[http://dx.doi.org/10.1016/j.ceb.2008.10.001] [PMID: 18955139]

[12]    Zeng Q, Hong W. The emerging role of the hippo pathway in cell contact inhibition, organ size control, and cancer development in mammals. Cancer Cell 2008; 13(3): 188-92.
[http://dx.doi.org/10.1016/j.ccr.2008.02.011] [PMID: 18328423]

[13]    Chan EHY, Nousiainen M, Chalamalasetty RB, Schäfer A, Nigg EA, Silljé HHW. The Ste20-like kinase Mst2 activates the human large tumor suppressor kinase Lats1. Oncogene 2005; 24(12): 2076-86.
[http://dx.doi.org/10.1038/sj.onc.1208445] [PMID: 15688006]

[14]    Callus BA, Verhagen AM, Vaux DL. Association of mammalian sterile twenty kinases, Mst1 and Mst2, with hSalvador *via* C-terminal coiled-coil domains, leads to its stabilization and

phosphorylation. FEBS J 2006; 273(18): 4264-76.
[http://dx.doi.org/10.1111/j.1742-4658.2006.05427.x] [PMID: 16930133]

[15] Praskova M, Xia F, Avruch J. MOBKL1A/MOBKL1B phosphorylation by MST1 and MST2 inhibits cell proliferation. Curr Biol 2008; 18(5): 311-21.
[http://dx.doi.org/10.1016/j.cub.2008.02.006] [PMID: 18328708]

[16] Ho KC, Zhou Z, She YM, Chun A, Cyr TD, Yang X. Itch E3 ubiquitin ligase regulates large tumor suppressor 1 stability. Proc Natl Acad Sci USA 2011; 108(12): 4870-5.
[http://dx.doi.org/10.1073/pnas.1101273108] [PMID: 21383157]

[17] Huang J, Wu S, Barrera J, Matthews K, Pan D. The Hippo signaling pathway coordinately regulates cell proliferation and apoptosis by inactivating Yorkie, the Drosophila Homolog of YAP. Cell 2005; 122(3): 421-34.
[http://dx.doi.org/10.1016/j.cell.2005.06.007] [PMID: 16096061]

[18] Lei QY, Zhang H, Zhao B, et al. TAZ promotes cell proliferation and epithelial-mesenchymal transition and is inhibited by the hippo pathway. Mol Cell Biol 2008; 28(7): 2426-36.
[http://dx.doi.org/10.1128/MCB.01874-07] [PMID: 18227151]

[19] Zhao B, Wei X, Li W, et al. Inactivation of YAP oncoprotein by the Hippo pathway is involved in cell contact inhibition and tissue growth control. Genes Dev 2007; 21(21): 2747-61.
[http://dx.doi.org/10.1101/gad.1602907] [PMID: 17974916]

[20] Kanai F, Marignani PA, Sarbassova D, et al. TAZ: a novel transcriptional co-activator regulated by interactions with 14-3-3 and PDZ domain proteins. EMBO J 2000; 19(24): 6778-91.
[http://dx.doi.org/10.1093/emboj/19.24.6778] [PMID: 11118213]

[21] Ren F, Zhang L, Jiang J. Hippo signaling regulates Yorkie nuclear localization and activity through 14-3-3 dependent and independent mechanisms. Dev Biol 2010; 337(2): 303-12.
[http://dx.doi.org/10.1016/j.ydbio.2009.10.046] [PMID: 19900439]

[22] Liu AM, Xu MZ, Chen J, Poon RT, Luk JM. Targeting YAP and Hippo signaling pathway in liver cancer. Expert Opin Ther Targets 2010; 14(8): 855-68.
[http://dx.doi.org/10.1517/14728222.2010.499361] [PMID: 20545481]

[23] Zhao B, Li L, Tumaneng K, Wang CY, Guan KL. A coordinated phosphorylation by Lats and CK1 regulates YAP stability through SCF $^{\beta-TRCP}$. Genes Dev 2010; 24(1): 72-85.
[http://dx.doi.org/10.1101/gad.1843810] [PMID: 20048001]

[24] Vassilev A, Kaneko KJ, Shu H, Zhao Y, DePamphilis ML. TEAD/TEF transcription factors utilize the activation domain of YAP65, a Src/Yes-associated protein localized in the cytoplasm. Genes Dev 2001; 15(10): 1229-41.
[http://dx.doi.org/10.1101/gad.888601] [PMID: 11358867]

[25] Goulev Y, Fauny JD, Gonzalez-Marti B, Flagiello D, Silber J, Zider A. SCALLOPED interacts with YORKIE, the nuclear effector of the hippo tumor-suppressor pathway in Drosophila. Curr Biol 2008; 18(6): 435-41.
[http://dx.doi.org/10.1016/j.cub.2008.02.034] [PMID: 18313299]

[26] Wu S, Liu Y, Zheng Y, Dong J, Pan D. The TEAD/TEF family protein Scalloped mediates transcriptional output of the Hippo growth-regulatory pathway. Dev Cell 2008; 14(3): 388-98.
[http://dx.doi.org/10.1016/j.devcel.2008.01.007] [PMID: 18258486]

[27] Alarcón C, Zaromytidou AI, Xi Q, et al. Nuclear CDKs drive Smad transcriptional activation and turnover in BMP and TGF-beta pathways. Cell 2009; 139(4): 757-69.
[http://dx.doi.org/10.1016/j.cell.2009.09.035] [PMID: 19914168]

[28] Varelas X, Sakuma R, Samavarchi-Tehrani P, et al. TAZ controls Smad nucleocytoplasmic shuttling and regulates human embryonic stem-cell self-renewal. Nat Cell Biol 2008; 10(7): 837-48.
[http://dx.doi.org/10.1038/ncb1748] [PMID: 18568018]

[29] Ferrigno O, Lallemand F, Verrecchia F, et al. Yes-associated protein (YAP65) interacts with Smad7

and potentiates its inhibitory activity against TGF-β/Smad signaling. Oncogene 2002; 21(32): 4879-84.
[http://dx.doi.org/10.1038/sj.onc.1205623] [PMID: 12118366]

[30]    Yagi R, Chen LF, Shigesada K, Murakami Y, Ito Y. A WW domain-containing Yes-associated protein (YAP) is a novel transcriptional co-activator. EMBO J 1999; 18(9): 2551-62.
[http://dx.doi.org/10.1093/emboj/18.9.2551] [PMID: 10228168]

[31]    Strano S, Munarriz E, Rossi M, *et al.* Physical interaction with Yes-associated protein enhances p73 transcriptional activity. J Biol Chem 2001; 276(18): 15164-73.
[http://dx.doi.org/10.1074/jbc.M010484200] [PMID: 11278685]

[32]    Omerovic J, Puggioni EMR, Napoletano S, *et al.* Ligand-regulated association of ErbB-4 to the transcriptional co-activator YAP65 controls transcription at the nuclear level. Exp Cell Res 2004; 294(2): 469-79.
[http://dx.doi.org/10.1016/j.yexcr.2003.12.002] [PMID: 15023535]

[33]    Tapon N, Harvey KF, Bell DW, *et al.* salvador Promotes both cell cycle exit and apoptosis in Drosophila and is mutated in human cancer cell lines. Cell 2002; 110(4): 467-78.
[http://dx.doi.org/10.1016/S0092-8674(02)00824-3] [PMID: 12202036]

[34]    Kosaka Y, Mimori K, Tanaka F, Inoue H, Watanabe M, Mori M. Clinical significance of the loss of MATS1 mRNA expression in colorectal cancer. Int J Oncol 2007; 31(2): 333-8.
[http://dx.doi.org/10.3892/ijo.31.2.333] [PMID: 17611689]

[35]    Hisaoka M, Tanaka A, Hashimoto H. Molecular alterations of h-warts/LATS1 tumor suppressor in human soft tissue sarcoma. Lab Invest 2002; 82(10): 1427-35.
[http://dx.doi.org/10.1097/01.LAB.0000032381.68634.CA] [PMID: 12379777]

[36]    Jiménez-Velasco A, Román-Gómez J, Agirre X, *et al.* Downregulation of the large tumor suppressor 2 (LATS2/KPM) gene is associated with poor prognosis in acute lymphoblastic leukemia. Leukemia 2005; 19(12): 2347-50.
[http://dx.doi.org/10.1038/sj.leu.2403974] [PMID: 16208412]

[37]    Chakraborty S, Khare S, Dorairaj SK, Prabhakaran VC, Prakash DR, Kumar A. Identification of genes associated with tumorigenesis of retinoblastoma by microarray analysis. Genomics 2007; 90(3): 344-53.
[http://dx.doi.org/10.1016/j.ygeno.2007.05.002] [PMID: 17604597]

[38]    Takahashi Y, Miyoshi Y, Takahata C, *et al.* Down-regulation of LATS1 and LATS2 mRNA expression by promoter hypermethylation and its association with biologically aggressive phenotype in human breast cancers. Clin Cancer Res 2005; 11(4): 1380-5.
[http://dx.doi.org/10.1158/1078-0432.CCR-04-1773] [PMID: 15746036]

[39]    Jiang Z, Li X, Hu J, *et al.* Promoter hypermethylation-mediated down-regulation of LATS1 and LATS2 in human astrocytoma. Neurosci Res 2006; 56(4): 450-8.
[http://dx.doi.org/10.1016/j.neures.2006.09.006] [PMID: 17049657]

[40]    Minoo P, Zlobec I, Baker K, *et al.* Prognostic significance of mammalian sterile20-like kinase 1 in colorectal cancer. Mod Pathol 2007; 20(3): 331-8.
[http://dx.doi.org/10.1038/modpathol.3800740] [PMID: 17277767]

[41]    Seidel C, Schagdarsurengin U, Blümke K, *et al.* Frequent hypermethylation of *MST1* and *MST2* in soft tissue sarcoma. Mol Carcinog 2007; 46(10): 865-71.
[http://dx.doi.org/10.1002/mc.20317] [PMID: 17538946]

[42]    Zhou D, Conrad C, Xia F, *et al.* Mst1 and Mst2 maintain hepatocyte quiescence and suppress hepatocellular carcinoma development through inactivation of the Yap1 oncogene. Cancer Cell 2009; 16(5): 425-38.
[http://dx.doi.org/10.1016/j.ccr.2009.09.026] [PMID: 19878874]

[43]    Baldwin C, Garnis C, Zhang L, Rosin MP, Lam WL. Multiple microalterations detected at high

frequency in oral cancer. Cancer Res 2005; 65(17): 7561-7.
[http://dx.doi.org/10.1158/0008-5472.CAN-05-1513] [PMID: 16140918]

[44]    Snijders AM, Schmidt BL, Fridlyand J, *et al.* Rare amplicons implicate frequent deregulation of cell fate specification pathways in oral squamous cell carcinoma. Oncogene 2005; 24(26): 4232-42.
[http://dx.doi.org/10.1038/sj.onc.1208601] [PMID: 15824737]

[45]    Modena P, Lualdi E, Facchinetti F, *et al.* Identification of tumor-specific molecular signatures in intracranial ependymoma and association with clinical characteristics. J Clin Oncol 2006; 24(33): 5223-33.
[http://dx.doi.org/10.1200/JCO.2006.06.3701] [PMID: 17114655]

[46]    Fernandez-L A, Northcott PA, Dalton J, *et al.* YAP1 is amplified and up-regulated in hedgehog-associated medulloblastomas and mediates Sonic hedgehog-driven neural precursor proliferation. Genes Dev 2009; 23(23): 2729-41.
[http://dx.doi.org/10.1101/gad.1824509] [PMID: 19952108]

[47]    Overholtzer M, Zhang J, Smolen GA, *et al.* Transforming properties of *YAP*, a candidate oncogene on the chromosome 11q22 amplicon. Proc Natl Acad Sci USA 2006; 103(33): 12405-10.
[http://dx.doi.org/10.1073/pnas.0605579103] [PMID: 16894141]

[48]    Zender L, Spector MS, Xue W, *et al.* Identification and validation of oncogenes in liver cancer using an integrative oncogenomic approach. Cell 2006; 125(7): 1253-67.
[http://dx.doi.org/10.1016/j.cell.2006.05.030] [PMID: 16814713]

[49]    Steinhardt AA, Gayyed MF, Klein AP, *et al.* Expression of Yes-associated protein in common solid tumors. Hum Pathol 2008; 39(11): 1582-9.
[http://dx.doi.org/10.1016/j.humpath.2008.04.012] [PMID: 18703216]

[50]    Matallanas D, Romano D, Yee K, *et al.* RASSF1A elicits apoptosis through an MST2 pathway directing proapoptotic transcription by the p73 tumor suppressor protein. Mol Cell 2007; 27(6): 962-75.
[http://dx.doi.org/10.1016/j.molcel.2007.08.008] [PMID: 17889669]

[51]    Oka T, Mazack V, Sudol M. Mst2 and Lats kinases regulate apoptotic function of Yes kinase-associated protein (YAP). J Biol Chem 2008; 283(41): 27534-46.
[http://dx.doi.org/10.1074/jbc.M804380200] [PMID: 18640976]

[52]    Yuan M, Tomlinson V, Lara R, *et al.* Yes-associated protein (YAP) functions as a tumor suppressor in breast. Cell Death Differ 2008; 15(11): 1752-9.
[http://dx.doi.org/10.1038/cdd.2008.108] [PMID: 18617895]

[53]    Lee KP, Lee JH, Kim TS, *et al.* The Hippo–Salvador pathway restrains hepatic oval cell proliferation, liver size, and liver tumorigenesis. Proc Natl Acad Sci USA 2010; 107(18): 8248-53.
[http://dx.doi.org/10.1073/pnas.0912203107] [PMID: 20404163]

[54]    Luo X. Snapshots of a hybrid transcription factor in the Hippo pathway. Protein Cell 2010; 1(9): 811-9.
[http://dx.doi.org/10.1007/s13238-010-0105-z] [PMID: 21203923]

[55]    Hilman D, Gat U. The evolutionary history of YAP and the hippo/YAP pathway. Mol Biol Evol 2011; 28(8): 2403-17.
[http://dx.doi.org/10.1093/molbev/msr065] [PMID: 21415026]

[56]    Kang W, Tong JHM, Chan AWH, *et al.* Yes-associated protein 1 exhibits oncogenic property in gastric cancer and its nuclear accumulation associates with poor prognosis. Clin Cancer Res 2011; 17(8): 2130-9.
[http://dx.doi.org/10.1158/1078-0432.CCR-10-2467] [PMID: 21346147]

[57]    Zender L, Xue W, Cordón-Cardo C, *et al.* Generation and analysis of genetically defined liver carcinomas derived from bipotential liver progenitors. Cold Spring Harb Symp Quant Biol 2005; 70(0): 251-61.

[http://dx.doi.org/10.1101/sqb.2005.70.059] [PMID: 16869761]

[58] Zhao B, Lei Q, Guan KL. Mst out and HCC in. Cancer Cell 2009; 16(5): 363-4.
[http://dx.doi.org/10.1016/j.ccr.2009.10.008] [PMID: 19878866]

[59] Hiemer SE, Varelas X. Stem cell regulation by the Hippo pathway. Biochim Biophys Acta, Gen Subj 2013; 1830(2): 2323-34.
[http://dx.doi.org/10.1016/j.bbagen.2012.07.005] [PMID: 22824335]

[60] Tufail R, Jorda M, Zhao W, Reis I, Nawaz Z. Loss of Yes-associated protein (YAP) expression is associated with estrogen and progesterone receptors negativity in invasive breast carcinomas. Breast Cancer Res Treat 2012; 131(3): 743-50.
[http://dx.doi.org/10.1007/s10549-011-1435-0] [PMID: 21399893]

[61] Urtasun R, Latasa MU, Demartis MI, *et al.* Connective tissue growth factor autocriny in human hepatocellular carcinoma: Oncogenic role and regulation by epidermal growth factor receptor/yes-associated protein-mediated activation. Hepatology 2011; 54(6): 2149-58.
[http://dx.doi.org/10.1002/hep.24587] [PMID: 21800344]

[62] Zheng T, Wang J, Jiang H, Liu L. Hippo signaling in oval cells and hepatocarcinogenesis. Cancer Lett 2011; 302(2): 91-9.
[http://dx.doi.org/10.1016/j.canlet.2010.12.008] [PMID: 21247686]

[63] Clevers H. Wnt/beta-catenin signaling in development and disease. Cell 2006; 127(3): 469-80.
[http://dx.doi.org/10.1016/j.cell.2006.10.018] [PMID: 17081971]

[64] MacDonald BT, Tamai K, He X. Wnt/beta-catenin signaling: components, mechanisms, and diseases. Dev Cell 2009; 17(1): 9-26.
[http://dx.doi.org/10.1016/j.devcel.2009.06.016] [PMID: 19619488]

[65] Varelas X, Miller BW, Sopko R, *et al.* The Hippo pathway regulates Wnt/beta-catenin signaling. Dev Cell 2010; 18(4): 579-91.
[http://dx.doi.org/10.1016/j.devcel.2010.03.007] [PMID: 20412773]

[66] Heallen T, Zhang M, Wang J, *et al.* Hippo pathway inhibits Wnt signaling to restrain cardiomyocyte proliferation and heart size. Science 2011; 332(6028): 458-61.
[http://dx.doi.org/10.1126/science.1199010] [PMID: 21512031]

[67] Attisano L, Wrana JL. Signal transduction by the TGF-beta superfamily. Science 2002; 296(5573): 1646-7.
[http://dx.doi.org/10.1126/science.1071809] [PMID: 12040180]

[68] Feng XH, Derynck R. Specificity and versatility in tgf-β signaling through smads. Annu Rev Cell Dev Biol 2005; 21(1): 659-93.
[http://dx.doi.org/10.1146/annurev.cellbio.21.022404.142018] [PMID: 16212511]

[69] Heldin CH, Landström M, Moustakas A. Mechanism of TGF-β signaling to growth arrest, apoptosis, and epithelial–mesenchymal transition. Curr Opin Cell Biol 2009; 21(2): 166-76.
[http://dx.doi.org/10.1016/j.ceb.2009.01.021] [PMID: 19237272]

[70] Varelas X, Samavarchi-Tehrani P, Narimatsu M, *et al.* The Crumbs complex couples cell density sensing to Hippo-dependent control of the TGF-β-SMAD pathway. Dev Cell 2010; 19(6): 831-44.
[http://dx.doi.org/10.1016/j.devcel.2010.11.012] [PMID: 21145499]

[71] Jang SW, Yang SJ, Srinivasan S, Ye K. Akt phosphorylates MstI and prevents its proteolytic activation, blocking FOXO3 phosphorylation and nuclear translocation. J Biol Chem 2007; 282(42): 30836-44.
[http://dx.doi.org/10.1074/jbc.M704542200] [PMID: 17726016]

[72] Basu S, Totty NF, Irwin MS, Sudol M, Downward J. Akt phosphorylates the Yes-associated protein, YAP, to induce interaction with 14-3-3 and attenuation of p73-mediated apoptosis. Mol Cell 2003; 11(1): 11-23.
[http://dx.doi.org/10.1016/S1097-2765(02)00776-1] [PMID: 12535517]

[73]   Camargo FD, Gokhale S, Johnnidis JB, *et al.* YAP1 increases organ size and expands undifferentiated progenitor cells. Curr Biol 2007; 17(23): 2054-60.
[http://dx.doi.org/10.1016/j.cub.2007.10.039] [PMID: 17980593]

[74]   Nguyen-Lefebvre AT, Selzner N, Wrana JL, Bhat M. The hippo pathway: A master regulator of liver metabolism, regeneration, and disease. FASEB J 2021; 35(5): e21570.
[http://dx.doi.org/10.1096/fj.202002284RR] [PMID: 33831275]

[75]   Patel SH, Camargo FD, Yimlamai D. Hippo signaling in the liver regulates organ size, cell fate, and carcinogenesis. Gastroenterology 2017; 152(3): 533-45.
[http://dx.doi.org/10.1053/j.gastro.2016.10.047] [PMID: 28003097]

[76]   Perumal N, Perumal M, Halagowder D, Sivasithamparam N. Morin attenuates diethylnitrosamine-induced rat liver fibrosis and hepatic stellate cell activation by co-ordinated regulation of Hippo/Yap and TGF-β1/Smad signaling. Biochimie 2017; 140: 10-9.
[http://dx.doi.org/10.1016/j.biochi.2017.05.017] [PMID: 28552397]

[77]   Zhang N, Bai H, David KK, *et al.* The Merlin/NF2 tumor suppressor functions through the YAP oncoprotein to regulate tissue homeostasis in mammals. Dev Cell 2010; 19(1): 27-38.
[http://dx.doi.org/10.1016/j.devcel.2010.06.015] [PMID: 20643348]

[78]   Song H, Mak KK, Topol L, *et al.* Mammalian Mst1 and Mst2 kinases play essential roles in organ size control and tumor suppression. Proc Natl Acad Sci USA 2010; 107(4): 1431-6.
[http://dx.doi.org/10.1073/pnas.0911409107] [PMID: 20080598]

[79]   Zhao B, Li L, Tumaneng K, Wang CY, Guan KL. A coordinated phosphorylation by Lats and CK1 regulates YAP stability through SCF [β-TRCP]. Genes Dev 2010; 24(1): 72-85.
[http://dx.doi.org/10.1101/gad.1843810] [PMID: 20048001]

[80]   Wu H, Xiao Y, Zhang S, *et al.* The Ets transcription factor GABP is a component of the hippo pathway essential for growth and antioxidant defense. Cell Rep 2013; 3(5): 1663-77.
[http://dx.doi.org/10.1016/j.celrep.2013.04.020] [PMID: 23684612]

[81]   Yang J, Zhang X, Liu L, Yang X, Qian Q, Du B. c-Src promotes the growth and tumorigenesis of hepatocellular carcinoma *via* the Hippo signaling pathway. Life Sci 2021; 264: 118711.
[http://dx.doi.org/10.1016/j.lfs.2020.118711] [PMID: 33186566]

[82]   Or Y, Chow AKM, Ng L, *et al.* Survivin depletion inhibits tumor growth and enhances chemosensitivity in hepatocellular carcinoma. Mol Med Rep 2014; 10(4): 2025-30.
[http://dx.doi.org/10.3892/mmr.2014.2413] [PMID: 25070628]

[83]   Su C. Survivin in survival of hepatocellular carcinoma. Cancer Lett 2016; 379(2): 184-90.
[http://dx.doi.org/10.1016/j.canlet.2015.06.016] [PMID: 26118774]

[84]   Mao B, Hu F, Cheng J, *et al.* SIRT1 regulates YAP2-mediated cell proliferation and chemoresistance in hepatocellular carcinoma. Oncogene 2014; 33(11): 1468-74.
[http://dx.doi.org/10.1038/onc.2013.88] [PMID: 23542177]

[85]   Paramasivam M, Sarkeshik A, Yates JR III, Fernandes MJG, McCollum D. Angiomotin family proteins are novel activators of the LATS2 kinase tumor suppressor. Mol Biol Cell 2011; 22(19): 3725-33.
[http://dx.doi.org/10.1091/mbc.e11-04-0300] [PMID: 21832154]

[86]   Mana-Capelli S, McCollum D. Angiomotins stimulate LATS kinase autophosphorylation and act as scaffolds that promote Hippo signaling. J Biol Chem 2018; 293(47): 18230-41.
[http://dx.doi.org/10.1074/jbc.RA118.004187] [PMID: 30266805]

[87]   Lee NH, Kim SJ, Hyun J. MicroRNAs Regulating Hippo-YAP Signaling in Liver Cancer. Biomedicines 2021; 9(4): 347.
[http://dx.doi.org/10.3390/biomedicines9040347] [PMID: 33808155]

[88]   Li L, Wang J, Zhang Y, *et al.* MEK1 promotes YAP and their interaction is critical for tumorigenesis

in liver cancer. FEBS Lett 2013; 587(24): 3921-7.
[http://dx.doi.org/10.1016/j.febslet.2013.10.042] [PMID: 24211253]

[89] Dan I, Watanabe NM, Kusumi A. The Ste20 group kinases as regulators of MAP kinase cascades. Trends Cell Biol 2001; 11(5): 220-30.
[http://dx.doi.org/10.1016/S0962-8924(01)01980-8] [PMID: 11316611]

[90] Harvey KF, Zhang X, Thomas DM. The Hippo pathway and human cancer. Nat Rev Cancer 2013; 13(4): 246-57.
[http://dx.doi.org/10.1038/nrc3458] [PMID: 23467301]

[91] Qin F, Tian J, Zhou D, Chen L. Mst1 and Mst2 kinases: regulations and diseases. Cell Biosci 2013; 3(1): 31.
[http://dx.doi.org/10.1186/2045-3701-3-31] [PMID: 23985272]

[92] Lu L, Li Y, Kim SM, *et al.* Hippo signaling is a potent *in vivo* growth and tumor suppressor pathway in the mammalian liver. Proc Natl Acad Sci USA 2010; 107(4): 1437-42.
[http://dx.doi.org/10.1073/pnas.0911427107] [PMID: 20080689]

[93] Perumal N, Perumal M, Kannan A, Subramani K, Halagowder D, Sivasithamparam N. Morin impedes Yap nuclear translocation and fosters apoptosis through suppression of Wnt/β-catenin and NF-κB signaling in Mst1 overexpressed HepG2 cells. Exp Cell Res 2017; 355(2): 124-41.
[http://dx.doi.org/10.1016/j.yexcr.2017.03.062] [PMID: 28366538]

[94] Saxena S, Shukla S, Kakkar P. Berberine induced modulation of PHLPP2-Akt-MST1 kinase signaling is coupled with mitochondrial impairment and hepatoma cell death. Toxicol Appl Pharmacol 2018; 347: 92-103.
[http://dx.doi.org/10.1016/j.taap.2018.03.033] [PMID: 29626488]

[95] Rawla P, Sunkara T, Muralidharan P, Raj JP. Update in global trends and aetiology of hepatocellular carcinoma. Contemp Oncol (Pozn) 2018; 22(3): 141-50.
[http://dx.doi.org/10.5114/wo.2018.78941] [PMID: 30455585]

[96] Li H, Wolfe A, Septer S, *et al.* Deregulation of Hippo kinase signalling in Human hepatic malignancies. Liver Int 2012; 32(1): 38-47.
[http://dx.doi.org/10.1111/j.1478-3231.2011.02646.x] [PMID: 22098159]

[97] Zhao B, Ye X, Yu J, *et al.* TEAD mediates YAP-dependent gene induction and growth control. Genes Dev 2008; 22(14): 1962-71.
[http://dx.doi.org/10.1101/gad.1664408] [PMID: 18579750]

[98] Tao J, Calvisi DF, Ranganathan S, *et al.* Activation of β-catenin and Yap1 in human hepatoblastoma and induction of hepatocarcinogenesis in mice. Gastroenterology 2014; 147(3): 690-701.
[http://dx.doi.org/10.1053/j.gastro.2014.05.004] [PMID: 24837480]

[99] Kew MC. Hepatitis B virus x protein in the pathogenesis of hepatitis B virus-induced hepatocellular carcinoma. J Gastroenterol Hepatol 2011; 26(s1) (Suppl. 1): 144-52.
[http://dx.doi.org/10.1111/j.1440-1746.2010.06546.x] [PMID: 21199526]

[100] Wu H, Xiao Y, Zhang S, *et al.* The Ets transcription factor GABP is a component of the hippo pathway essential for growth and antioxidant defense. Cell Rep 2013; 3(5): 1663-77.
[http://dx.doi.org/10.1016/j.celrep.2013.04.020] [PMID: 23684612]

[101] Danovi SA, Rossi M, Gudmundsdottir K, Yuan M, Melino G, Basu S. Yes-Associated Protein (YAP) is a critical mediator of c-Jun-dependent apoptosis. Cell Death Differ 2008 151. 2007, 7; 15(1): 217-9.
[http://dx.doi.org/10.1038/sj.cdd.4402226]

[102] Liu AM, Poon RTP, Luk JM. MicroRNA-375 targets Hippo-signaling effector YAP in liver cancer and inhibits tumor properties. Biochem Biophys Res Commun 2010; 394(3): 623-7.
[http://dx.doi.org/10.1016/j.bbrc.2010.03.036] [PMID: 20226166]

[103] Chen M, Wu L, Tu J, *et al.* miR-590-5p suppresses hepatocellular carcinoma chemoresistance by targeting YAP1 expression. EBioMedicine 2018; 35: 142-54.

[http://dx.doi.org/10.1016/j.ebiom.2018.08.010] [PMID: 30111512]

[104]   Zhao B, Li L, Tumaneng K, Wang CY, Guan KL. A coordinated phosphorylation by Lats and CK1 regulates YAP stability through SCF $^{\beta\text{-TRCP}}$. Genes Dev 2010; 24(1): 72-85.
[http://dx.doi.org/10.1101/gad.1843810] [PMID: 20048001]

[105]   Zhang X, Qiao Y, Wu Q, Chen Y, Zou S, Liu X, *et al.* The essential role of YAP O-GlcNAcylation in high-glucose-stimulated liver tumorigenesis. Nat Commun 2017, 8(1): 1–15.
[http://dx.doi.org/10.1038/ncomms15280]

[106]   Zhang S, Zhou D. Role of the transcriptional coactivators YAP/TAZ in liver cancer. Curr Opin Cell Biol 2019; 61: 64-71.
[http://dx.doi.org/10.1016/j.ceb.2019.07.006] [PMID: 31387016]

[107]   Carter SL, Eklund AC, Kohane IS, Harris LN, Szallasi Z. A signature of chromosomal instability inferred from gene expression profiles predicts clinical outcome in multiple human cancers. Nat Genet 2006 389. 2006, 20; 38(9): 1043–8.
[http://dx.doi.org/10.1038/ng1861]

[108]   Cox AG, Hwang KL, Brown KK, *et al.* Yap reprograms glutamine metabolism to increase nucleotide biosynthesis and enable liver growth. Nat Cell Biol 2016 188. 2016, 18; 18(8): 886–96.
[http://dx.doi.org/10.1038/ncb3389]

[109]   Cox AG, Tsomides A, Yimlamai D, *et al.* Yap regulates glucose utilization and sustains nucleotide synthesis to enable organ growth. EMBO J 2018; 37(22): e100294.
[http://dx.doi.org/10.15252/embj.2018100294] [PMID: 30348863]

[110]   Li W, Xiao J, Zhou X, *et al.* STK4 regulates TLR pathways and protects against chronic inflammation–related hepatocellular carcinoma. J Clin Invest 2015; 125(11): 4239-54.
[http://dx.doi.org/10.1172/JCI81203] [PMID: 26457732]

[111]   Kim W, Khan SK, Gvozdenovic-Jeremic J, *et al.* Hippo signaling interactions with Wnt/β-catenin and Notch signaling repress liver tumorigenesis. J Clin Invest 2016; 127(1): 137-52.
[http://dx.doi.org/10.1172/JCI88486] [PMID: 27869648]

[112]   Xu MZ, Yao TJ, Lee NPY, *et al.* Yes-associated protein is an independent prognostic marker in hepatocellular carcinoma. Cancer 2009; 115(19): 4576-85.
[http://dx.doi.org/10.1002/cncr.24495] [PMID: 19551889]

[113]   Moon H, Cho K, Shin S, Kim DY, Han KH, Ro SW. High risk of hepatocellular carcinoma development in fibrotic liver: Role of the Hippo-YAP/TAZ signaling pathway. Int J Mol Sci 2019; 20(3): 581.
[http://dx.doi.org/10.3390/ijms20030581]

[114]   Perumal N, Perumal M, Halagowder D, Sivasithamparam N. Morin attenuates diethylnitrosamine-induced rat liver fibrosis and hepatic stellate cell activation by co-ordinated regulation of Hippo/Yap and TGF-β1/Smad signaling. Biochimie 2017; 140: 10-9.
[http://dx.doi.org/10.1016/j.biochi.2017.05.017] [PMID: 28552397]

[115]   Li M, Chen J, Yu X, *et al.* Myricetin suppresses the propagation of hepatocellular carcinoma *via* down-regulating expression of YAP. Cells 2019; 8(4): 358.
[http://dx.doi.org/10.3390/cells8040358]

[116]   Wang L, Zhu Z, Han L, *et al.* A curcumin derivative, WZ35, suppresses hepatocellular cancer cell growth *via* downregulating YAP-mediated autophagy. Food Funct 2019; 10(6): 3748-57.
[http://dx.doi.org/10.1039/C8FO02448K] [PMID: 31172987]

[117]   Jia M, Xiong Y, Li M, Mao Q. Corosolic acid inhibits cancer progress through inactivating YAP in hepatocellular carcinoma. Oncol Res 2020; 28(4): 371-83.
[http://dx.doi.org/10.3727/096504020X15853075736554] [PMID: 32220262]

[118]   Zhang C, Niu Y, Wang Z, Xu X, Li Y, Ma L, *et al.* Corosolic acid inhibits cancer progression by decreasing the level of CDK19-mediated O-GlcNAcylation in liver cancer cells. Cell Death Dis

2021;12(10):889.
[http://dx.doi.org/10.1038/s41419-021-04164-y]

[119] Furth N, Aylon Y. The LATS1 and LATS2 tumor suppressors: beyond the Hippo pathway. Cell Death Differ 2017; 24(9): 1488-501.
[http://dx.doi.org/10.1038/cdd.2017.99] [PMID: 28644436]

[120] Jie L, Fan W, Weiqi D, *et al.* The hippo-yes association protein pathway in liver cancer. Gastroenterol Res Pract 2013; 2013: 1-7.
[http://dx.doi.org/10.1155/2013/187070] [PMID: 23986776]

[121] Liu AM, Xu Z, Luk JM. An update on targeting Hippo-YAP signaling in liver cancer. Expert Opin Ther Targets 2012; 16(3): 243-7.
[http://dx.doi.org/10.1517/14728222.2012.662958] [PMID: 22335485]

[122] Ma S, Meng Z, Chen R, Guan KL. The hippo pathway: Biology and pathophysiology. Annu Rev Biochem 2019; 88(1): 577-604.
[http://dx.doi.org/10.1146/annurev-biochem-013118-111829] [PMID: 30566373]

[123] Boopathy GTK, Hong W. Role of hippo pathway-YAP/TAZ signaling in angiogenesis. Front Cell Dev Biol 2019; 7: 49.
[http://dx.doi.org/10.3389/fcell.2019.00049] [PMID: 31024911]

[124] Plouffe SW, Hong AW, Guan KL. Disease implications of the Hippo/YAP pathway. Trends Mol Med 2015; 21(4): 212-22.
[http://dx.doi.org/10.1016/j.molmed.2015.01.003] [PMID: 25702974]

[125] Wang S, Zhou L, Ling L, *et al.* The crosstalk between hippo-yap pathway and innate immunity. Front Immunol 2020; 11: 323.
[http://dx.doi.org/10.3389/fimmu.2020.00323] [PMID: 32174922]

[126] Johnson R, Halder G. The two faces of Hippo: targeting the Hippo pathway for regenerative medicine and cancer treatment. Nat Rev Drug Discov 2014; 13(1): 63-79.
[http://dx.doi.org/10.1038/nrd4161] [PMID: 24336504]

[127] Hayashi H, Higashi T, Yokoyama N, *et al.* An imbalance in TAZ and YAP expression in hepatocellular carcinoma confers cancer stem cell–like behaviors contributing to disease progression. Cancer Res 2015; 75(22): 4985-97.
[http://dx.doi.org/10.1158/0008-5472.CAN-15-0291] [PMID: 26420216]

[128] Liu H, Li J, Yuan W, *et al.* Bioactive components and mechanisms of poplar propolis in inhibiting proliferation of human hepatocellular carcinoma HepG2 cells. Biomed Pharmacother 2021; 144: 112364.
[http://dx.doi.org/10.1016/j.biopha.2021.112364] [PMID: 34700230]

[129] Chen YL, Yen IC, Lin KT, Lai FY, Lee SY. 4-Acetylantrocamol LT3, a New Ubiquinone from *Antrodia cinnamomea*, Inhibits Hepatocellular Carcinoma HepG2 Cell Growth by Targeting YAP/TAZ, mTOR, and WNT/β-Catenin Signaling. Am J Chin Med 2020; 48(5): 1243-61.
[http://dx.doi.org/10.1142/S0192415X20500615] [PMID: 32668963]

# CHAPTER 8

# Immunotoxin: A New Generation Agent for Cancer Treatment

**Subha Ranjan Das**[1]**, Dibyendu Giri**[1]**, Tamanna Roy**[1]**, Surya Kanta Dey**[1]**, Rumi Mahata**[1]**, Angsuman Das Chaudhuri**[1]**, Suman Mondal**[1] **and Sujata Maiti Choudhury**[1,*]

[1] *Department of Human Physiology, Vidyasagar University, Midnapore 721102, West Bengal, Pin-721102, India*

**Abstract:** According to WHO/ Pan American Health Organization, 10 million global cancer deaths have been estimated in 2023. The International Agency for Research on Cancer (IARC) declares that over the ensuing two decades, the burden of cancer will augment by about 60%. For several years, the main treatment modalities for cancer were entailing chemotherapy, radiotherapy, and surgery. Conventional chemotherapies were not tumor-tissue specific and presented a large toll of toxicities for normal cells. But in the last two decades, the idea of targeted therapy, where drug or protein molecules are delivered to specific cells, is a captivating approach to treating malignancy. Immunotoxins comprising a toxin together with an antibody or growth factor hinder the growth and progression of cancer by disrupting specific genes that employ tumor growth and development. With further advances, it is expected that immunotoxins will exhibit a brilliant role and will bring a new era in the treatment of malignancy.

**Keywords:** Antibodies, Cancer, Immunotoxin, Malignancy, Toxins.

## INTRODUCTION

According to the World Health Organization (WHO) estimate, there were over 18 million new cases of cancer and around 10 million deaths from cancer-related causes in 2018 [1]. It is predicted that by 2040, the rate of cancer mortality will get nearly doubled due to the increasing pace of industrialization [2]. Radiotherapy, chemotherapy, and surgical excrescence excision are conventional treatment modalities for cancer and these not only eradicate malignant cells, but also disrupt healthy cells leading to numerous uninvited health hazards, like loss of appetite, anemia, internal bleeding, and fatigue [3].

[*] **Corresponding author Sujata Maiti Choudhury:** Department of Human Physiology, Vidyasagar University, Midnapore 721102, West Bengal, Pin-721102, India; E-mail: sujata_vu@mail.vidyasagar.ac.in

**Ashok Kumar Pandurangan (Ed.)**

Early in the 1980s, when monoclonal antibodies that responded to cancer cells were widely accessible, the first immunotoxins were created. Numerous bacterium and protein toxins from different sources were investigated [4]. The production of immunotoxins using *Pseudomonas exotoxin* A (PE) has drawn the attention of numerous researchers. Immunotoxins directed against CD22 have the potential to induce complete remissions in individuals with refractory hairy cell leukemia (HCL) [2]. In several instances of advanced chemotherapy-resistant mesothelioma, recombinant immunotoxins directed against the mesothelin protein resulted in significant excrescence retrogressions [3].

One of the key medications to fight against cancer is monoclonal antibodies (mAbs) [4-6]. Generally speaking, the mAbs bind to cell face receptors and invade through their signal transduction pathways, inducing cell death and apoptosis [7, 8]. Because of their big size (150 kDa), tumor penetration and mAb dispersion are limited [9, 10]. As an example, antigen-list scrap (Fab), single-chain variable scrap (scFv), and disulphide stabilised Fv (dsFv) are used to generate mAbs fractions in order to overcome the problem [11 - 13].

According to mAbs resistance and the need into cancer treatment, immunotoxins (ITs), a novel class of anticancer drugs, are produced [14, 15]. ITs are anticancer medications made up of two distinct pathways: the cytotoxic half and the targeted half. The receptor binding sphere of native poison replaces the targeting half in the formation of ITs, guiding the IT to the target cell [16, 17]. Usually, mAbs (or antibody fractions) make up the targeted halves. Targeting peptides like affibody [22], growth factors [20, 21], protein ligands resembling interleukins (ILs) [18, 19], and designed ankyrin repeat proteins (DARPins) [23] have all been employed. Generally, the cytotoxic half causes both cell death and suppression of growth. The source of the cytotoxic portion is bacteria that are found in insects, plants, and invertebrates.

After processing, the cytotoxic half enters the cytosol and generally inhibits protein coalescence, and induces apoptosis [2, 24]. Antibody-medicine conjugates (ADCs) are other vehicles for the delivery of cytotoxic half [25, 26]. The cytotoxic halves of ADCs are small patch composites that conjugate to the targeted half by a chemical or enzymatic response [27]. Due to the non-specific nature of chemotherapy medications and the resistance that the solid dosage forms induce, additional poisons may result. Immunotherapy snappily came as one of the smart styles of cancer treatment, along with chemotherapy and radiation [28]. In the end, despite clinical aspirations centered around the creation of innovative cancer therapies, a great deal has been learned about intracellular pathways and toxin action. As a result, poisons are viewed as both diagnostic tools for cellular function and medications for treating fatal ailments.

## Mechanism of Action

In immunotoxins, plant and bacterial poisons are employed to stop cellular protein coalescence and kill cells. For anticancer activity, intracellular transport to the cytosol is required. The patch is internalized to the endocytic cube when the immunotoxin targeting half binds to the face of the cancer cell. As these specks are processed and transported in a target- and poison-specific manner, an enzymatically active part of the poison is eventually delivered to the cytosol.

Diphtheria toxin (DT) and PE cause irreversible modification and inactivation of eukaryotic extension factor 2 (eEF2), an essential part of the protein synthesis machinery [29, 30]. Plant poisons that are similar to ricin and gelonin also stop proteins from fusing together, but they accomplish this by blocking the ribosomal enzyme instead of eEF2 [31, 32]. Variations mediated by poison activate the apoptotic pathway, resulting in cell death.

### *Diptheria Toxin (DT)*

The prototype for the class of ADP-ribosylating poisons is DT, a single-chain 58 kD protein produced by the bacterial disease of *Corynebacterium diphtheria*. Diphtheria toxin consists of two subunits connected by disulfide bridges, recognized as an A-B toxin. It comprises a B subunit (amino acids 482–535) and an enzymatic A subunit (amino acids 1–193, catalytic C domain). Subunit B controls cell entrance while subunit A intoxicates the cell *via* its class of enzymatic action. A third domain, called the translocation or trans-membrane (T) domain, is located in the center of the patch. It is sometimes referred to as the part of the B subunit. The C domain blocks protein synthesis through the transfer of ADP-ribose (from NAD) to a diphthamide residue (of eukaryotic elongation factor 2, eEF-2). The T domain or TM domain is assumed to perform the cytoplasmic transfer of the C domain. The C-terminal receptor-binding R domain allows the toxin to get entry into the cell through the process of receptor-mediated endocytosis.

In order to destroy the cells, DT goes through the following processes, which are supported by the 3-D structure of the DTs in reality and the absence of NAD [33 - 35]:

• Cell-face furin or furin-like proteases intracellularly disrupt native DT between residues Arg193 and Ser194, located within a disulfide circle formed by Cys186 and Cys201. This results in a complex of CD9 *via* its residues 482 to 535 on the receptor list sphere and heparin-binding EGF precursor on the cell membrane.

• Later, the di-chain DT internalizes into specks covered in clathrin, travels to the lumen of endosomes that are about to expire and unfolds at low pH by breaking down a disulfide link between amino acids 186 and 201. This forms a hairpin that aligns the translocational subunit's hydrophobic residues TH8 (amino acids 326-347) and TH9 (amino acids 358-376).

• Before protein fusion and programmed cell death, the eukaryotic restatement extension factor (eEF-2) converts NAD's ADP ribose to a modified histidine residue (diphthamide) at position 715 when the active-point crack of DT (amino acids 34-52) contacts NAD in the cytosol [33 - 38].

Poisons for tagging mAbs are moved to prevent their distribution to normal cells in order to develop specificity. When imitation DTs are employed to produce immunotoxins, their C- boundary is either partially or totally canceled (as in the case of DT388, DAB389, or DAB486), but they nonetheless display the translocation and ADP-ribosylation activities of DTs.

### Pseudomonas Exotoxin A

Pseudomonas exotoxin A from *Pseudomonas aeruginosa* is a single-chain 66-kDa patch with three main domains and each domain performs a distinct role. Nominated as the binding sphere, the N-terminal domain Ia (amino acids 1-252) facilitates interaction with the α2-macroglobulin receptor. Little domain Ib is situated between domains II and III and serves no use. The translocation of domain III, the carboxyl-terminal ADP-ribosylating domain comprising amino acids 400–613, into the cytoplasm of target cells is mediated by domain II (amino acids 253–364). Translocation occurs through a number of unique processes after poison internalization, such as a reductive process that disengages the amino and carboxyl fractions, proteolytic fractionalization at a particular location in domain II, and pH-driven conformational change. Ultimately, the carboxyl domain of PE from the endoplasmic reticulum is translocated into the cytoplasm, where the ADP-ribosylating enzyme inactivates it (at amino acids 400–602), promoting apoptosis [33, 39].

### Immunoconjugates for Cancer Therapy

More than 70 mAbs have been reported, the majority of which are used for treatments related to cancer. Nevertheless, one reasonable design that would increase the efficacy of the targeted treatment would be immunoconjugates with cytotoxic drugs. Protein poisons, chemotherapeutic drugs, radionuclides, or other cytotoxic agents can all result in the production of radioimmunoconjugates (RICs), immunotoxins, or ADCs [40, 41]. The targeting half of immunoconjugates, which is often an antibody or cytokine, is the most important component. Delivering and enhancing the conjugated load buildup, especially to the targeted locations, is the hallmark of an excellent antibody. Selection of the right targeted antigen or receptor is the most crucial stage in creating an immunoconjugate. Other factors that need careful consideration include the relation strategy, the linker, and the connection of the loads to the targeting half. It is important that the linker maintains its affinity for the targets while being stable in the circulation and labile within the targeted cells, releasing the loads in their active state. To meet this demand, a number of regioselective linking techniques have been created. The cytotoxic loads are the third component of an immunoconjugate. Protein poisoning, radionuclide, or chemotherapeutic medication are examples of loads.

## *Antibody-drug Conjugates*

Antibody-drug conjugates (ADCs) contain an mAb conjugated with a cytotoxic medicine *via* a linker. Beforehand ADCs were composed of whole murine antibodies conjugated to traditional chemotherapeutic medicine. These attempts failed because of immunogenicity, limited internalization, insufficient anticancer energy of conjugated cytotoxic agents, and rapid-fire concurrence caused by the nonspecific toxin to normal cells and napkins. As a result, the amount of effector accumulated in the targeted cells was insufficient to cause cell death [40, 42, 43]. Based on early studies, several advancements were introduced in developing new ADCs. Gemtuzumab ozogamicin (Mylotarg), a humanized CD33-targeting IgG4 linked to calicheamicin *via* an acid-labile hydrazine linker, was the first authorized ADC [43, 44]. It was approved to treat CD33-positive acute myeloid leukemia (AML) in the time 2000 but was withdrawn from the request in 2010. In August 2011, the U.S. FDA approved methodical anaplastic large cell carcinoma (ALCL) treatment with benuximab vedotin (Adcetris or SGN-35), an antiCD30 ADC conjugated to the auristatin secondary monomethyl auristatin E (MMAE) *via* the cleavable valine – citrulline dipeptide (vc) linker treating Hodgkin cancer after autologous stem cell transplant and multi-agent therapy failed [45]. The first ADC authorized for the treatment of solid excrescences was trastuzumab emtansine (Kadcyla) [46], a humanized HER-2-targeted antibody conjugated to maytansinoid *via* a thioether linker (Table **1**). Other ADCs that target other multitudinous malices were developed after the success of Adcetris and Kadcyla [47, 48].

**Table 1. ADCs currently under clinical investigation [118].**

| Cytotoxic Payload | ADC | Target | mAb | Linker | Payload/ Payload Class | Disease Indication (Year of Approval) |
|---|---|---|---|---|---|---|
| DNA cleavage | Mylotarg® (gemtuzumab ozogamicin) | CD33 | IgG4 | acid cleavable | Ozogamicin/ calicheamicin | CD33+ R/R AML (2000) |
| | Besponsa® (inotuzumab ozogamicin) | CD22 | IgG4 | acid cleavable | Ozogamicin/ calicheamicin | R/R B-ALL (2017) |
| | Zynlonta® (loncastuximab tesirine-lpyl) | CD19 | IgG1 | Enzyme cleavable | SG3199/PBD dimer | R/R large B-cell lymphoma, high-grade B-cell lymphoma, and DLBCL not otherwise defined following two or more lines of systemic treatment (2021). |
| microtubule inhibitor | Adcetris® (brentuximab vedotin) | CD30 | IgG1 | enzyme cleavable | MMAE/ auristatin | sALCL or cHL in R/R (2011)R/R cHL, sALCL, or CD30+ PTCL (2018); pcALCL or CD30+ MF (2017) |
| | Kadcyla® (adotrastuzumab emtansine) | HER2 | IgG1 | noncleavable | DM1/ maytansinoid | HER2+ early breast cancer following neoadjuvant taxane & trastuzumab-based therapy (2013); HER2+ metastatic breast cancer previously treated with trastuzumab & a taxane (2019). |
| | Polivy® (polatuzumab vedotin-piiq) | CD79b | IgG1 | enzyme cleavable | MMAE/ auristatin | R/R DLBCL in 2019. |
| | Padcev® (enfortumab vedotin-ejfv) | Nectin4 | IgG1 | enzyme cleavable | MMAE/ auristatin | PD-1 or PD-L1 inhibitor with Pt-containing chemotherapy for locally advanced or metastatic urothelial cancer(2019) or are not eligible for cisplatin-containing chemotherapy and have already had one or more lines of treatment (2021). |

*(Table 1) cont.....*

| Cytotoxic Payload | ADC | Target | mAb | Linker | Payload/ Payload Class | Disease Indication (Year of Approval) |
|---|---|---|---|---|---|---|
| - | Blenrep® (belantamab mafodotinblmf) | BCMA | IgG1 | noncleavable | MMAF/ auristatin | R/R multiple myeloma following at least four previous treatments with an immunomodulatory drug, a proteasome inhibitor, and an anti-CD38 mAb (2020). |
| - | Tivdak® (tisotumab vedotin-tftv) | Tissue Factor | IgG1 | enzyme cleavable | MMAE/ auristatin | Cervical cancer that has returned or spread, either during or following treatment (2021). |
| TOP1 Inhibitor | Enhertu® (famtrastuzumab deruxtecannxki) | HER2 | IgG1 | enzyme cleavable | DXd/ camptothecin | After two or more anti-HER2 treatments, unresectable or metastatic HER2+ breast cancer (2019) d; following a trastuzumab-based treatment, locally progressed or metastatic HER2+ gastric or gastroesophageal junction cancer (2021). |
| - | Trodelvy® (sacituzumab govitecanhziy) | TROP2 | IgG1 | acid cleavable | SN-38/ camptothecin | Localized metastatic or advanced triple-negative breast cancer following two or more previous treatments (2020); locally advanced or metastatic urothelial carcinoma following PT-containing chemotherapy and PD-1 or PD-L1 inhibitor (2021). |

## *Radioimmunoconjugates (RICs)*

When a large dose of radiation is administered, a cancer cell is destroyed. Researchers created RICs with high energy for treating cancer by fusing the advantages of radiation curves with the specificity of antibodies [41]. Monoclonal antibodies RICs bear the names of therapeutic radionuclides that are capable of precisely delivering radiation to excrescence cells or cells that exhibit heterogeneous antigen presentation. As of now, 90Y-ibritumomab tiuxetan and 131I-tositumomab, two RICs that target CD20, have been licensed for the treatment of haematological disorders. Although RICs were successful in treating haematological malignancies, solid excrescences did not respond as well; this may be because these excrescences had poor radio sensitivity and could not deliver enough boluses to the targets. To increase the effectiveness of RICs, adjustments to the absorption of antibodies could be made [47]. For the time being, many other RICs are being developed to treat solid excrescence [49]. These developments open up a number of opportunities for treating tumours with a variety of colours, where radiolabeled antibodies may be especially helpful for immune-specific phenotypic imaging, such as companion diagnostics. Regarding corrective procedures, RICs have been effective in treating both haematological malignancy and solid excrescences [41, 47]. Different types of immunoconjugates are displayed in Table **2**.

**Table 2. Different types of immunoconjugates.**

| Trade Name | Generic Name | Radio Nucleotide | Target Antigen | Antibody Type | Cancer | Year |
|---|---|---|---|---|---|---|
| OncoScint | Satumonab pendetide | 111In | Anti-TAG-72 | Murine IgG | Colorectal and ovarian | 1992 |
| Verluma | Nofetumomab merpentan | 99mTc | Anti-EGP-1 | Murine fab | Small cell lung | 1996 |
| CEA-scan | Arcitumomab | 99mTc | Anti-CEA | Murine fab | Colorectal | 1996 |
| ProstaScint | Capromab pendetide | 111In | Anti-PSMA | Murine IgG | Prostate | 1996 |
| Zevalin | Ibritumomab tiuxetan | 90Y | Anti-CD20 | Murine IgG+rituximab | B-cell lymphoma | 2002 |
| Bexxar | Tositumomab | 131I | Anti-CD20 | Murine IgG+``cold" tositumomab | B-cell lymphoma | 2003 |

Source: https://www.clinicaltrials.gov, Octobor 15, 2009.

## The Antibody as a Targeting Moiety

Excluding the undesirable cells is the goal of the antibody-mediated reward for cancer rectifiers. The complaint target, as determined by the findings of preliminary investigations, will influence the antibody choice. In general, targets that are expressed on harmful cells rather than on healthy critical tissues are specialised antigens or receptors. In order to ensure that the poison or drug reaches the inside the cell, breaks free from the antibody, and kills the cell, these antigens and receptors should be internalized after the antibody list. It is crucial to remember that poorly verified targeting antigens provide a risk to target selection. If the clinical outcomes of using mAb to target an antigen are available, the threat is mitigated. The targeting component of immunotoxins can be either a ligand (like cytokines, growth factors, and hormone peptides) or an antibody (like mimics like mAb, scFv, and single-sphere antibodies) that binds widely to an antigen or a receptor expressed on the surface of target cells.

## Ligand as a Target and Cytokine Receptor as a Targeting Moiety

The IL-2R complex consists of three subunits, which are expressed by T lymphocytes and natural killer (NK) cells: CD25, CD122, and CD132 [49]. The first 388 amino acids of DT are joined to IL-2 to form the emulsion protein known as ontak. It targets and kills cells in the same way as an immunotoxin, except instead of an Fv, it has IL-2. Compactly binding to IL-2, Ontak lowers to the α subunit. The T cell malice exhibits a significant overexpression of the α subunit because of the attempt by a novel immunotoxin to bind the lower-affinity-2 receptor α subunit (CD25) [50, 51]. The Fv component of an antibody to CD25, the α chain of the IL-2 receptor, is joined to PE38 to form the emulsion protein known as LMB2 (anti-Tac (Fv) – PE38). Gliomas have been reported to overexpress IL receptors. Excrescence cells were used to target gliomas because they overexpress cytokines IL-4 and IL-13. The IL4-PE toxin also showed evidence of *in vivo* anticancer efficacy and the regression of deadly glioma excrescences, which led to the current phase I/II clinical studies [52]. Utilizing the anti-melanoma antibody (scFvMEL), immunotoxins based on excretion necrosis factor (TNF) were produced, and untreated mice demonstrated cytotoxicity from these agents [53].

## Growth Factor Receptors as Targets

Growth factor receptors usually overexpressed in solid excrescences, have made them effective remedial targets. ErbB has advanced expressions in numerous excrescences; ErbB2/ Her2 was targeted by ScFv (FRP5)-ETA for solid excrescences [53]. It consists of a truncated PE genetically linked to an N-terminal ScFv. Epidermal growth factor receptor (EGFR) is another growth factor that is frequently used for solid excrescences. In an athymic rat model of neoplastic meningitis, anti-ScFv EGFRvIII-PE38 was shown to improve median survival. TP-38 is a recombinant fantastic-targeted toxin that is composed of TGF-α, an EGFR binding ligand, and PE-38 [54, 55].

## Targeting Antigens Associated with Tumors

The recombinant emulsion protein VB4-845 (also known as oportuzumab monatox, Proxinium) combines the particularity of an anti-EpCAM ScFv with the toxin of PE 40. EpCAM, the excrescence-associated face antigen, has been used to target solid excrescences and has demonstrated retrogression of large excrescence xenografts deduced from lung, colon, or scaled cell lymphomas using ScFv against EpCAM with PE [56-58]. Mesothelin, a plant that has a synergistic impact with chemotherapeutic treatments, has been targeted with PE poison and is expressed on mesotheliomas, and pancreatic, ovarian, and lung tumors [59 - 61]. Furthermore, a bivalent recombinant immunotoxin grounded in diphtheria has been obtained, which targets CD19 and CD22 (DT2219ARL). The expression of CD22, a lineage-confined isolation antigen, is seen on B cells and the most malignant B cells. Because it is only momentarily absorbed after binding, immunotoxins and ADCs find it to be a tempting target. CD30 is expressed by a variety of hematopoietic excrescence types, particularly HL and ALCL. To create SGN-35, also known as brentuximab vedotin, the antiCD30 mAb cAC10 was attached to MMAE *via* a valine citrulline peptide linker [62, 63].

## The Antibody as a Targeting Moiety

As targeting halves, antibodies can be humanised, full-length murine, single-sphere, ScFv, or full-length antibodies. Full mouse mAbs have a substantial molecular weight (MW) of around 150 kDa, which may be difficult to diffuse and access into solid excrescence cells. Therefore, haematological excrescences often utilised these immunotoxins. Antibodies composed of similar full-size mAbs are cytotoxic, which makes them difficult to produce in host cells and extremely immunogenic. With a molecular weight (MW) of about 25 kDa, the ScFv combines a light-chain variable scrap (VL) and a heavy-chain variable scrap (VH) *via* a flexible linker peptide, maintaining the full-length mAb's specificity and affinity. Its MW is roughly half that of ScFv, although it nevertheless possesses almost the same antigen-binding capacity [64]. While still having a lengthy half-life and strong affinity, humanized antibodies are less immunogenic than murine antibodies. However, the drawbacks of high MW and low permeability still exist. The humanized antibody has also been used as an ADC targeting partner. Although it is an ADC medicine, it is veritably analogous to humanized immunotoxin. It was made by a chemical coupling system and using a humanized antibody as the targeting half [64].

## HER2 Specific Immunotoxins

In immunotoxins, the recombinant proteins have an excrescence-specific ligand and a modified poison (Table **3**). A scrap is usually a part of an mAb that hits cell face receptors. Recombinant immunotoxin (rIT) binds to excrescence cell face receptors through the excrescence-specific ligand, which also enters the cell by endocytosis [65]. To overcome these constraints, recombinant DNA technology, also known as inheritable engineering, is used to create rITs through the emulsion of modified toxins and cell targeting fractions. In order to create rITs, modified poisons are genetically joined to the variable scrap of anti-TAA antibodies, while simultaneously removing the poisons' cell-binding sphere [66]. The targeted component of HER2-grounded rectifiers is these humanized anti-HER2 antibodies, which were generated from murine antibodies linked to 4D5, FRP5, and E23 [67 - 69]. The Fc sphere prevents ScFv specks from interacting with Fc receptors in normal cells [70]. 4D5scFv binds to HER2 extremely firmly and is very thermodynamically stable in serum [71]. In addition to antibodies, non-immunoglobulin altar proteins like Designed Ankyrin Reprise Proteins (DARPins) can also be used in this targeted therapy [72]. Small single-chain altar proteins called DARPins can be created utilising protein engineering techniques to bind to particular targets [73]. Similar to scFv, DARPins' smaller size enhances their ability to penetrate cells more effectively than antibodies. Furthermore, DARPins' structure lacks free cysteine, which effectively greases their product in bacterial cells. Additionally, they do not seem to trigger T cell-independent susceptible responses and are less immunogenic [74]. Other non-immunoglobulin altar proteins called antibodies have the ability to precisely engage with a number of excrescence antigens, including HER2, IGF-1R, and EGFR [75, 76]. Because HER2-expressing excrescences are easily engineered, have molecular sizes less than 10 kDa, and have short tube half-lives of antibodies, they may now be observed individually after being labeled with near-infrared fluorescence tests and radioactive essence [77]. Nevertheless, the modest size of antibodies (58 amino acids, 7 kDa) causes renal buildup of rectifiers and rapid glomerular filtration [78]. Another class of affinity proteins that conform to 46 amino acids (5 kDa) are called ABD-deduced affinity proteins (ADAPTs). With a KD of 0.5 nM, ADAPT6 is the most HER2-targeted medication version obtained from many research laboratories [79]. It binds to the ECD IV of HER2. Because ADAPTs and antibodies are smaller and accumulate in solid excrescences more efficiently.

**Table 3. HER2-based immunotoxins in cancer therapy [119].**

| Immunotoxin | Targeting Moiety | Toxic Moiety | Origin of Toxic Moiety | Mechanism of Action |
|---|---|---|---|---|
| *PEA-based rIT* | | | | |
| 4D5scFv-PE40 | 4D5scFv | PEA, PE40 | *Pseudomonas aeruginosa* | Mono-ADP ribosyltransferases |
| HER2-PE25-X7 | ZHER2:2891 | PEA, PE25-X7 | *Pseudomonas aeruginosa* | Mono-ADP-ribosyltransferases |
| ADAPT6-ABD-PE38X8 | ADAPT6 | PEA, PE38X8 | *Pseudomonas aeruginosa* | Mono-ADP-ribosyltransferases |
| ZHER2:2891-ABD-PE38X8 | ZHER2:2891 Affibody | PEA, PE38X8 | *Pseudomonas aeruginosa* | Mono-ADP-ribosyltransferases |
| ZHER2:2891-ADAPT6-ABD- PE25 | ZHER2:2891 Affibody, ADAPT6 | PEA, PE25 | *Pseudomonas aeruginosa* | Mono-ADP-ribosyltransferases |

*(Table 3) cont.....*

| Immunotoxin | Targeting Moiety | Toxic Moiety | Origin of Toxic Moiety | Mechanism of Action |
|---|---|---|---|---|
| 5F7-PE24 X7 | 5F7 sdAb | PEA, PE24 X7 | *Pseudomonas aeruginosa* | Mono-ADP-ribosyltransferases |
| 11A4-PE24 X7 | 11A4 sdAb | PEA, PE24X7 | *Pseudomonas aeruginosa* | Mono-ADP-ribosyltransferase |
| 47D5-PE24X | 47D5 sdAb | PEA, PE24X7 | *Pseudomonas aeruginosa* | Mono-ADP-ribosyltransferase |
| DARPin-LoPE | DARPin | LoPE | *Pseudomonas aeruginosa* | Mono-ADP-ribosyltransferase |
| *RIP-based rIT* | | | | |
| RTA-4D5-KDEL | | Ricin | *Ricinus communis* | *N*-Glycosidase |
| 4D5/rGel | 4D5scFv | Gelonin | *Gelonium multiflorum* | *N*-Glycosidase |
| Fab–Gelonin | Trastuzumab Fab | Gelonin | *Gelonium multiflorum* | *N*-Glycosidase |
| Trastuzumab–saporin | Trastuzumab | Saporin | *Saponaria officinalis* | *N*-Glycosidase |
| T-CUS245C | Trastuzumab | CUS245C | *Cucurbita moschata* | *N*-Glycosidase |
| *ImmunoRNase* | | | | |
| ScFv 4D5-dibarnase | 4D5scFv | Barnase | *Bacillus amyloliquefac* | RNase activity |
| hERB-hRNase | anti-ErbB-2 scFv | HP-RNase | *iens* Human | RNase activity |
| Erb-hcAb-RNase– | Erb-hcAb | HP-RNase | Human | RNase activity, ADCC,CDC |
| ERB–HP-DDADD-RNase | Erbicin scFv | HP-RNase | Human | RNase activity |
| *Immunoapoptotin* | | | | |
| GrbR201K- | scFv | GrB | Human | Serine protease |
| scFv1711 | 4D5 scFv | GrB | Human | Serine protease |
| GrB-4D5-26 | 4D5 scFv | GrB | Human | Serine protease |
| GrB-Fc-4D5 | FRP5 scFv | GrB | Human | Serine protease |
| GrB-FRP5 | FRP5 scFv | AIF | Human | Apoptosis effector |
| Immunotoxin | Targeting moiety | Toxic moiety | Origin of toxic moiety | Mechanism of action |
| *PEA-based rIT* | | | | |
| 4D5scFv-PE40 | 4D5scFv | PEA, PE40 | *Pseudomonas aeruginosa* | Mono-ADP ribosyltransferases |

*(Table 3) cont.....*

| Immunotoxin | Targeting Moiety | Toxic Moiety | Origin of Toxic Moiety | Mechanism of Action |
|---|---|---|---|---|
| HER2-PE25-X7 | ZHER2:2891 | PEA, PE25-X7 | *Pseudomonas aeruginosa* | Mono-ADP-ribosyltransferases |
| ADAPT6-ABD-PE38X8 | ADAPT6 | PEA, PE38X8 | *Pseudomonas aeruginosa* | Mono-ADP-ribosyltransferases |
| ZHER2: 2891-ABD-PE38X8 | ZHER2:2891 Affibody | PEA, PE38X8 | *Pseudomonas aeruginosa* | Mono-ADP-ribosyltransferases |
| ZHER2: 2891-ADAPT6-ABD- PE25 | ZHER2:2891 Affibody, ADAPT6 | PEA, PE25 | *Pseudomonas aeruginosa* | Mono-ADP-ribosyltransferases |
| 5F7-PE24 X7 | 5F7 sdAb | PEA, PE24 X7 | *Pseudomonas aeruginosa* | Mono-ADP-ribosyltransferases |
| 11A4-PE24 X7 | 11A4 sdAb | PEA, PE24X7 | *Pseudomonas aeruginosa* | Mono-ADP-ribosyltransferase |
| 47D5-PE24X | 47D5 sdAb | PEA, PE24X7 | *Pseudomonas aeruginosa* | Mono-ADP-ribosyltransferase |
| DARPin-LoPE | DARPin | LoPE | *Pseudomonas aeruginosa* | Mono-ADP-ribosyltransferase |
| **RIP-based rIT** | | | | |
| RTA-4D5-KDEL | | Ricin | *Ricinus communis* | *N*-Glycosidase |
| 4D5/rGel | 4D5scFv | Gelonin | *Gelonium multiflorum* | *N*-Glycosidase |
| Fab–Gelonin | Trastuzumab Fab | Gelonin | *Gelonium multiflorum* | *N*-Glycosidase |
| Trastuzumab–saporin | Trastuzumab | Saporin | *Saponaria officinalis* | *N*-Glycosidase |
| T-CUS245C | Trastuzumab | CUS245C | *Cucurbita moschata* | *N*-Glycosidase |
| **ImmunoRNase** | | | | |
| ScFv 4D5-dibarnase | 4D5scFv | Barnase | *Bacillus amyloliquefac* | RNase activity |
| hERB-hRNase | anti-ErbB-2 scFv | HP-RNase | *iens* Human | RNase activity |
| Erb-hcAb-RNase– | Erb-hcAb | HP-RNase | Human | RNase activity, ADCC,CDC |
| ERB–HP-DDADD-RNase | Erbicin scFv | HP-RNase | Human | RNase activity |
| **Immunoapoptotin** | | | | |
| GrbR201K- | scFv | GrB | Human | Serine protease |
| scFv1711 | 4D5 scFv | GrB | Human | Serine protease |

*(Table 3) cont.....*

| Immunotoxin | Targeting Moiety | Toxic Moiety | Origin of Toxic Moiety | Mechanism of Action |
|---|---|---|---|---|
| GrB-4D5-26 | 4D5 scFv | GrB | Human | Serine protease |
| GrB-Fc-4D5 | FRP5 scFv | GrB | Human | Serine protease |
| GrB-FRP5 | FRP5 scFv | AIF | Human | Apoptosis effector |

The tiny size of ADAPTs reduces their half-life in blood circulation similar to antibodies, which makes them more effective for excrescence imaging [80]. However, the emulsion proteins' brief half-life and rapid blood concurrence require additional injections for therapeutic purposes. The rITs that contain toxins and ADAPTs can quickly be removed from rotation because of their modest size. These target molecules have longer half-lives in the blood when an ABD is added, which links them to albumin. Recently, bioinformatics approaches have been adopted to improve their efficacy and decrease unwanted poison parcels and immunotoxin targets [81].

### Immunotoxins Against Hepatocellular Carcinoma (HCC)

The antigens recognized in HCC are those encoded by shifting Ras proto-oncogenes genes. The mutation in K-Ras codon 12; the N-Ras codon 61 [82], and the H-Ras codon 12 [83] are the most generally delved mutations in HCC. It was noticed that because the majority of shifting antigens and viral antigens are cytosolically confined, they are poor targets for immunotoxins. The expression on the cell faces of the overexpressed antigens makes them more fascinating. The internalisation process is emphasised for the immunotoxin's efficacy and energy when the immunotoxin lists cancer cells as its target. The rate of internalisation into the cells is said to be significantly correlated with the immunotoxin energy and cytotoxicity [84]. These two targeted poisons are similar in receptor and targeted cancer, interleukin-3 receptor (IL-3Ralpha, CD123), and acute myeloid leukemia (AML), independently, despite the difference in the kind of poison and the last half. DT388IL3, which is similar to (Fv)-PE38KDEL, but its cytotoxicity is 50 times lower [85]. The antigen-binding affinity, epitope location, the type of amino acid on an antibody paratope, and the frequency of the target antigen on the cell face are just a few other factors that might affect how effective an immunotoxin is [86, 87].

Their results suggest that immunotoxins may be a promising general therapy option for HCC [88]. Numerous excrescence markers on HCC cells, including EGFR, FGFR, PDGFR, MUC1, and mesothelin, have not yet been addressed. (Table **4**).

Table 4. HCC-specific immunotoxins [120].

| Label Year | Targeting Moiety | Toxin Moiety | Receptor Type |
|---|---|---|---|
| hscFv25-TNFα | scFv | TNFα | Unknown |
| hscFv25-mTNFα | scFv | Mutant TNFα | Unknown |
| mut1 | SM5-1 single | PE38KDEL | p230 |
| - | chain antibody | - | - |
| - | (SMFv) | - | - |
| C1M | scFv of anti- | Melittin | ASGPR |
| - | ASGPR | - | - |
| anti-c- | ScFv | PE38KDEL | c-Met |
| Met/PE38KDEL | - | - | - |
| VB4-845 | scFv | PE | EpCAM |
| APE | scFv | PE38KDEL PE38 | EpCAM |
| HN3-PE38 | VH domain | PE38 | GPC3 |
| YP7-PE38 | ScFv | PE38 | GPC3 |
| HS20-PE38 | ScFv | PE38 | GPC3 |
| YP7-PE38 | ScFv | PE38 | GPC3 |
| Humanized | scFv | - | GPC3 |
| YP7-PE38 | - | PE38 | - |
| YP9.1-PE38 | scFv | PE38 | GPC3 |
| Humanized | scFv | - | GPC3 |
| YP9.1-PE38 | - | mPE24 | - |
| HN3-mPE24 | VH domain | mPE24 | GPC3 |
| HN3- HN3-mPE24 | VH domain | - | GPC3 |
| HN3-T20 | - | mPE24 | - |
| HN3-ABD-T20 | VH domain | mPE24 | GPC3 |
| - | VH domain | - | GPC3 |

## *Immunotoxin Therapy for Lung Cancer*

MAb L6 is an immunotoxin that targets antigens expressed in mortal lung, bone, colon, and ovarian cancers. The antibody and the whole ricin structure are chemically linked. In lung adenocarcinoma xenograft fatality, mAb L6 showed advantages for cell payoff [89]. Mesothelin is expressed weakly in mesothelium but strongly in a variety of solid excrescences, such as lung adenocarcinoma and mesothelioma [90 - 99]. The immunotoxin RG 7787, the humanized Fv scrap of

SS1, and a modified PE scrap have been demonstrated to decrease the size of excrescence in a xenograft mesothelin-expressing lung model [100, 101]. Numerous epithelial excrescences have high Lewis Y antigen (Ley) expression. In one instance, an immunohistochemical investigation revealed that the Ley antigen was expressed in 42 scaled cell lung lymphomas and 80 lung adenocarcinomas [102]. When the Ley antigen is encountered, the mAb B3 and PE38 create the immunotoxin LMB 1 [103]. Because of the toxin's limited selectivity for endothelial cells, it is effective against both bone and colon tumors [104]. The SCLC cluster 1 antigen is CD56, a member of the family of neural cell adhesion patches. According to reports, the immunotoxin N901 bR, which was created by fusing modified ricin with the anti-CD56 antibody N901, is effective against SCLC that expresses CD56 [105].

### Immunotoxins for Leukemia

Monoclonal antibodies (mAbs) are being used more frequently to treat hematologic malignancies [106]. T lymphocytes and natural killer cells express the interleukin-2 receptor (IL-2R) complex, which has three subunits: a (CD25), b (CD122), and g (CD132) [107]. The protein denileukin diftitox (DD) consists of the first 388 amino acids of DT joined to IL-2. It targets and performs like an immunotoxin despite having IL-2 rather than an Fv. DD is an effective treatment for adults with cutaneous T-cell carcinoma. Exertion has also been connected to other hematologic disorders, such as leukemia, which expresses the IL-2R [108]. More recent constructions have been developed in an attempt to target this IL2 receptor a (CD25) with reduced affinity [21]. BL22 (CAT-3888), a recombinant immunotoxin, with the anti-CD22 antibody RFB4's Fv is connected to PE38 [109]. A modified medication with increased affinity called uxetumomab pasudotox (HA22; CAT-8015) was developed to lessen the exertion of BL22 by altering 3 amino acids in Fv heavy chain CDR3 region from serine-serine-tyrosine (SSY) to threonine-histidine-tryptophan (THW) [110, 111]. On the surface of T-cell aggression, CD3 is highly expressed. An anti-CD3 recombinant immunotoxin-A dmDT390-bisFv (UCHT1) is made using a divalent patch made of two single-chain antibody fractions reactive with the extracellular sphere of CD3e connected to the catalytic and translocation disciplines of DT [112]. The list of immunotoxins for leukemia is displayed in Table **5**.

### Immunotoxins for Colorectal Cancer Therapy

Advanced colorectal cancer (CRC) patients have access to a variety of therapy options, including monoclonal antibodies (mAbs) (Table **6**). Still, while these mAbs effectively target cancer cells, they may have limited clinical exertion. Small molecules and monoclonal antibodies (mAbs) directed against excrescence-associated antigens (TAA), angiogenic pathways, and susceptible checkpoints are examples of targeted curatives that are a priori pickier and have fewer adverse effects. At least nine of these curatives—many of which have different snooping routes—have been licensed for use in the treatment of colorectal cancer patients [113]. Two mAbs that have received FDA clearance target the epidermal growth factor receptor (EGFR), which is the TAA in colorectal cancer (CRC): cetuximab and panitumumab. Both are indicated for cases with wild-type KRAS, since mutations in this gene, present in 36 CRC cases, avert clinical benefit [114].

**Table 5. Immunotoxins for leukemia**

| Antigen | Target Leukemia | Agent | Conjugate | ClinicalTrials.gov Identifier(12/2013) |
|---|---|---|---|---|
| CD3 | T-lineage ALL | A-dmDT390-bisFv(UCHT1) Combotox (mixture of | Diphtheria toxin | A NCT00611208 |
| - | B-lineage ALL, | HD37-dgA and | - | - |
| CD19, CD22 | CLL | RFB4-dgA) | Ricin-dgA | NCT00450944 |
| - | - | DT2219ARL(bispecific) | - | NCT01408160 |
| - | - | - | Diphtheria toxin Pseudomonas exotoxin A | - |
| - | B-lineage ALL, | Moxetumomab pasudotox, | - | NCT00889408 |
| - | CLL, HCL | (HA22, CAT- 8015) | Pseudomonas exotoxin A Pseudomonas exotoxin A | - |
| CD22 | - | BL22 (CAT-3888) | Ricin-dgA | NCT01891981 |
| - | - | - | - | NCT01829711 |
| - | ALL, ATL | LMB-2 | IL-2 conjugated to | NCT00659425 |
| - | - | - | diphtheria toxin | - |
| - | - | RFT5-dgA (IMTOX-25) | Gelonin | - |
| CD25 | - | Denileukin diftitox (Ontak)* | - | NCT00924170 |
| - | ALL, ATL | - | - | NCT00321555 NCT01378871 |
| - | - | HUM-195/rGEL | - | - |
| CD25, CD122, | - | - | - | - |

*(Table 5) cont.....*

| Antigen | Target Leukemia | Agent | Conjugate | ClinicalTrials.gov Identifier(12/2013) |
|---------|-----------------|-------|-----------|----------------------------------------|
| CD132 | AML, CML | - | - | - |
| CD33 | - | - | - | - |

**Table 6. Immunotoxins tested in colorectal cancer patients.**

| ITX | Toxin | Antibody Format | Target | Clinical Trial |
|-----|-------|-----------------|--------|----------------|
| Xomazyme-791 | Ricin | mo IgG2b | 72kDa | N/A |
| Anti-CEA-bR | Blocked ricin | mo IgG | CEA | N/A |
| LMB-1 | PE38 | mo IgG1 | Lewis Y | NCT00001805 NCT00019435 NCT00005858 |
| LMB-9 | PE38 | dsFv | Lewis Y | N/A |
| - | - | - | - | NCT01061645 NCT02219893 NCT04550897 |
| SGN-10 | PE40 | scFv | Lewis Y | - |
| MOC31PE | PE | mo IgG1 | EpCAM(CD326) | - |
| BM7PE | PE | mo IgG1 | MUC-1 | - |

The murine mAb791/36, obtained from animals vaccinated with the 791T sarcoma cell line, is coupled *via* a disulfide bond to ricin toxin A chain (RTA) to form 791T/36-RTA (XomaZyme-791). The 791T/36 antibody binds to an excrescence-associated antigen (gp72) expressed on a range of deadly excrescences, in addition to osteogenic sarcoma and CRC [115].

## *Immunotoxin Therapy of Glioblastoma*

A type of recombinant protein-grounded rectifiers known as recombinant immunotoxins (RITs) consists of two parts: a deadly scrap that, upon internalization, destroys the target cells and an antibody variable scrap that functions as a particular ligand to allow RITs to attach to target cells with precision. Recombinant immunotoxins (RITs) are a potential method of treating GBM because of their benefits over conventional chemotherapeutics and monoclonal antibodies (mAbs) [116 - 118]. It is well known that DT- and PE-grounded RITs can kill specific cells directly by preventing cell protein aggregation *via* ADP ribosylation of the extension factor 2. Furthermore, current studies have demonstrated that RIT results in excrescence retrogression and delayed cytotoxic effects [119]. The clinical development of RITs for glioblastoma therapy is represented in Table **7**.

**Table 7. Clinical development of RITs for glioblastoma therapy.**

| RITs | Clinical Trials | Status | Outcome and Side Effects | Refs. |
|---|---|---|---|---|
| D2C7(scdsFv)-PE38 (D2C7-IT) | Phase I/II | Ongoing | N/A | NCT02303678 |
| IL-4(38-37)-PE38KDEL (cpIL4-PE) | - | - | - | - |
| - | Phase I/II | Ongoing | MS☐: 4.7 months; 36% survive during six months | NCT00014677 |
| - | - | - | seizures, headaches, weakening, hydrocephalus, and dysphasia MS: phase II lasted 42.7 weeks, whereas phase III lasted 36.4 weeks. Headache, weakness, seizures, dysphasia, and pulmonary embolism | - |
| - | - | - | MS: 28 weeks (4.1–45.1, 95% CI) Hemiparesis in grade 3, exhaustion in grade 4, headache, and dysphasia Ineffective for more than 80% of intracranial infusions | - |
| - | - | - | N/A | - |
| IL13-PE38QQR (IL-13PE) | - | - | Minimal accretion | - |
| - | Phase I/II/III | Not Active | - | - |
| TGF☐-PE38 (TP38) | - | - | - | - |
| DAB389EGF | - | - | - | - |
| MR1-1(Fv)-PE38 (MR1-1) | - | - | - | - |
| - | Phase I | Discontinued | - | - |
| - | Phase I/II | Discontinued Discontinued | - | - |
| - | Phase I | - | - | - |

## CONCLUSION

Overall, the market share for antibody-based cancer treatments has steadily increased from clinical and preclinical pipelines. Chimeric proteins known as immunotoxins combine the benefits of protein toxins' powerful cytotoxicity with the selectivity of their targeting components. And the extent of immunotoxin improvement is in quick extension. ITX is a promising new therapeutic option for cancer, having been explored for the past 30 years on a range of targets and toxins. Some of the immunotoxins that were introduced appear to be highly amenable to future research. Clinical trials of ITX in cancer therapy were not successful, but they did open up a new path for the development of ITX with better qualities. There are still several difficulties, namely with regard to cytosolic administration, pharmacokinetics, and, in particular, the immunogenicity of non-human poisons. Deimmunization techniques that show promise for improving endolysosomal escape and extending serum half-life are being actively studied. Next-generation antibody engineering, production, conjugation, and administration technologies alongside revolutionary combination treatments personalized to cancer patients will endure fueling the victory of these pharmaceuticals. The development of immunotoxins with high specificity that kill target cells with less toxicity and immunogenicity is made possible by recent developments in genetic engineering and efforts to identify novel tumor markers that are unique to cancer cells.

## REFERENCES

[1]     Duan H, Liu Y, Gao Z, Huang W. Recent advances in drug delivery systems for targeting cancer stem cells. Acta Pharm Sin B 2021; 11(1): 55-70.
[http://dx.doi.org/10.1016/j.apsb.2020.09.016] [PMID: 33532180]

[2]     World Health Organization. WHO report on cancer: setting priorities, investing wisely and providing care for all. 2020.

[3]     Asghari F, Khademi R, Esmaeili Ranjbar F, Veisi Malekshahi Z, Faridi Majidi R. Application of nanotechnology in targeting of cancer stem cells: a review. Int J Stem Cells 2019; 12(2): 227-39.
[http://dx.doi.org/10.15283/ijsc19006] [PMID: 31242721]

[4]     Antignani A, FitzGerald D. Immunotoxins: the role of the toxin. Toxins (Basel) 2013; 5(8): 1486-502.
[http://dx.doi.org/10.3390/toxins5081486] [PMID: 23965432]

[2]     Kreitman RJ, Tallman MS, Robak T, *et al.* Phase I trial of anti-CD22 recombinant immunotoxin moxetumomab pasudotox (CAT-8015 or HA22) in patients with hairy cell leukemia. J Clin Oncol 2012; 30(15): 1822-8.
[http://dx.doi.org/10.1200/JCO.2011.38.1756] [PMID: 22355053]

[3]     Hassan R, Miller AC, Sharon E, *et al.* Major cancer regressions in mesothelioma after treatment with an anti-mesothelin immunotoxin and immune suppression. Sci Transl Med 2013; 5(208): 208ra147.
[http://dx.doi.org/10.1126/scitranslmed.3006941] [PMID: 24154601]

[4]     Coulson A, Levy A, Gossell-Williams M. Monoclonal antibodies in cancer therapy: mechanisms, successes and limitations. West Indian Med J 2014; 63(6): 650-4.
[PMID: 25803383]

[5]     Ludwig DL, Pereira DS, Zhu Z, Hicklin DJ, Bohlen P. Monoclonal antibody therapeutics and apoptosis. Oncogene 2003; 22(56): 9097-106.
[http://dx.doi.org/10.1038/sj.onc.1207104] [PMID: 14663488]

[6]     Jain M, Chauhan SC, Singh AP, Venkatraman G, Colcher D, Batra SK. Penetratin improves tumor retention of single-chain antibodies: a novel step toward optimization of radioimmunotherapy of solid tumors. Cancer Res 2005; 65(17): 7840-6.
[http://dx.doi.org/10.1158/0008-5472.CAN-05-0662] [PMID: 16140953]

[7]     Chames P, Van Regenmortel M, Weiss E, Baty D. Therapeutic antibodies: successes, limitations and hopes for the future. Br J Pharmacol 2009; 157(2): 220-33.
        [http://dx.doi.org/10.1111/j.1476-5381.2009.00190.x] [PMID: 19459844]

[8]     Bell A, Wang ZJ, Arbabi-Ghahroudi M, *et al*. Differential tumor-targeting abilities of three single-domain antibody formats. Cancer Lett 2010; 289(1): 81-90.
        [http://dx.doi.org/10.1016/j.canlet.2009.08.003] [PMID: 19716651]

[9]     Bates A, Power CA. David vs. Goliath: the structure, function, and clinical prospects of antibody fragments. Antibodies (Basel) 2019; 8(2): 28.
        [http://dx.doi.org/10.3390/antib8020028] [PMID: 31544834]

[10]    Akbari B, Farajnia S, Zarghami N, *et al*. Design, expression and evaluation of a novel humanized single chain antibody against epidermal growth factor receptor (EGFR). Protein Expr Purif 2016; 127: 8-15.
        [http://dx.doi.org/10.1016/j.pep.2016.06.001] [PMID: 27298212]

[11]    Pastan I, Hassan R, FitzGerald DJ, Kreitman RJ. Immunotoxin treatment of cancer. Annu Rev Med 2007; 58(1): 221-37.
        [http://dx.doi.org/10.1146/annurev.med.58.070605.115320] [PMID: 17059365]

[12]    Reslan L, Dalle S, Dumontet C. Understanding and circumventing resistance to anticancer monoclonal antibodies. InMAbs 2009 May 1 (Vol. 1, No. 3, pp. 222-229). Taylor & Francis.
        [http://dx.doi.org/10.4161/mabs.1.3.8292]

[13]    Becker N, Benhar I. Antibody-based immunotoxins for the treatment of cancer. Antibodies (Basel) 2012; 1(1): 39-69.
        [http://dx.doi.org/10.3390/antib1010039]

[14]    Simon N, FitzGerald D. Immunotoxin therapies for the treatment of epidermal growth factor receptor-dependent cancers. Toxins (Basel) 2016; 8(5): 137.
        [http://dx.doi.org/10.3390/toxins8050137] [PMID: 27153091]

[15]    Kunwar S, Prados MD, Chang SM, *et al*. Direct intracerebral delivery of cintredekin besudotox (IL13-PE38QQR) in recurrent malignant glioma: a report by the Cintredekin Besudotox Intraparenchymal Study Group. J Clin Oncol 2007; 25(7): 837-44.
        [http://dx.doi.org/10.1200/JCO.2006.08.1117] [PMID: 17327604]

[16]    Antignani A, Ho ECH, Bilotta MT, Qiu R, Sarnvosky R, FitzGerald DJ. Targeting receptors on cancer cells with protein toxins. Biomolecules 2020; 10(9): 1331.
        [http://dx.doi.org/10.3390/biom10091331] [PMID: 32957689]

[17]    Leshem Y, Pastan I. Pseudomonas exotoxin immunotoxins and anti-tumor immunity: from observations at the patient's bedside to evaluation in preclinical models. Toxins (Basel) 2019; 11(1): 20.
        [http://dx.doi.org/10.3390/toxins11010020] [PMID: 30621280]

[18]    Cohen K, Liu T, Bissonette R, Puri R, Frankel A. DAB389EGF fusion protein therapy of refractory glioblastoma multiforme. Curr Pharm Biotechnol 2003; 4(1): 39-49.
        [http://dx.doi.org/10.2174/1389201033378039] [PMID: 12570681]

[19]    Zielinski R, Lyakhov I, Jacobs A, *et al*. Affitoxin--a novel recombinant, HER2-specific, anticancer agent for targeted therapy of HER2-positive tumors. J Immunother 2009; 32(8): 817-25.
        [http://dx.doi.org/10.1097/CJI.0b013e3181ad4d5d] [PMID: 19752752]

[20]    Martin-Killias P, Stefan N, Rothschild S, Plückthun A, Zangemeister-Wittke U. A novel fusion toxin derived from an EpCAM-specific designed ankyrin repeat protein has potent antitumor activity. Clin Cancer Res 2011; 17(1): 100-10.
        [http://dx.doi.org/10.1158/1078-0432.CCR-10-1303] [PMID: 21075824]

[21]    Weidle UH, Tiefenthaler G, Schiller C, Weiss EH, Georges G, Brinkmann U. Prospects of bacterial and plant protein-based immunotoxins for treatment of cancer. Cancer Genomics Proteomics 2014;

11(1): 25-38.
[PMID: 24633317]

[22]    Alewine C, Hassan R, Pastan I. Advances in anticancer immunotoxin therapy. Oncologist 2015; 20(2): 176-85.
[http://dx.doi.org/10.1634/theoncologist.2014-0358] [PMID: 25561510]

[23]    Fuchs H, Weng A, Gilabert-Oriol R. Augmenting the efficacy of immunotoxins and other targeted protein toxinsby endosomal escape enhancers. Toxins (Basel) 2016; 8(7): 200.
[http://dx.doi.org/10.3390/toxins8070200] [PMID: 27376327]

[24]    Khirehgesh MR, Sharifi J, Safari F, Akbari B. Immunotoxins and nanobody-based immunotoxins: review and update. J Drug Target 2021; 29(8): 848-62.
[http://dx.doi.org/10.1080/1061186X.2021.1894435] [PMID: 33615933]

[25]    Weldon JE, Pastan I. A guide to taming a toxin – recombinant immunotoxins constructed from *Pseudomonas* exotoxin A for the treatment of cancer. FEBS J 2011; 278(23): 4683-700.
[http://dx.doi.org/10.1111/j.1742-4658.2011.08182.x] [PMID: 21585657]

[26]    Stirpe F, Olsnes S, Pihl A. Gelonin, a new inhibitor of protein synthesis, nontoxic to intact cells. Isolation, characterization, and preparation of cytotoxic complexes with concanavalin A. J Biol Chem 1980; 255(14): 6947-53.
[http://dx.doi.org/10.1016/S0021-9258(18)43667-8] [PMID: 7391060]

[27]    Walsh MJ, Dodd JE, Hautbergue GM. Ribosome-inactivating proteins. Virulence 2013; 4(8): 774-84.
[http://dx.doi.org/10.4161/viru.26399] [PMID: 24071927]

[28]    Shapira A, Benhar I. Toxin-based therapeutic approaches. Toxins (Basel) 2010; 2(11): 2519-83.
[http://dx.doi.org/10.3390/toxins2112519] [PMID: 22069564]

[29]    Potala S, Verma RS. A novel fusion protein diphtheria toxin-stem cell factor (DT-SCF)-purification and characterization. Appl Biochem Biotechnol 2010; 162(5): 1258-69.
[http://dx.doi.org/10.1007/s12010-009-8896-1] [PMID: 20084469]

[30]    Antignani A, FitzGerald D. Immunotoxins: the role of the toxin. Toxins (Basel) 2013; 5(8): 1486-502.
[http://dx.doi.org/10.3390/toxins5081486] [PMID: 23965432]

[31]    Choe S, Bennett MJ, Fujii G, *et al.* The crystal structure of diphtheria toxin. Nature 1992; 357(6375): 216-22.
[http://dx.doi.org/10.1038/357216a0] [PMID: 1589020]

[32]    Tsuneoka M, Nakayama K, Hatsuzawa K, Komada M, Kitamura N, Mekada E. Evidence for involvement of furin in cleavage and activation of diphtheria toxin. J Biol Chem 1993; 268(35): 26461-5.
[http://dx.doi.org/10.1016/S0021-9258(19)74337-3] [PMID: 8253774]

[33]    Yamaizumi M, Mekada E, Uchida T, Okada Y. One molecule of diphtheria toxin fragment a introduced into a cell can kill the cell. Cell 1978; 15(1): 245-50.
[http://dx.doi.org/10.1016/0092-8674(78)90099-5] [PMID: 699044]

[34]    Iglewski BH, Kabat D. NAD-dependent inhibition of protein synthesis by Pseudomonas aeruginosa toxin. Proc Natl Acad Sci USA 1975; 72(6): 2284-8.
[http://dx.doi.org/10.1073/pnas.72.6.2284] [PMID: 166383]

[35]    Donaghy H. Effects of antibody, drug and linker on the preclinical and clinical toxicities of antibody-drug conjugates. MAbs 2016; 8(4): 659-71.
[http://dx.doi.org/10.1080/19420862.2016.1156829] [PMID: 27045800]

[36]    Bourgeois M, Bailly C, Frindel M, *et al.* Radioimmunoconjugates for treating cancer: recent advances and current opportunities. Expert Opin Biol Ther 2017; 17(7): 813-9.
[http://dx.doi.org/10.1080/14712598.2017.1322577] [PMID: 28438082]

[37]    Sahota S, Vahdat LT. Sacituzumab govitecan: an antibody–drug conjugate. Expert Opin Biol Ther

2017; 17(8): 1027-31.
[http://dx.doi.org/10.1080/14712598.2017.1331214] [PMID: 28503956]

[38] Lambert JM, Morris CQ. Antibody-drug conjugates(ADCs) for personalized treatment of solid tumors: a review. Adv Ther 2017; 34(5): 1015-35.
[http://dx.doi.org/10.1007/s12325-017-0519-6] [PMID: 28361465]

[39] Sassoon I, Blanc V. Antibody-drug conjugate (ADC) clinical pipeline: a review. Methods Mol Biol 2013; 1045: 1-27.
[http://dx.doi.org/10.1007/978-1-62703-541-5_1] [PMID: 23913138]

[40] Minich SS. Brentuximab vedotin: a new age in the treatment of Hodgkin lymphoma and anaplastic large cell lymphoma. Ann Pharmacother 2012; 46(3): 377-83.
[http://dx.doi.org/10.1345/aph.1Q680] [PMID: 22395252]

[41] Arannilewa AJ, Alakanse OS, Adeleye AO, *et al.* Molecular docking analysis of Cianidanol from Ginkgo biloba with HER2+ breast cancer target. Bioinformation 2018; 14(9): 482-7.
[http://dx.doi.org/10.6026/97320630014482] [PMID: 31223207]

[42] Aghevlian S, Boyle AJ, Reilly RM. Radioimmunotherapy of cancer with high linear energy transfer (LET) radiation delivered by radionuclides emitting α-particles or Auger electrons. Adv Drug Deliv Rev 2017; 109: 102-18.
[http://dx.doi.org/10.1016/j.addr.2015.12.003] [PMID: 26705852]

[43] Steiner M, Neri D. Antibody-radionuclide conjugates for cancer therapy: historical considerations and new trends. Clin Cancer Res 2011; 17(20): 6406-16.
[http://dx.doi.org/10.1158/1078-0432.CCR-11-0483] [PMID: 22003068]

[44] Malek TR, Castro I. Interleukin-2 receptor signaling: at the interface between tolerance and immunity. Immunity 2010; 33(2): 153-65.
[http://dx.doi.org/10.1016/j.immuni.2010.08.004] [PMID: 20732639]

[45] Powell DJ Jr, Felipe-Silva A, Merino MJ, *et al.* Administration of a CD25-directed immunotoxin, LMB-2, to patients with metastatic melanoma induces a selective partial reduction in regulatory T cells *in vivo*. J Immunol 2007; 179(7): 4919-28.
[http://dx.doi.org/10.4049/jimmunol.179.7.4919] [PMID: 17878392]

[46] Kaplan G, Mazor R, Lee F, Jang Y, Leshem Y, Pastan I. Improving the *in vivo* efficacy of an anti-Tac (CD25) immunotoxin by Pseudomonas exotoxin A domain II engineering. Mol Cancer Ther 2018; 17(7): 1486-93.
[http://dx.doi.org/10.1158/1535-7163.MCT-17-1041] [PMID: 29695631]

[47] Shimamura T, Husain SR, Puri RK. The IL-4 and IL-13 pseudomonas exotoxins: new hope for brain tumor therapy. Neurosurg Focus 2006; 20(4): E11.
[http://dx.doi.org/10.3171/foc.2006.20.4.6] [PMID: 16709016]

[48] Sokolova E, Guryev E, Yudintsev A, Vodeneev V, Deyev S, Balalaeva I. HER2-specific recombinant immunotoxin 4D5scFv-PE40 passes through retrograde trafficking route and forces cells to enter apoptosis. Oncotarget 2017; 8(13): 22048-58.
[http://dx.doi.org/10.18632/oncotarget.15833] [PMID: 28423549]

[49] Rainov N, Söling A. Clinical studies with targeted toxins in malignant glioma. Rev Recent Clin Trials 2006; 1(2): 119-31.
[http://dx.doi.org/10.2174/157488706776876454] [PMID: 18473963]

[50] MacDonald GC, Rasamoelisolo M, Entwistle J, *et al.* A phase I clinical study of VB4-845: weekly intratumoral administration of an anti-EpCAM recombinant fusion protein in patients with squamous cell carcinoma of the head and neck. Drug Des Devel Ther 2009; 2: 105-14.
[PMID: 19920898]

[51] Hassan R, Ho M. Mesothelin targeted cancer immunotherapy. Eur J Cancer 2008; 44(1): 46-53.
[http://dx.doi.org/10.1016/j.ejca.2007.08.028] [PMID: 17945478]

[52]    Hosseinian SA, Haddad-Mashadrizeh A, Dolatabadi S. Simulation and stability assessment of anti-EpCAM immunotoxin for cancer therapy. Adv Pharm Bull 2018; 8(3): 447-55.
[http://dx.doi.org/10.15171/apb.2018.052] [PMID: 30276141]

[53]    Lv M, Qiu F, Li T, *et al.* Construction, expression, and characterization of a recombinant immunotoxin targeting EpCAM. Mediators Inflamm 2015; 2015(1): 460264.
[http://dx.doi.org/10.1155/2015/460264] [PMID: 25960617]

[54]    Vallera DA, Chen H, Sicheneder AR, Panoskaltsis-Mortari A, Taras EP. Genetic alteration of a bispecific ligand-directed toxin targeting human CD19 and CD22 receptors resulting in improved efficacy against systemic B cell malignancy. Leuk Res 2009; 33(9): 1233-42.
[http://dx.doi.org/10.1016/j.leukres.2009.02.006] [PMID: 19327829]

[55]    Hassan R, Thomas A, Alewine C, Le DT, Jaffee EM, Pastan I. Mesothelin immunotherapy for cancer: Ready for prime time. J Clin Oncol 2016; 34(34): 4171-9.
[http://dx.doi.org/10.1200/JCO.2016.68.3672] [PMID: 27863199]

[56]    Robak T. Hairy-cell leukemia variant: Recent view on diagnosis, biology and treatment. Cancer Treat Rev 2011; 37(1): 3-10.
[http://dx.doi.org/10.1016/j.ctrv.2010.05.003] [PMID: 20558005]

[57]    Younes A, Bartlett NL, Leonard JP, *et al.* Brentuximab vedotin (SGN-35) for relapsed CD30-positive lymphomas. N Engl J Med 2010; 363(19): 1812-21.
[http://dx.doi.org/10.1056/NEJMoa1002965] [PMID: 21047225]

[58]    Borthakur G, Rosenblum MG, Talpaz M, *et al.* Phase 1 study of an anti-CD33 immunotoxin, humanized monoclonal antibody M195 conjugated to recombinant gelonin (HUM-195/rGEL), in patients with advanced myeloid malignancies. Haematologica 2013; 98(2): 217-21.
[http://dx.doi.org/10.3324/haematol.2012.071092] [PMID: 22875630]

[59]    Vallera DA, Kreitman RJ. Immunotoxins targeting B cell malignancy- progress and problems with immunogenicity. Biomedicines 2018; 7(1): 1.
[http://dx.doi.org/10.3390/biomedicines7010001] [PMID: 30577664]

[60]    Alewine C, Hassan R, Pastan I. Advances in anticancer immunotoxin therapy. Oncologist 2015; 20(2): 176-85.
[http://dx.doi.org/10.1634/theoncologist.2014-0358] [PMID: 25561510]

[61]    Choudhary S, Mathew M, Verma RS. Therapeutic potential of anticancer immunotoxins. Drug Discov Today 2011; 16(11-12): 495-503.
[http://dx.doi.org/10.1016/j.drudis.2011.04.003] [PMID: 21511052]

[62]    Kubetzko S, Balic E, Waibel R, Zangemeister-Wittke U, Plückthun A. PEGylation and multimerization of the anti-p185HER-2 single chain Fv fragment 4D5: effects on tumor targeting. J Biol Chem 2006; 281(46): 35186-201.
[http://dx.doi.org/10.1074/jbc.M604127200] [PMID: 16963450]

[63]    von Minckwitz G, Harder S, Hövelmann S, *et al.* Phase I clinical study of the recombinant antibody toxin scFv(FRP5)-ETA specific for the ErbB2/HER2 receptor in patients with advanced solid malignomas. Breast Cancer Res 2005; 7(5): R617-26.
[http://dx.doi.org/10.1186/bcr1264] [PMID: 16168106]

[64]    Guo R, Yang Y, Zhang D, *et al.* A bispecific immunotoxin (IHPP) with a long half-life targeting HER2 and PDGFRβ exhibited improved efficacy against HER2-positive tumors in a mouse xenograft model. Int J Pharm 2021; 592: 120037.
[http://dx.doi.org/10.1016/j.ijpharm.2020.120037] [PMID: 33161038]

[65]    Wels W, Biburger M, Müller T, *et al.* Recombinant immunotoxins and retargeted killer cells: employing engineered antibody fragments for tumor-specific targeting of cytotoxic effectors. Cancer Immunol Immunother 2004; 53(3): 217-26.
[http://dx.doi.org/10.1007/s00262-003-0482-8] [PMID: 14704833]

[66]  Boersma YL, Plückthun A. DARPins and other repeat protein scaffolds: advances in engineering and applications. Curr Opin Biotechnol 2011; 22(6): 849-57.
[http://dx.doi.org/10.1016/j.copbio.2011.06.004] [PMID: 21715155]

[67]  Stumpp MT, Binz HK, Amstutz P. DARPins: A new generation of protein therapeutics. Drug Discov Today 2008; 13(15-16): 695-701.
[http://dx.doi.org/10.1016/j.drudis.2008.04.013] [PMID: 18621567]

[68]  Caputi AP, Navarra P. Beyond antibodies: ankyrins and DARPins. From basic research to drug approval. Curr Opin Pharmacol 2020; 51: 93-101.
[http://dx.doi.org/10.1016/j.coph.2020.05.004] [PMID: 32674998]

[69]  Sokolova E, Proshkina G, Kutova O, *et al.* Recombinant targeted toxin based on HER2-specific DARPin possesses a strong selective cytotoxic effect *in vitro* and a potent antitumor activity *in vivo*. J Control Release 2016; 233: 48-56.
[http://dx.doi.org/10.1016/j.jconrel.2016.05.020] [PMID: 27178808]

[70]  Li J, Lundberg E, Vernet E, Larsson B, Höidén-Guthenberg I, Gräslund T. Selection of affibody molecules to the ligand-binding site of the insulin-like growth factor-1 receptor. Biotechnol Appl Biochem 2010; 55(2): 99-109.
[http://dx.doi.org/10.1042/BA20090226] [PMID: 20088825]

[71]  Tolmachev V, Rosik D, Wållberg H, *et al.* Imaging of EGFR expression in murine xenografts using site-specifically labelled anti-EGFR 111In-DOTA-ZEGFR:2377 Affibody molecule: aspect of the injected tracer amount. Eur J Nucl Med Mol Imaging 2010; 37(3): 613-22.
[http://dx.doi.org/10.1007/s00259-009-1283-x] [PMID: 19838701]

[72]  Frejd FY, Kim KT. Affibody molecules as engineered protein drugs. Exp Mol Med 2017; 49(3): e306-6.
[http://dx.doi.org/10.1038/emm.2017.35] [PMID: 28336959]

[73]  Tolmachev V, Orlova A, Pehrson R, *et al.* Radionuclide therapy of HER2-positive microxenografts using a 177Lu-labeled HER2-specific Affibody molecule. Cancer Res 2007; 67(6): 2773-82.
[http://dx.doi.org/10.1158/0008-5472.CAN-06-1630] [PMID: 17363599]

[74]  Liu H, Lindbo S, Ding H, *et al.* Potent and specific fusion toxins consisting of a HER2-binding, ABD-derived affinity protein, fused to truncated versions of Pseudomonas exotoxin-A. Int J Oncol 2019; 55(1): 309-19.
[http://dx.doi.org/10.3892/ijo.2019.4814] [PMID: 31180549]

[75]  Sörensen J, Velikyan I, Sandberg D, *et al.* Measuring HER2-receptor expression in metastatic breast cancer using [68Ga] ABY-025 Affibody PET/CT. Theranostics 2016; 6(2): 262-71.
[http://dx.doi.org/10.7150/thno.13502] [PMID: 26877784]

[76]  Garousi J, Lindbo S, Nilvebrant J, *et al.* ADAPT, a novel scaffold protein-based probe for radionuclide imaging of molecular targets that are expressed in disseminated cancers. Cancer Res 2015; 75(20): 4364-71.
[http://dx.doi.org/10.1158/0008-5472.CAN-14-3497] [PMID: 26297736]

[77]  Vafadar A, Taheri-Anganeh M, Movahedpour A, *et al. In silico* design and evaluation of scFv-CdtBas a novel immunotoxin for breast cancer treatment. Int J Cancer Manag 2020; 13(1): e96094.
[http://dx.doi.org/10.5812/ijcm.96094]

[78]  Vigneron N. Human tumor antigens and cancer immunotherapy. BioMed Res Int 2015; 2015: 1-17.
[http://dx.doi.org/10.1155/2015/948501] [PMID: 26161423]

[79]  Cerutti P, Hussain P, Pourzand C, Aguilar F. Mutagenesis of the H-ras protooncogene and the p53 tumor suppressor gene. Cancer Res 1994; 54(7) (Suppl.): 1934s-8s.
[PMID: 7907948]

[80]  Wargalla UC, Reisfeld RA. Rate of internalization of an immunotoxin correlates with cytotoxic activity against human tumor cells. Proc Natl Acad Sci USA 1989; 86(13): 5146-50.

[http://dx.doi.org/10.1073/pnas.86.13.5146] [PMID: 2544891]

[81]   Fu Liu T, Urieto JO, Moore JE, *et al.* Diphtheria toxin fused to variant interleukin-3 provides enhanced binding to the interleukin-3 receptor and more potent leukemia cell cytotoxicity. Exp Hematol 2004; 32(3): 277-81.
[http://dx.doi.org/10.1016/j.exphem.2003.11.010] [PMID: 15003313]

[82]   Hexham JM, Dudas D, Hugo R, *et al.* Influence of relative binding affinity on efficacy in a panel of anti-CD3 scFv immunotoxins. Mol Immunol 2001; 38(5): 397-408.
[http://dx.doi.org/10.1016/S0161-5890(01)00070-0] [PMID: 11684296]

[83]   Hou SC, Chen HS, Lin HW, *et al.* High throughput cytotoxicity screening of anti-HER2 immunotoxins conjugated with antibody fragments from phage-displayed synthetic antibody libraries. Sci Rep 2016; 6(1): 31878.
[http://dx.doi.org/10.1038/srep31878] [PMID: 27550798]

[84]   Zhang J, Liu YF, Yang SJ, *et al.* Primary targeting of recombinant Fv-immunotoxin hscFv $_{25}$ -mTNFα against hepatocellular carcinoma. World J Gastroenterol 2004; 10(13): 1872-5.
[http://dx.doi.org/10.3748/wjg.v10.i13.1872] [PMID: 15222026]

[85]   Schmidberger H, King L, Lasky LC, Vallera DA. Antitumor activity of L6-ricin immunotoxin against the H2981-T3 lung adenocarcinoma cell line *in vitro* and *in vivo.* Cancer Res 1990; 50(11): 3249-56.
[PMID: 1692258]

[86]   Ho M, Bera TK, Willingham MC, *et al.* Mesothelin expression in human lung cancer. Clin Cancer Res 2007; 13(5): 1571-5.
[http://dx.doi.org/10.1158/1078-0432.CCR-06-2161] [PMID: 17332303]

[87]   Thomas A, Chen Y, Steinberg SM, *et al.* High mesothelin expression in advanced lung adenocarcinoma is associated with *KRAS* mutations and a poor prognosis. Oncotarget 2015; 6(13): 11694-703.
[http://dx.doi.org/10.18632/oncotarget.3429] [PMID: 26028668]

[88]   Hassan R, Ho M. Mesothelin targeted cancer immunotherapy. Eur J Cancer 2008; 44(1): 46-53.
[http://dx.doi.org/10.1016/j.ejca.2007.08.028] [PMID: 17945478]

[89]   Miettinen M, Sarlomo-Rikala M. Expression of calretinin, thrombomodulin, keratin 5, and mesothelin in lung carcinomas of different types: an immunohistochemical analysis of 596 tumors in comparison with epithelioid mesotheliomas of the pleura. Am J Surg Pathol 2003; 27(2): 150-8.
[http://dx.doi.org/10.1097/00000478-200302000-00002] [PMID: 12548160]

[90]   Argani P, Iacobuzio-Donahue C, Ryu B, *et al.* Mesothelin is overexpressed in the vast majority of ductal adenocarcinomas of the pancreas: identification of a new pancreatic cancer marker by serial analysis of gene expression (SAGE). Clin Cancer Res 2001; 7(12): 3862-8.
[PMID: 11751476]

[91]   Hassan R, Laszik ZG, Lerner M, Raffeld M, Postier R, Brackett D. Mesothelin is overexpressed in pancreaticobiliary adenocarcinomas but not in normal pancreas and chronic pancreatitis. Am J Clin Pathol 2005; 124(6): 838-45.
[http://dx.doi.org/10.1309/F1B64CL7H8VJKEAF] [PMID: 16416732]

[92]   Hassan R, Kreitman RJ, Pastan I, Willingham MC. Localization of mesothelin in epithelial ovarian cancer. Appl Immunohistochem Mol Morphol 2005; 13(3): 243-7.
[http://dx.doi.org/10.1097/01.pai.00000141545.36485.d6] [PMID: 16082249]

[93]   Einama T, Homma S, Kamachi H, *et al.* Luminal membrane expression of mesothelin is a prominent poor prognostic factor for gastric cancer. Br J Cancer 2012; 107(1): 137-42.
[http://dx.doi.org/10.1038/bjc.2012.235] [PMID: 22644300]

[94]   Baba K, Ishigami S, Arigami T, *et al.* Mesothelin expression correlates with prolonged patient survival in gastric cancer. J Surg Oncol 2012; 105(2): 195-9.
[http://dx.doi.org/10.1002/jso.22024] [PMID: 21780126]

[95]    Tchou J, Wang LC, Selven B, *et al.* Mesothelin, a novel immunotherapy target for triple negative breast cancer. Breast Cancer Res Treat 2012; 133(2): 799-804.
[http://dx.doi.org/10.1007/s10549-012-2018-4] [PMID: 22418702]

[96]    https://www.clinicaltrials.gov/ct2/show/NCT01362790

[97]    Alewine C, Hassan R, Pastan I. Advances in anticancer immunotoxin therapy. Oncologist 2015; 20(2): 176-85.
[http://dx.doi.org/10.1634/theoncologist.2014-0358] [PMID: 25561510]

[98]    Hassan R, Alewine C, Pastan I. New life for immunotoxin cancer therapy. Clin Cancer Res 2016; 22(5): 1055-8.
[http://dx.doi.org/10.1158/1078-0432.CCR-15-1623] [PMID: 26463707]

[99]    Westwood JA, Murray WK, Trivett M, *et al.* The Lewis-Y carbohydrate antigen is expressed by many human tumors and can serve as a target for genetically redirected T cells despite the presence of soluble antigen in serum. J Immunother 2009; 32(3): 292-301.
[http://dx.doi.org/10.1097/CJI.0b013e31819b7c8e] [PMID: 19242371]

[100]   Pastan I, Lovelace ET, Gallo MG, Rutherford AV, Magnani JL, Willingham MC. Characterization of monoclonal antibodies B1 and B3 that react with mucinous adenocarcinomas. Cancer Res 1991; 51(14): 3781-7.
[PMID: 1648444]

[101]   Derbyshire EJ, Wawrzynczak EJ. An anti-mucin immunotoxin BrE-3-ricin A-chain is potently and selectively toxic to human small-cell lung cancer. Int J Cancer 1992; 52(4): 624-30.
[http://dx.doi.org/10.1002/ijc.2910520422] [PMID: 1328073]

[102]   Sheets SS. Lung and Bronchus Cancer. National Cancer Institute. Last accessed on. 2016.

[103]   Kreitman RJ, Batra JK, Seetharam S, Chaudhary VK, FitzGerald DJ, Pastan I. Single-chain immunotoxin fusions between anti-tac and Pseudomonas exotoxin: Relative importance of the two toxin disulfide bonds. Bioconjug Chem 1993; 4(2): 112-20.
[http://dx.doi.org/10.1021/bc00020a002] [PMID: 7873642]

[104]   Williams DP, Snider CE, Strom TB, Murphy JR. Structure/function analysis of interleukin-2-toxin (DAB486-IL-2). Fragment B sequences required for the delivery of fragment A to the cytosol of target cells. J Biol Chem 1990; 265(20): 11885-9.
[http://dx.doi.org/10.1016/S0021-9258(19)38482-0] [PMID: 2195027]

[105]   Gould BJ, Borowitz MJ, Groves ES, *et al.* Phase I study of an anti-breast cancer immunotoxin by continuous infusion: report of a targeted toxic effect not predicted by animal studies. J Natl Cancer Inst 1989; 81(10): 775-81.
[http://dx.doi.org/10.1093/jnci/81.10.775] [PMID: 2785605]

[106]   Gould BJ, Borowitz MJ, Groves ES, *et al.* Phase I study of an anti-breast cancer immunotoxin by continuous infusion: report of a targeted toxic effect not predicted by animal studies. J Natl Cancer Inst 1989; 81(10): 775-81.
[http://dx.doi.org/10.1093/jnci/81.10.775] [PMID: 2785605]

[107]   Hassan R, Alewine C, Pastan I. New life for immunotoxin cancer therapy. Clin Cancer Res 2016; 22(5): 1055-8.
[http://dx.doi.org/10.1158/1078-0432.CCR-15-1623] [PMID: 26463707]

[108]   Xie YH, Chen YX, Fang JY. Comprehensive review of targeted therapy for colorectal cancer. Signal Transduct Target Ther 2020; 5(1): 22.
[http://dx.doi.org/10.1038/s41392-020-0116-z] [PMID: 32296018]

[109]   Wilson CY, Tolias P. Recent advances in cancer drug discovery targeting RAS. Drug Discov Today 2016; 21(12): 1915-9.
[http://dx.doi.org/10.1016/j.drudis.2016.08.002] [PMID: 27506872]

[110]  Byers VS, Rodvien R, Grant K, *et al.* Phase I study of monoclonal antibody-ricin A chain immunotoxin XomaZyme-791 in patients with metastatic colon cancer. Cancer Res 1989; 49(21): 6153-60.
[PMID: 2790828]

[111]  Li YM, Hall WA. Targeted toxins in brain tumor therapy. Toxins (Basel) 2010; 2(11): 2645-62.
[http://dx.doi.org/10.3390/toxins2112645] [PMID: 22069569]

[112]  Pastan I, Hassan R, FitzGerald DJ, Kreitman RJ. Immunotoxin therapy of cancer. Nat Rev Cancer 2006; 6(7): 559-65.
[http://dx.doi.org/10.1038/nrc1891] [PMID: 16794638]

[113]  Hernández-Pedro NY, Rangel-López E, Vargas Félix G, Pineda B, Sotelo J. An update in the use of antibodies to treat glioblastoma multiforme. Autoimmune Dis 2013; 2013: 1-14.
[http://dx.doi.org/10.1155/2013/716813] [PMID: 24294521]

[114]  Tong JTW, Harris PWR, Brimble MA, Kavianinia I. An Insight into FDA Approved Antibody-Drug Conjugates for Cancer Therapy. Molecules 2021; 26(19): 5847.
[http://dx.doi.org/10.3390/molecules26195847] [PMID: 34641391]

[115]  Mahmoudi R, Dianat-Moghadam H, Poorebrahim M, *et al.* Recombinant immunotoxins development for HER2-based targeted cancer therapies. Cancer Cell Int 2021; 21(1): 470.
[http://dx.doi.org/10.1186/s12935-021-02182-6] [PMID: 34488747]

[116]  Heiat M, Hashemi Yeganeh H, Alavian SM, Rezaie E. Immunotoxins immunotherapy against hepatocellular carcinoma: a promising prospect. Toxins (Basel) 2021; 13(10): 719.
[http://dx.doi.org/10.3390/toxins13100719] [PMID: 34679012]

[117]  Wayne AS, FitzGerald DJ, Kreitman RJ, Pastan I. Immunotoxins for leukemia. Blood 2014; 123(16): 2470-7.
[http://dx.doi.org/10.1182/blood-2014-01-492256] [PMID: 24578503]

[118]  Sanz L, Ibáñez-Pérez R, Guerrero-Ochoa P, Lacadena J, Anel A. Antibody-based immunotoxins for colorectal cancer therapy. Biomedicines 2021; 9(11): 1729.
[http://dx.doi.org/10.3390/biomedicines9111729] [PMID: 34829955]

[119]  Zhu S, Liu Y, Wang PC, Gu X, Shan L. Recombinant immunotoxin therapy of glioblastoma: smart design, key findings, and specific challenges. BioMed Res Int 2017; 2017: 1-18.
[http://dx.doi.org/10.1155/2017/7929286] [PMID: 28752098]

# Multifactorial Drug - A Revolution in the Treatment of Cancer by Inhibiting Hedgehog Pathway

**M. Santosh Kumar[1,*], Poornima D. Vijendra[2], Pratap G. Kenchappa[1] and A. Gowtami[1]**

*[1] Department of Studies in Biochemistry, Davangere University Shivagangothri, Davangere-577007, Karnataka, India*

*[2] Department of Studies in Biochemistry and Food Technology, Davangere University Shivagangothri, Davangere – 577007, Karnataka, India*

**Abstract:** In the human body, Hedgehog (Hh) signaling is an essential pathway and plays a major role in embryo development, tumorigenesis, distant metastasis, poor prognosis, and tissue patterning. The Hh pathway has three ligands in mammals: Sonic Hedgehog (SHh), Desert Hedgehog (DHh), and Indian Hedgehog (IHh). Malfunctions of this pathway are associated with diseases that include cancer. Cancer is one of the leading causes of death worldwide and factors like dietary habits, family history, obesity, environmental conditions, tobacco, and genetic factors affect the likelihood of developing cancer. The Hh signaling pathway through sporadic mutations is explicitly associated with cancer development and progression in various solid malignancies. Abnormal expression of the Hh signaling cascade has been reported in the development of basal cell carcinoma, breast, liver, prostate, colon, pancreas, and stomach cancer. Most researchers target the inhibition of the Hh signaling pathway and therefore it has emerged as a popular and validated therapeutic for the treatment of a wide range of cancers. A novel class of drugs such as sonidegib and vismodegib inhibits the Hedgehog pathway. There has been significant progress regarding the development of multifactorial drugs blocking Hh signaling. The discovery of multifactorial drugs to block the pathway has led to a new treatment that may significantly improve clinical outcomes in cancer patients. Several of these molecules have been included in the clinical testing stage. Yet finding a sustainable multifactorial inhibitor is still a challenge. This book chapter describes the Hh signaling pathway as a vital and multifactorial therapeutic target for cancer.

**Keywords:** Cancer therapy, Hedgehog pathway, Multifactorial drug, Sonidegib, Vismodigeb.

---

*** Corresponding author M. Santosh Kumar:** Department of Studies in Biochemistry, Davangere University Shivagangothri, Davangere-577007, Karnataka, India; E-mail: santoshmudde@gmail.com

**Ashok Kumar Pandurangan (Ed.)**

# INTRODUCTION

Cancer is a disease in which some of the body's cells grow uncontrollably and spread to other parts of the body, cancer is one of the leading causes of mortality worldwide, in both developed and developing nations due to changes in lifestyle and eating habits. Around 7.6 million people die from cancer each year, according to current estimates [1, 2]. The Hedgehog (Hh) pathway is a signalling mechanism that drives patterning and is required for appropriate development. At the molecular level, Hh ligands cause cell proliferation in some cell types while inducing differentiation in others. It is most active during embryogenesis, and its aberrant reactivation in adult tissue has been linked to the development of cancer [1]. Hedgehog gets its name from a polypeptide ligand identified in the *Drosophila* genus named Hedgehog (Hh). Christiane Nusslein-Volhard and Eric F. Weischaus found the Hh gene in 1980 [3]. The Hh signalling pathway's key target genes are PTCH1, PTCH2, and GLI1. Deregulation of the Hh signalling pathway has been linked to sporadic malignancies such as basal cell carcinoma, medulloblastoma, pancreatic, breast, colon, ovarian, and small-cell lung carcinomas, as well as developmental defects and cancers like Gorlin syndrome [4]. In humans inflicted with cancer, the Hh pathway boosts stem cell DNA synthesis. Many signalling pathways involved in the developmental process, including Hedgehog, Wnt, and Notch, have a critical role in carcinogenesis as well as resistance to various anticancer medicines. Understanding how cancer uses these developmental pathways to resist multi-therapeutic approaches can lead to new insights into anti-therapy resistance mechanisms that can be investigated for the creation of a new therapeutic method [5].

According to some evidence, Hh ligand binding to PTCH1 regulates the cell cycle by facilitating the transition from Gap 2 to mitosis by binding to a cyclin B1 and CDK-1 complex. PTCH1 functions as a tumour suppressor. The pathophysiology of cancers such as breast, lung, pancreatic, prostate, and haematological malignancies is linked to abnormal activation of Hh signalling [6]. The first Hh pathway inhibitor is cyclopamine, a naturally occurring plant alkaloid. The active cyclopamine chemical found in corn lilies was later discovered to block the Hh pathway by binding to and inactivating the Smoothened (SMO) transmembrane receptor protein [3]. Hedgehog pathway inhibitors were found by researchers, and the Vismodegib advance medication was authorised by the FDA for use in basal cell carcinomas [7].

Cancer resistance is influenced by the Hedgehog signalling system. Different cancer treatment options include immunotherapy, chemotherapy, molecular targeted therapy, and radiation [5]. As a result, Hh signalling has become a therapeutic target for cancer treatment. The topic of Hh signalling and the principal molecular actors engaged in suppressing the Hh pathway modulator, as well as a current description of what natural and synthetic chemicals affect Hh signalling in cancer treatment, will be discussed in the framework of this chapter.

## CANCER AND Hh PATHWAY

Hedgehog (Hh) is a short- or long-range morphogen that affects a variety of tissue types. Sonic Hh, Indian Hh, and Desert Hh are the three Hh proteins found in mammals. Newly produced Hh enters the secretory system and undergoes auto-processing and lipid modifications resulting in the addition of a palmitoyl group to the $NH_2$ terminus and cholesterol to the COOH terminus in cells to produce Hh [8]. The Hh protein is involved in various developmental processes in Drosophila, including gonadal formation and function [9]. The Hedgehog (Hh) signaling pathway, also known as Hedgehog-Patched (Hh-PTCH), Hedgehog-GLI (Hh-GLI), or Hedgehog-Patched-Smoothened (Hh-Patch-Smo), is an evolutionarily conserved signaling pathway that transmits from the cell membrane to the nucleus [10]. This pathway involves inhibition of the twelve transmembrane protein Pathed1 (PTCH1) by binding Hh protein, activation of the seven-transmembrane protein Smoothened (SMO), the release of the five-zinc finger transcription factor GLI forms a large protein complex, and is involved in the nuclear translocation of GLI, and transcription of target genes. GLI makes a large protein complex with Costal2, Fused, and suppressor fused in the absence of sonic Hh (SHh) and are sequestered in the cytoplasm. A full-length GLI3 produced from the big protein complex is transported into the nucleus in the presence of SHh to activate Hh target genes. GLI1 is one of the GLI3's target genes. As a result, GLI1 is a marker for the activation of the Hh pathway [11]. The role of Hedgehog signaling is to control cell proliferation and differentiation in the embryonic development stage and when it is altered or misregulated, it can lead to cancer [10].

Hh signalling has been implicated in various stages of carcinogenesis in various cancers, according to several research. The activation of this signalling system is seen in the early stages of pancreatic and oesophageal cancers, as well as in metastatic tumors. The activation of the Hh signalling system has been linked to tissue invasion and enhanced metastatic potential in various cancers, such as gastric cancer and prostate cancer. Inhibition of the Hh signalling pathway suppresses tumour cell proliferation in prostate and gastric cancer, according to research studies [4]. In cancer, abnormal Hh pathway activation is caused by both ligand-dependent and ligand-independent pathways. Loss-of-function PTCH or SUFU mutations (Fig. **1**), as well as gain-of-function SMO mutations, promote ligand-independent Hh signalling and drive the development of basal cell carcinoma (BCC), medulloblastoma (MB), rhabdomyosarcoma, and meningioma tumors [12]. Studies on Gorlin syndrome, an autosomal dominant illness characterised by craniofacial and skeletal deformities as well as a significantly elevated risk of advanced basal cell carcinoma (BCC) and medulloblastoma, provided the first evidence for a role for Hh signalling in cancer [13]. The Hh pathway assists in the clonal development of cell lines originating from human ovarian cancer. *In vitro*, treatment with cyclopamine, a selective inhibitor of the HH pathway, inhibits proliferation and clonal expansion of all ovarian cancer cell lines, and *in vivo*, it suppresses tumor growth [9].

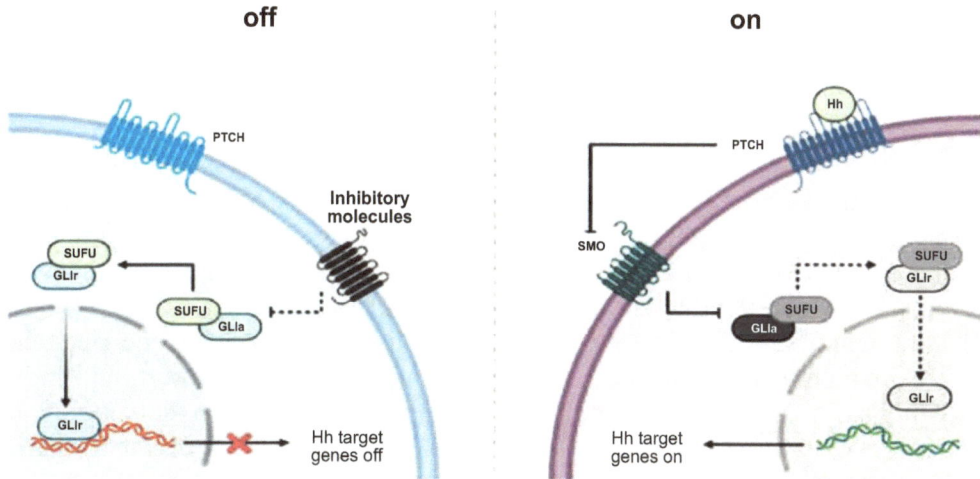

**Fig. [1].** Role of Hedgehog signaling pathways involved in the acquisition of resistance to molecular targeted therapies in cancer.

Patched receptor (PTCH), a 12-transmembrane protein receptor, and Smoothened (SMO, a 7-transmembrane protein linked to G protein-coupled receptors) protein make up the hedgehog signalling pathways in vertebrates. PTCH 1 and PTCH 2 are two other PTCH genes. PTCH 2 has a 54 percent sequence similarity to PTCH 1. Because all three mammalian hedgehogs bind both receptors with identical affinity, PTCH 1 and PTCH 2 are unable to differentiate between the ligands, although each of them has unique downstream signalling functions. GLIoma-associated oncogene-GLI 1, GLI 2, and GLI 3 are the oncogenes that signal downstream of SMO in mammals. GLI 1 and GLI 2 are transcriptional activators, while GLI 3 is a repressor [7, 14].

PTCH, which is present on the cell membrane at the base of primary cilia, a cellular structure seen in most mammalian cells, prevents the SMO from entering the cilium in the absence of hedgehog ligand, blocking downstream signalling processes. PTCH serves as a sterol pump, removing oxysterols produced by 7-dehydrocholesterol reductase and therefore inhibiting the SMO-initiated pathway [3] GLI 1 activators, in combination with SUFU (Suppressor of fused), a negative suppressor, inhibit GLI 1 target genes from being transcribed, thereby shutting down the pathway [7] (Fig. **1**).

The Hedgehog pathway is started when the Hedgehog ligand binds to the PTCH 1 receptor. The sterol pumps are switched off as a result of PTCH 1 translocation and internalisation, enabling oxysterols to accumulate around SMO, reducing its inhibitory function. Activated SMO then travels to the cilium's cell membrane, where it promotes the activation of the GLI family of transcription factors by cleaving it from the inhibitory SUFU protein. These active GLI proteins reach the nucleus and bind to GLI-promoters, causing mammalian target genes to be transcribed (Fig. **1**) [7].

## HEDGEHOG SIGNALING AND HUMAN DISEASES

Hedgehog is the secreted signal molecule that acts as a local mediator and morphogen in various tissues' development in both vertebrates and invertebrates. At first, these hedgehog proteins were discovered in *D.melanogaster* [15]. These proteins were found on the larvae of the drosophila as denticles, which resemble the small mammals called Hedgehogs. Three drosophila genes encode Hedgehog proteins, which were identified in vertebrates that are Sonic, Desert, and Indian Hedgehogs. In invertebrates, the Hedgehog pathway helps in developing the embryos, skeleton, limbs, lungs, skin, hairs, *etc.* Disruption of the signaling causes various defects in the organisms [16].

The hedgehog effects are mediated by a transcriptional regulator - Cubitus interruptus (Ci protein). Hedgehog ligands, patched receptor, smoothened receptor, suppressor of a fused homolog, kinesin protein Kif7, protein kinase A, and cyclic adenosine monophosphate (cAMP) are the components of the hedgehog signaling pathway involved in the transfer of the signal to the GLIoma transcription factors, which were identified through genetic analysis over a decade. PTCH1, PTCH2, and GLI1 are the main targets of the hedgehog signaling pathway. Overexpression of Hedgehog signalling molecules or mutations in genes can cause the Hedgehog signalling pathway to be activated abnormally [14].

There are various diseases caused by the mutations in the Hedgehog signaling pathway. Sonic hedgehog is responsible for the major effects on the development of the brain, spinal cord, lungs, axial skeleton, regulating pulmonary branching, mesenchyme differentiation, and limbs. Indian hedgehog is responsible for cartilage differentiation in the growth of long bones. Desert hedgehogs are responsible for the development of the germline and Schwann cells of the peripheral nervous system.

Colon cancer is a tumour caused by a subset of cancer stem cells. Canonical GLI-dependent hedgehog signalling is a negative modulator of Wnt signalling in intestinal cancers. Hedgehog signalling is autocrine sonic hedgehog dependent, noncanonical PTCH1 dependent, and GLI independent in colon cancer stem cells. Non-canonical Hedgehog signalling is a positive regulator of Wnt signalling [17].

Meningiomas are the most common primary intracranial tumors. A small percentage of meningiomas harbor somatic variants in the Hedgehog pathway, a conserved gene expression program that is essential for development and adult stem cell homeostasis. Hedgehog signals are transduced through primary cilia, and misactivation of the Hedgehog pathway is known to underlie cancer. The expression of Smoothened alleles that are oncogenic in other contexts fails to activate the Hedgehog transcriptional program or promote proliferation in primary meningioma cells. These data reveal that meningiomas can express the subcellular structure necessary for canonical Hedgehog signalling but suggest that they do not transduce ciliary Hedgehog signals [18].

Hedgehog signalling is required for bone development and skeletal mineralization. SLIT and NTRK-like protein-5 are the transmembrane proteins that act as osteoblasts hedgehog signaling negative regulators. Slitrk5 is selectively expressed in osteoblasts and loss of Slitrk5 enhanced osteoblast differentiation *in vitro* and *in vivo*. Loss of SLITRK5 *in vitro* leads to increased hedgehog signaling and overexpression of Slitrk5 in osteoblasts inhibits the induction of targets downstream of hedgehog signaling. Mechanistically, Slitrk5 binds to hedgehog ligands *via* its extracellular domain and interacts with PTCH1 *via* its intracellular domain. Slitrk5 is present in the primary cilium, and loss of Slitrk5 enhances SMO ciliary enrichment upon SHH stimulation. Thus, SLITRK5 is a negative regulator of hedgehog signaling in osteoblasts that may be attractive as a therapeutic target to enhance bone formation [19].

VACTERL syndrome is the non-random association of malformations in the heart, fistula, renal abnormalities, anal atresia, limb anomalies, and diaphragmatic hernia. The Pallister-Hall syndrome and Gorlin syndrome share some of the abnormalities of VACTERL syndrome. GLI2 and GLI3 are the genes that are associated with this syndrome, which were identified in the mouse model as the loss of function. Where the combination of the GLI2 and GLI3 genes leads to a phenotype with all components of the human syndrome. Pallister-Hall syndrome is also associated with the GLI3 gene in dominant [20].

Gorlin syndrome is the autosomal dominant disorder associated with the skin, medulloblastomas, ovarian fibromas, and neoplasms that include fibrosarcomas, meningiomas, rhabdomyosarcomas, and cardiac fibromas. This Gorlin syndrome,

Spordiac basal cell carcinoma is associated with the loss of function of the PTCH gene, whereas Holoprosencephaly is associated with the gain of the function of the PTCH gene [21].

The developmental abnormalities and cancers such as basal cell nevus syndrome (BCNS), also known as Gorlin syndrome, sporadic basal cell carcinoma (BCC), medulloblastomas (MBs), rhabdomyosarcomas, meningiomas [22], and others are linked to dysfunction or abnormal activation of the Hh signalling pathway [23]. The Hh signalling pathway is thought to contribute to the formation of one-third of all malignant tumors, according to recent estimates [24]. Any component of the Hh pathway that is downregulated causes it to activate abnormally, resulting in malignant transformation. In various cancer types, three pathways of abnormal Hh signalling activation have been proposed such as, [3]. Ligand-independent, autonomous type of Hh signaling (Type I), Ligand-dependent oncogenic Hh signaling in autocrine/juxtacrine manner (Type II), and Ligand-dependent Hh signaling in paracrine or reverse paracrine manner (Type IIIa/b).

## Type I- Ligand-Independent Hedgehog Signaling

Tumors of type 1 origin have genetic mutations in components of the Hh pathway, which increase tumour cell-intrinsic growth and survival. Inactivating mutations, such as deletions, mRNA splice-site and nonsense mutations in PTCH1, SUFU [25, 26] or activating missense mutations in SMO, SmoM2 (Trp535Leu), or gene amplifications and translocations of GLI1 or GLI2 [27], usually in combination with the inactivation of additional tumour suppressor genes, are sufficient to form a variety of sporadic tumours. According to the analysis of human cancer tissue, this is notably true for basal cell carcinomas (BCCs), which are keratinocyte-based skin tumours, medulloblastoma, a pediatric cerebellar cancer, and rhabdomyosarcoma [25].

## Type II- Ligand-Dependent Autocrine/Juxtacrine Signalling

Type II is autocrine/juxtacrine ligand-dependent, which responds to Hh, resulting in tumour development and proliferation. Hh ligand is generated and taken up by the same or neighboring tumour cells because the Hh pathway is activated in a cell-autonomous manner [28]. Overexpression of the ligand-dependent autocrine/juxtacrine Hh signalling pathway has been observed in esophageal, stomach, pancreatic, colorectal, ovarian, and endometrial tumours, melanomas, prostate, lung, breast, GLIomas, and other extracutaneous tumours, among others.

Other than Hh ligand overexpression, the majority of these cancers had ectopic PTCH1 and GLI expression [14].

## Type IIIa/b: Ligand-Dependent Hh Signaling in Paracrine Manner

The importance of Hh signalling in the promotion of the tumour microenvironment was recently highlighted by Yauch and colleagues, who discovered that tumour Hh signalling can be mediated through paracrine pathways. Paracrine Hh signalling is required for the formation and maintenance of different epithelial structures, including the small intestine, according to Theunissen and de Sauvage (2009). The Hh ligand secreted by the epithelium reaches the mesenchymal stroma, where it has a direct influence on and stimulates proliferation in the mesenchyme. When the Hh target gene is active, the mesenchyme produces additional molecules that feedback to the epithelium [3].

## HH SIGNALING PATHWAY TARGETS AND MULTIFACTORIAL DRUGS

The PTCH1, PTCH2, and GLI1 genes are the key target genes of the Hh signalling pathway, and their activation leads to increased levels of the respective mRNAs and proteins. Increased expression of the PTCH1, PTCH2, and GLI1 genes is a highly reliable indicator of an activated signalling pathway, and it regulates Hh signalling *via* negative (PTCH1) and positive (GLI1) feedback loop processes [29].

Hedgehog-interacting protein (Hhip), cell cycle regulators (CCND2 and CCNE1), apoptosis regulator (BCL2), MYCN, VEGFA, PAX6, PAX7, PAX9, FOXM1, JAG1, and components of the link between the Wnt and Hh signalling pathways and list of target genes are among the other target genes listed in Table **1**. The activation and deactivation of these Hh genes may have a role in cancer as well as the development of normal tissues and organs [30].

Recent findings of the Hh signalling system and its role in carcinogenesis have ushered in a new era of Hh pathway molecular targeting and tumour prevention. Targeted Hh signalling pathway inhibition (HPI) has garnered specific interest as a treatment for locally aggressive and metastatic BCCs when radiotherapy and surgery are ineffective [31]. At varying levels, more than 50 HPI molecules are engaged in the Hh signalling pathway. Atypical protein kinase C (aPKC) inhibitors, Hh ligand inhibitors, Smo antagonists, GLI inhibitors, BET family protein inhibitors, and phosphodiesterase inhibitors are all examples of HPIs [32] (Table **2**).

Table 1. Hh signaling pathway target genes.

| Gene | Full Name of the Protein | Effect of the Gene Product | References |
|---|---|---|---|
| PTCH1 | Patched 1 | Indicator of an active signalling system | |
| PTCH2 | Patched 2 | Negative feedback | |
| GLI1 | GLIoma-associated oncogene 1 | Indicator of an active signaling pathway, Positive feedback | |
| Hhip | Hedgehog-interacting protein | Hh signaling pathway regulation | |
| CCND2 | G1/S-specific cyclin-D2 | Cell cycle regulator | |
| CCNE1 | G1/S-specific cyclin-E1 | | |
| MYCN | N-myc proto-oncogene protein | Cell proliferation and tumorigenesis | [14] |
| BCL2 | B-cell lymphoma 2 | Apoptosis regulator | |
| VEGFA | Vascular endothelial growth factor A | Angiogenesis, vasculogenesis, endothelial cell growth | |
| PAX6, PAX7, PAX9 | Paired box protein Pax-6, 7 and 9 | Transcription factors during embryogenesis | |
| JAG1 | Jagged 1 | Notch ligand and Wnt signaling pathway | |
| FOXM1 | Forkhead box protein M1 | Transcription factor | |

The hedgehog pathway has been discovered to be blocked by the use of two novel SMO inhibitors, Sonidegib (LDE225) and Vismodegib (GDC-0449). Both drugs are hedgehog pathway antagonists, meaning they bind to SMO and prevent downstream hedgehog target genes from being activated. Vismodegib has been approved by the US Food and Drug Administration (FDA) for the treatment of metastatic or locally advanced non-resectable basal cell carcinoma (BCC) [34]. Vismodegib suppressed SMO and was discovered by screening cyclopamine derivatives on a GLI luciferase reporter cell line. Vismodegib directly binds to SMO, according to competitive binding assays and molecular docking prediction studies. In addition to revealing that vismodegib binds to SMO, it was observed in patient samples and animal models that exposure to the medicine induced mutations in SMO, which prevented the medication from binding with the protein and resulting in vismodegib adaptive resistance [35, 36].

**Table 2. Targeted tumor therapy associated with the Hh signaling pathway.**

| Group | Drug | Mechanism of Action | References |
|---|---|---|---|
| Hh ligand inhibitors | Robotnikinin Cyclopamine Saridegib Vismodegib BMS 833923 Sonidegib Glasdegib | Robotnikinin is the first recognised inhibitor of SHh protein, binding to PTCH and removing its inhibitory action on Smo, allowing for uninterrupted cellular signalling. Saridegib, Vismodegib, and BMS 833923 are selective Hh pathway inhibitors that bind to Smo and prevent downstream Hh target genes from being activated. | |
| Smo antagonists | Taladegib LEQ506 TAK- 441 XL-139 Itraconazole HPI-1 HPI-2 | Smo antagonists attach to the Smo drug-binding pocket, blocking the Hh signalling cascade from being activated downstream. | |
| | GANT-56 GANT-61 ATO JK 184 GANT-58 | GLI inhibitors | [14] |
| BET inhibitors | JQ1 | Tumour cells' viability and proliferation are reduced in Smo-resistant malignancies. | |
| aPKC inhibitors | PSI | Effective in the treatment of resistant BCCs. | |
| Phosphodiesterase inhibitors | NVP-ABE171 Cilomilast Deguelin | *In vivo*, phosphodiesterase inhibitors proved effective in treating Smo-resistant MB. | |
| Natural products | *Siegesbeckiaglabrescens* extracts Vitamin D3 | Reduce transcriptional activity and proliferation in human pancreatic cells mediated by GLI. | |
| | Physalin B | Inhibits transcription in HaCaT cells mediated by GLI1,2, PTCH1 and BCL2 | [33] |
| | Physalin F | | |

Vismodegib is a small synthetic drug molecule and it is used for the treatment of hedgehog inhibitors. Vismodegib is the first FDA-approved pharmacologic agent that targets the Hedgehog signaling pathway. It is supposed to play an important role in regulating stem cell function in adults. Hedgehog pathway in adults is concerned with the development of different types of cancers, including Basal Cell Carcinoma (BCC) and medulloblastoma. Vismodegib drug suppresses hedgehog signaling by binding to the smoothened (SMO) transmembrane protein that provides activating downstream signals to the pathway, providing a strong validation for its use in the treatment of cancers. The Hedgehog pathway regulates cell growth and differentiation in embryogenesis. This pathway is not active in adult tissue. SMO is a G-protein-coupled transmembrane receptor involved in the signal transduction of the SHH pathway. Vismodegib is a selective Hedgehog pathway inhibitor that binds to and competitively inhibits SMO. Inhibition of SMO results in transcription factors GLI1 and GLI2 remaining inactive; this prevents the expression of tumor-mediating genes within the Hedgehog pathway [34]. Some other studies preclinical studies demonstrated the antitumor activity of Vismodegib in mouse models of medulloblastoma (MB) and xenograft models of colorectal and pancreatic cancer. Phase I and II clinical trials in patients with various carcinomas have shown a positive objective response to Vismodegib [7]. Vismodegib inhibits the hedgehog signalling pathway and is indicated for the treatment of adult basal cell carcinoma.

Sonidegib is a highly successful medication because of its pharmacokinetic features. Sonidegib is being studied for use in the treatment of MB, renal, lung, pancreatic, and ovarian carcinomas, as well as hematologic malignancies like myeloid leukaemia and lymphoma. Vismodegib has a comparable safety profile as sonidegib, but it has lower therapeutic efficacy and more serious adverse effects, including considerable fatigue, hyponatremia, hypocalcemia, muscle spasms, and atrial fibrillation [34]. Although Smo inhibitors have a lot of promise for treating BCC, tumour cells may develop resistance to them due to mutations in the drug-binding pocket [37].

BET inhibitors can also reduce the viability and proliferation of tumour cells in Smo-resistant malignancies due to abnormal Hh signalling activity. JQ1 is a BET inhibitor that is extensively utilised in research studies, among other inhibitors. BET inhibitors have been demonstrated to reduce the growth of MB and BCC as well as increase survival in mouse models. *In vivo* therapy of Smo-resistant MB with phosphodiesterase inhibitors was successful, and aPKC inhibitors may be effective in the treatment of resistant BCCs. Several natural compounds have also shown potential in the therapy of cancer. Deguelin, for example, is a flavonoid that has anticarcinogenic and antiproliferative properties. It inhibits blood vessel development and promotes apoptosis and cell cycle arrest. Many researchers have identified deguelin as a regulator of the Hh signalling system, and multiple studies have already demonstrated its efficacy in the treatment of various malignant tumours, including gastric, lung, and breast cancers, as well as, more recently, pancreatic cancer [38].

## Inhibitors of Hedgehog Pathway

Several Hh inhibitors are now being tested in clinical studies for various kinds of brain cancers (Table **3**). Although SMO is the primary target for SHh-pathway inhibitors, preclinical and clinical investigations have shown that using Smo inhibitors causes the formation of mutations that lead to treatment resistance [39]. Sesquiterpenes are a class of terpenes isolated from *Siegesbeckia glabrescens* and have also been reported to decrease GLI-mediated transcriptional activity and proliferation in human pancreatic cells. Smo protein can also be inhibited by the release of PTCH-dependent (pro-) Vitamin D3. [14].

Cyclopamine is the SHh pathway's prototypical inhibitor, attached to the SMO's hepta-helical bundle, which inactivates it. It is now being studied as an anticancer treatment in basal cell carcinoma, medulloblastoma, and rhabdomyosarcoma in both preclinical and clinical trials. In contrast to its anti-lanosterol action in fungi, this chemical works as an SMO antagonist (other azole drugs have not been found to have this effect). Novartis' LDE-225, Millennium Pharmaceuticals' TAK-441, Exelixis/ Bristol-Myers Squibb's BMS-833923 (XL139), and Pfizer's PF-04449913 are among the other prospects for future studies. The FDA has authorised Vismodegib for the treatment of advanced basal cell carcinoma. However, it, like other medications in the class, has a side effect profile. It is contraindicated during pregnancy due to its method of action since it is teratogenic, embryotoxic, and fetotoxic. Alopecia, muscular spasms, weight loss, exhaustion, GIT abnormalities, and arthralgias are some of the other side effects [40].

Table 3. Hh inhibitors are now being tested in clinical studies for various kinds of brain cancers.

| Inhibitors | Compound | Torget Pathway | References |
|---|---|---|---|
| Biological-based inhibitors | 3H8, 6D7 (antibody) | SHh pathway inhibitor | |
| | Cyclopamine | | |
| | 5E1 Antibody | | |
| | Isoflavon (Genistein) | | |
| | Curcumin | GLI 1 inhibitor | |
| | Resveratrol | | |
| | Epigallocatechin-3-gallate | | |
| | Physalin B and Physalin F | | |

*(Table 3) cont.....*

| | Jervine | SMO inhibitor | |
| --- | --- | --- | --- |
| | Zerumbone | GLI 1 inhibitor | |
| | Staurosporinone | | |
| | Vitamin D3 | SMO inhibitor | |
| Chemical Based inhibitors | GDC-0449 (Vismodegib/Erivedge™) | SMO inhibitor | [39] |
| | IPI-926 (Saridegib) | | |
| | NVP-LDE225 (Erismodegib) (Sonidegib) | | |
| | PF-04449913 (Glasdegib) | | |
| | BRD-6851 | | |
| | LY2940680 | | |
| | MK-5710 | | |
| | SEN450 | | |
| | PF-5274857 (A-116) | | |
| | MRT-10 and MRT-14 | | |
| | TAK-441 | | |
| | SANT1, SANT2, SANT3, SANT4, SANT74 and SANT75 | | |
| | MS-0022 | SMO inhibitor | |
| | Arsenic Trioxide (ATO) | GLI 1 inhibitor | |
| | Sodium Arsenite | | |
| | HPI-1, HPI-2, HPI-3 and HPI-4 | | |
| | AKI0532 | Probably Smo inhibitor | |
| | Itraconazole | SMO inhibitor | |
| | GANT 58, GANT 61 | GLI 1 inhibitor | |
| | KAAD-Cyclopamine | Smo inhibitor | |
| | Cur-61,414 | | |
| | Robotnikinin | SHh pathway inhibitor | |

*(Table 3) cont.....*

| | | |
|---|---|---|
| SAG | SMO inhibitor | |
| Purmorphamine | | |
| BMS-833923 (XL139) | | |
| LY2940680 (Taladegib) | | |
| MRT-92 | | |
| PF-5274857 | | |
| LEQ506 | | |
| RU-SKI 43 | SHh pathway inhibitor | |
| Imiquimod | | |
| Patidegib | | |

# CONCLUSION

Hh signalling has been implicated in various stages of carcinogenesis in various cancers, according to several research works. The activation of the Hh signalling system has been linked to tissue invasion and enhanced metastatic potential in various cancers. In cancer, abnormal Hh pathway activation is caused by both ligand-dependent and ligand-independent pathways. Evolutionary conserved developmental signaling pathways such as Notch, Hedgehog, and Wnt signaling are well recognized for their role in regulating many cellular functions that play key roles in tumor development and progression. These signaling pathways are often up-regulated in tumors, which often hijack these pathways to evolve continuously under the pressure induced by the therapy, thereby enabling them to become resistant to various therapies. The latest surprises on potential endogenous SMO modulators reminded us that, even after decades of research, many things about the Hh pathway are yet to be better understood. Several natural and synthetic medications are being studied for use in the treatment of renal, lung, pancreatic, and ovarian carcinomas, as well as hematologic malignancies such as myeloid leukaemia and lymphoma, due to their pharmacokinetic properties. Many inhibitors developed to target these signaling pathways have shown promising efficacy in preclinical cancer models, and some have even advanced to clinical trials with modest efficacy seen so far.

# REFERENCES

[1]  Thun MJ, DeLancey JO, Center MM, Jemal A, Ward EM. The global burden of cancer: priorities for prevention. Carcinogenesis 2010; 31(1): 100-10.
[http://dx.doi.org/10.1093/carcin/bgp263] [PMID: 19934210]

[2]  Society. AC. American cancer society. Glob cancer facts fig am cancer soc atlanta, GA [Internet] 2007; 48(7): 936-44.
[http://dx.doi.org/10.1016/j.cortex.2011.07.008]

[3] Gupta S, Takebe N, LoRusso P. Review: Targeting the Hedgehog pathway in cancer. Ther Adv Med Oncol 2010; 2(4): 237-50.
[http://dx.doi.org/10.1177/1758834010366430] [PMID: 21789137]

[4] Skoda1 AM, Simovic1 D, Karin1 V, * VK, Vranic3 S, Ljiljana Serman. The role of the Hedgehog signaling pathway in cancer: A comprehensive review. Bosn J Basic Med Sci 2009; 9(3): 173.
[PMID: 19754468]

[5] Kumar V, Vashishta M, Kong L, *et al.* The role of notch, hedgehog, and wnt signaling pathways in the resistance of tumors to anticancer therapies. Front Cell Dev Biol 2021; 9(April): 650772.
[http://dx.doi.org/10.3389/fcell.2021.650772] [PMID: 33968932]

[6] Cortes JE, Gutzmer R, Kieran MW, Solomon JA. Hedgehog signaling inhibitors in solid and hematological cancers. Cancer Treat Rev 2019; 76(76): 41-50.
[http://dx.doi.org/10.1016/j.ctrv.2019.04.005] [PMID: 31125907]

[7] Abidi A. Hedgehog signaling pathway: A novel target for cancer therapy: Vismodegib , a promising therapeutic option in treatment of basal cell carcinomas. Indian J Pharmacol 2014;46(1):3-12.
[http://dx.doi.org/10.4103/0253-7613.124884]

[8] Evangelista M, Tian H, de Sauvage FJ. The hedgehog signaling pathway in cancer. Clin Cancer Res 2006; 12(20): 5924-8.
[http://dx.doi.org/10.1158/1078-0432.CCR-06-1736] [PMID: 17062662]

[9] Bhattacharya R, Kwon J, Ali B, *et al.* Role of hedgehog signaling in ovarian cancer. Clin Cancer Res 2008; 14(23): 7659-66.
[http://dx.doi.org/10.1158/1078-0432.CCR-08-1414] [PMID: 19047091]

[10] Theunissen JW, de Sauvage FJ. Paracrine Hedgehog signaling in cancer. Cancer Res 2009; 69(15): 6007-10.
[http://dx.doi.org/10.1158/0008-5472.CAN-09-0756] [PMID: 19638582]

[11] Kubo M, Nakamura M, Tasaki A, *et al.* Hedgehog signaling pathway is a new therapeutic target for patients with breast cancer. Cancer Res 2004; 64(17): 6071-4.
[http://dx.doi.org/10.1158/0008-5472.CAN-04-0416] [PMID: 15342389]

[12] Justilien V, Fields AP. Molecular pathways: novel approaches for improved therapeutic targeting of Hedgehog signaling in cancer stem cells. Clin Cancer Res 2015; 21(3): 505-13.
[http://dx.doi.org/10.1158/1078-0432.CCR-14-0507] [PMID: 25646180]

[13] McMillan R, Matsui W. Molecular pathways: the hedgehog signaling pathway in cancer. Clin Cancer Res 2012; 18(18): 4883-8.
[http://dx.doi.org/10.1158/1078-0432.CCR-11-2509] [PMID: 22718857]

[14] Skoda AM, Simovic D, Karin V, Kardum V, Vranic S, Serman L. The role of the Hedgehog signaling pathway in cancer: A comprehensive review. Bosn J Basic Med Sci 2018; 18(1): 8-20.
[http://dx.doi.org/10.17305/bjbms.2018.2756] [PMID: 29274272]

[15] Sari IN, Phi LTH, Jun N, Wijaya YT, Lee S, Kwon HY. Hedgehog signaling in cancer: A prospective therapeutic target for eradicating cancer stem cells. Cells 2018; 7(11): 208.
[http://dx.doi.org/10.3390/cells7110208] [PMID: 30423843]

[16] Brennan D, Chen X, Cheng L, Mahoney M, Riobo NA. Noncanonical Hedgehog signaling. Vitam Horm 2012; 88: 55-72.
[http://dx.doi.org/10.1016/B978-0-12-394622-5.00003-1] [PMID: 22391299]

[17] Regan JL, Schumacher D, Staudte S, *et al.* Non-canonical hedgehog signaling is a positive regulator of the wnt pathway and is required for the survival of colon cancer stem cells. Cell Rep 2017; 21(10): 2813-2828.
[http://dx.doi.org/10.1016/j.celrep.2017.11.025]

[18] Findakly S, Choudhury A, Daggubati V, Pekmezci M, Lang UE, Raleigh DR. Meningioma cells

express primary cilia but do not transduce ciliary Hedgehog signals. Acta Neuropathol Commun 2020;8(1):114.
[http://dx.doi.org/10.1186/s40478-020-00994-7]

[19]  Sun J, Shin DY, Eiseman M, *et al.* SLITRK5 is a negative regulator of hedgehog signaling in osteoblasts. Nat Commun 2021; 12(1): 4611.
[http://dx.doi.org/10.1038/s41467-021-24819-w] [PMID: 34326333]

[20]  Demirdöven M, Yazgan H, Korkmaz M, G AG, Tonbul A. Case report smith-lemli-opitz syndrome: a case with annular pancreas. Case Rep Pediatr 2014: 2014:623926.
[http://dx.doi.org/10.1155/2014/623926]

[21]  Gailani MR, Bale AE. Developmental genes and cancer: role of patched in basal cell carcinoma of the skin. J Natl Cancer Inst 1997; 89(15): 1103-9.
[http://dx.doi.org/10.1093/jnci/89.15.1103] [PMID: 9262247]

[22]  Hahn H, Wicking C, Zaphiropoulos PG, *et al.* Mutations of the human homolog of Drosophila patched in the nevoid basal cell carcinoma syndrome. Cell 1996; 85(6): 841-51.
[http://dx.doi.org/10.1016/S0092-8674(00)81268-4] [PMID: 8681379]

[23]  Goodrich LV, Scott MP. Hedgehog and patched in neural development and disease. Neuron 1998; 21(6): 1243-57.
[http://dx.doi.org/10.1016/S0896-6273(00)80645-5] [PMID: 9883719]

[24]  Murone M, Rosenthal A, de Sauvage FJ. Hedgehog signal transduction: from flies to vertebrates. Exp Cell Res 1999; 253(1): 25-33.
[http://dx.doi.org/10.1006/excr.1999.4676] [PMID: 10579908]

[25]  Cochrane CR, Szczepny A, Watkins DN, Cain JE. Hedgehog signaling in the maintenance of cancer stem cells. Cancers (Basel) 2015; 1554–85.
[http://dx.doi.org/10.3390/cancers7030851]

[26]  Tostar U, Malm CJ, Meis-Kindblom JM, Kindblom LG, Toftgård R, Undén AB. Deregulation of the hedgehog signalling pathway: a possible role for the *PTCH* and *SUFU* genes in human rhabdomyoma and rhabdomyosarcoma development. J Pathol 2006; 208(1): 17-25.
[http://dx.doi.org/10.1002/path.1882] [PMID: 16294371]

[27]  Kinzler KW, Bigner SH, Bigner DD, Trent JM, Law ML, O'Brien SJ, *et al.* Identification of an amplified, highly expressed gene in a human GLIoma. Science (80- ). 1987; 236(4797): 70–3.
[http://dx.doi.org/10.1126/science.3563490]

[28]  Doheny D, Manore SG, Wong GL, Lo HW. Hedgehog Signaling and Truncated GLI1 in Cancer. Cells 2020; 9(9): 2114.
[http://dx.doi.org/10.3390/cells9092114] [PMID: 32957513]

[29]  Lee EY, Ji H, Ouyang Z, *et al.* Hedgehog pathway-regulated gene networks in cerebellum development and tumorigenesis. Proc Natl Acad Sci USA 2010; 107(21): 9736-41.
[http://dx.doi.org/10.1073/pnas.1004602107] [PMID: 20460306]

[30]  Duman-Scheel M, Weng L, Xin S, Du W. Hedgehog regulates cell growth and proliferation by inducing Cyclin D and Cyclin E. Nature 2002; 417(6886): 299-304.
[http://dx.doi.org/10.1038/417299a] [PMID: 12015606]

[31]  Skoda AM, Simovic D, Karin V, Kardum V, Vranic S, Serman L. The role of the Hedgehog signaling pathway in cancer: A comprehensive review. Bosn J Basic Med Sci 2018;18(1):8-20.
[http://dx.doi.org/10.17305/bjbms.2018.2756]

[32]  Alvarez-trotta A, Wang Z, Shersher E, Li B. The bromodomain inhibitor IBET-151 attenuates vismodegib- resistant esophageal adenocarcinoma growth through reduction of GLI signaling. Oncotarget 2020;11(33):3174-3187.
[http://dx.doi.org/10.18632/oncotarget.27699]

[33]  Stanton BZ, Peng LF, Stanton BZ, Stanton BZ. Small-molecule modulators of the Sonic Hedgehog

signaling pathway. Mol Biosyst 2010;6(1):44-54.
[http://dx.doi.org/10.1039/B910196A]

[34] Scharf. PMZANR. Vismodegib. StatPearls 2021; 7(1): 123.

[35] Carpenter RL, Ray H. Efficacy and safety of sonic hedgehog pathway inhibitors in cancer. Drug Saf 2019; 42(2): 263-79.
[http://dx.doi.org/10.1007/s40264-018-0777-5] [PMID: 30649745]

[36] An X, Bai Q, Bai F, Shi D, Liu H, Yao X. Deciphering the allosteric effect of antagonist vismodegib on smoothened receptor deactivation using metadynamics simulation preparation of simulation systems. Front Chem 2019; 7: 406.
[http://dx.doi.org/10.3332/ecancer.2018.824]

[37] Dong X, Wang C, Chen Z, Zhao W. Overcoming the resistance mechanisms of Smoothened inhibitors. Drug Discov Today 2018; 23(3): 704-10.
[http://dx.doi.org/10.1016/j.drudis.2018.01.012] [PMID: 29326074]

[38] Pantziarka P, Sukhatme V, Crispino S, Bouche G, Meheus L, Sukhatme VP. Repurposing drugs in oncology (ReDO) selective PDE5 inhibitors as anti-cancer agents. 1853; 1–22.

[39] Carballo GB, Honorato JR, de Lopes GPF, Spohr TCLS. A highlight on Sonic hedgehog pathway. Cell Commun Signal 2018; 16(1): 11.
[http://dx.doi.org/10.1186/s12964-018-0220-7] [PMID: 29558958]

[40] Sheikh A, Alvi AA, Aslam HM, Haseeb A. Hedgehog pathway inhibitors – current status and future prospects. Infect Agent Cancer 2012; 7(1): 29.
[http://dx.doi.org/10.1186/1750-9378-7-29] [PMID: 22214493]

# CHAPTER 10

# Promising Natural Agents for Targeting Micro-RNAs in Cancer

**Rumi Mahata¹, Subhabrata Das¹, Suman Mondal¹, Surya Kanta Dey¹, Anirban Majumder¹ and Sujata Maiti Choudhury¹,***

*¹ Biochemistry, Molecular Endocrinology and Reproductive Physiology Laboratory, Department of Human Physiology, Vidyasagar University, Midnapore, West Bengal, Pin-721102, India*

**Abstract:** Micro-RNAs, a family of small non-coding RNAs of 20-22 nucleotides, are evolutionarily preserved, and regulatory RNAs that negatively control gene expression also play an important role in all biological pathways in multicellular organisms by inducing feedback mechanisms that safeguard key biological processes including cell proliferation, differentiation, and apoptosis. The 3′ UTR of the target mRNAs is the binding site of micro-mRNAs, to induce translational repression by mRNA degradation or inhibition of protein synthesis from m-RNA while miRNA interaction with promoter region has been reported to induce transcription. Many natural products and dietary phytochemicals possess anti-cancer properties along with their tested antioxidant, anti-inflammatory, and anti-proliferative effects. Natural agents including (-)-resveratrol, curcumin, indole-3-carbinol, isoflavone, epigallocatechin-3-gallate, and 3,3'-diindolylmethane could modify miRNA expression, therefore reverse the epithelial-mesenchymal transition, causing the induction of apoptosis as well as the inhibition of cancer cell growth leading towards the advances of the efficacy of conventional cancer therapeutics. This review paper focuses on the precise targeting of mi-RNAs by natural agents that could open a newer line of attack for the complete eradication of tumors by killing drug-resistant cells to improve survival outcomes in patients with malignancy. In this chapter, we have paid attention to the use of natural products for mi-RN--mediated chemo-preventive and therapeutic approaches in various cancers, with the aim to extensively identify their pharmacological prospective.

**Keywords:** Chemo-preventive, Cancer therapeutics, Gene expression, Induction of Apoptosis, Micro-RNA, Natural Products.

## INTRODUCTION

Despite the advances in different cancer therapies, cancer is still the second leading cause of death worldwide. About 1,898,160 new cancer cases and 608,570

---
* **Corresponding author Sujata Maiti Choudhury:** Biochemistry, Molecular Endocrinology and Reproductive Physiology Laboratory, Department of Human Physiology, Vidyasagar University, Midnapore, West Bengal, Pin-721102, India; E-mail: sujata_vu@mail.vidyasagar.ac.in

**Ashok Kumar Pandurangan (Ed.)**

cancer deaths were expected to occur in 2021 in the United States. Among all incident cases in men, 46% constitute prostate, lung, bronchus, and colorectal cancers whereas prostate cancer alone accounts for 26%. In women, breast cancer, lung cancer, and CRCs account for 50% of all new diagnoses, while breast cancer alone accounts for 30% of female cancers [1]. The primary treatment of cancer includes surgery, chemotherapy, radiotherapy, and palliative care along with immunotherapy, stem cell therapy, hormonal therapy, and gene therapy. The treatment should be provided depending on the size, type, and location of the tumor, and also metastasis diagnosis depending on the health of the patient. Different approaches have been used for targeting cancer in three ways, one is by expressing a gene to encourage apoptosis or enhance tumor sensitivity to conservative drug-radiation therapy, the second one is by inserting a wild-type tumor suppressor gene to compensate for its damage and the third one is by blocking the expression of an oncogene by using antisense by RNA or DNA for enhancing the immunogenicity of the tumor to stimulate immune cell recognition [2].

Micro-RNAs are a highly conserved family of small non-coding RNAs of 20-22 nucleotides that can regulate a wide array of biological processes including cell proliferation, differentiation, apoptosis, and others [3]. Normally miRNAs belong to the heterogeneous class of non-coding RNAs, that can reduce translation by binding to the 3'- untranslated regions (UTRs) of target mRNA, thus triggering mRNA degradation and causing inhibition of protein translation [4]. They regulate gene expression both at the posttranslational and posttranscriptional levels [5]. Up to now, in humans, more than 2500 miRNAs have been isolated, and miRNA-conserved targets control around $1/3^{rd}$ of all human genes [4]. Individual miRNA plays a specific function in cells. miRNAs have been found to be severely dysregulated in cancer cells compared to normal healthy cells. miRNAs have different targets on genes by inhibiting or overexpressing the specific gene and miRNAs show a potential effect by inhibiting cancer [6]. Natural products could sensitize cancer cells to therapeutic agents by altering miRNA expression or function, therefore benefiting cancer patients [7]. As natural agents exercise their antineoplastic effects by targeting multiple signaling pathways, and miRNAs regulate various biological processes comprising cell proliferation and apoptosis or programmed cell death, it is assumed that miRNAs could take a key role in governing response towards natural agents. Hence, In the last few decades in cancer therapy, natural agents have gained attention for their applications in the modulation of miRNAs expression.

## miRNA Synthesis

It is well known that microRNAs (miRNAs), short non-coding regulatory RNAs are found to be dysregulated in almost all types of cancers and play significant roles in cancer growth and progression [8]. RNA interference (RNAi) has come into the limelight in the antisense world in the last few years in the therapeutic market. There has been a significant effort to investigate miRNAs' processing in animals and plants. The synthesis of miRNAs starts from DNA sequences, called miRNA genes, or the clusters, genes, or polycistronic transcripts, respectively. Alternatively, the miRNAs can be restricted within an intron or untranslated region (UTR) of a protein-coding gene [9]. From the miRNA gene, miRNAs are transcribed to a primary miRNA (pri-miRNA) by RNA pol-II that also possesses one or more hairpin structures within the miRNA [8]. In animal cells, the biogenesis of miRNA is Drosha and DGCR8 dependent, those are not found in plant cells. Drosha and Dicer, two RNase III enzymes can form mature miRNA in an evolutionary conserved process (Fig. **1**). Pri-miRNA is the substrate of DROSHA. The miRNA hairpins are acknowledged and cleaved by a heterotrimeric complex of DROSHA and two molecules of DGCR8 (DiGeorge syndrome critical region 8), a double-stranded RNA binding protein that releases precursor miRNAs (pre-miRNAs). Then exportin-5 (EXP-5) transports the pre-miRNA, connected with Ran-GTP into the cytoplasm where they are further processed by Dicer, an RNase III type protein to develop mature miRNAs and loaded onto the Argonaute (ago) protein to form the effector RNA-induced silencing complex (RISC) [10, 11]. Dicer, Argonaute2, and TRBP are vital components in the formation of the RISC-loading complex (RLC), thus contributing to the formation of short RNAs [12]. Another alternative pathway for miRNA biosynthesis is Dicer-independent. After the transcription and cleavage by Drosha, the precursor binds to Ago2. As it is a dicer-independent, the Ago2 splits the star strand [13]. Fig. (**1**) represents the overview of biosynthesis of microRNAs.

## MicroRNA (miRNAs) in the Development of Tumorigenesis and Carcinogenesis

Several research articles have been reported that are associated with the process of tumorigenesis and carcinogenesis (Fig. **2**). The exact role of miRNAs in the molecular mechanism of initiation, promotion, progression, and metastasis of some cancers was recognized previously. They employ a critical role in the mechanism of programmed cell death as well as cellular differentiation by regulating tumor suppressors and oncogenes. With the ability to regulate the expression of a lot of genes, miRNAs have the ability to modulate many cellular pathways. Different investigators have reported that about half of the miRNAs are related to the regions of the genome coding for oncogenes. To identify the role of miRNAs in cancer pathogenesis, specific miRNAs overexpression or misexpression are to be studied to explain the initiation and development of different types of malignancies that are involved in human cancers and further establish the role of miRNAs as biomarkers in cancer diagnostics [15]. miR-17-92 cluster includes six miRNAs (miR-17, miR-18a, miR-19a, miR-20a, miR-19b-1, and miR-92-1), which are overexpressed in a variety of solid tumors and different cancers of the breast, colon, lung, pancreas, prostate, and stomach as well as in lymphomas [16].

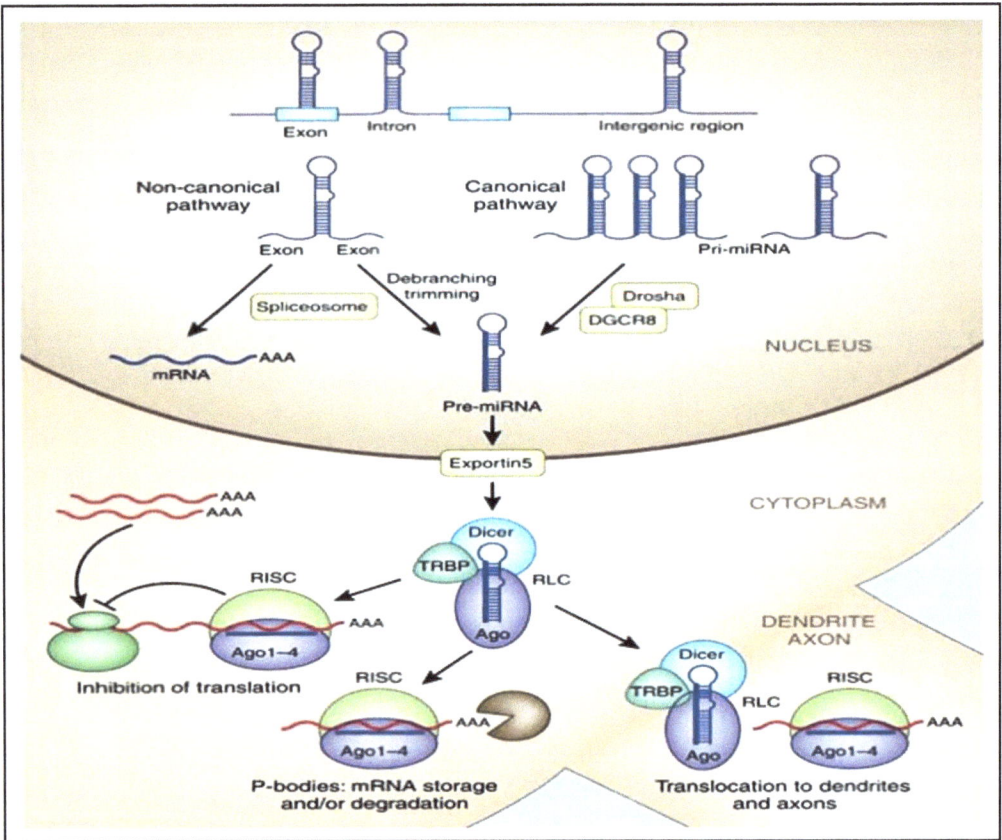

**Fig. (1).** Overview of biosynthesis of microRNAs [14]. After synthesis from the miRNA gene cluster, the pri-miRNA goes through two pathways one is **a**) Dorsha Dependent, where the long pri-miRNA is cleaved into short Pri-miRNA by the microprocessor of Dorsha and DGCR8. Another is **b**) Dorsha-independent where Pri-miRNA is cleaved by debranching enzymes instead of Dorsha. Then the pre-miRNA is transported to cytosol by Exportin5 and then processed by Dicer dependent or independent pathway to form the mature miRNA. Then this mature miRNA is loaded onto the RISC complex and mediates the gene suppression by mRNA degradation or translation inhibition.

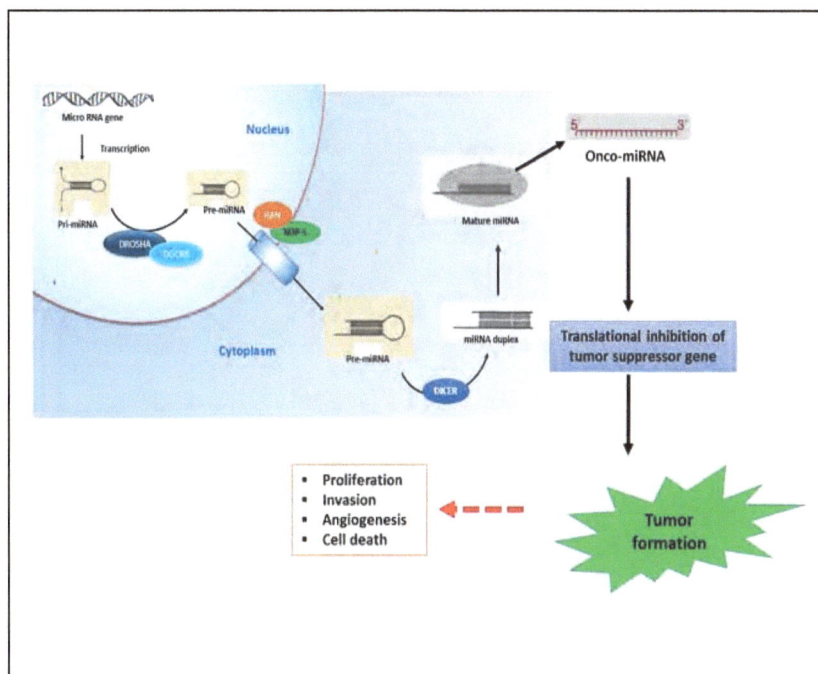

**Fig. (2).** Role of miRNA in tumorigenesis and carcinogenesis.

## Modulation of miRNA Expression in Cancer Using Phytocompounds

Natural phytocompounds and their derivatives have been widely used in various medicinal industries for the treatment of cancer, diabetes, gastrointestinal diseases, and obesity. Due to having chemical complexity, biological function, novel structure, and less deleterious effects on normal cells, some natural product compounds exhibit an anti-tumor potential by targeting cellular signaling pathways [17]. The multi-functional role of natural products offers a great advantage to deal with tumorigeneses; which is a multistage process that is triggered by the dysregulation of many cellular signaling pathways [18]. This is possibly one of the best believable explanations of why single chemotherapy often fails in the therapeutics of cancer. Exerting effects on numerous target sites, natural products are believed to be more effective in cancer therapy. Besides exhibiting other potential biological activities, the recent data demonstrated that natural products exhibit anti-proliferative properties by modulating cancer epigenetics [19]. Since natural compounds and miRNAs, both exert an impact on numerous cellular targets. So, there is a strong notion that natural products have the ability to modulate miRNAs and pave the way for future therapeutics for many diseases including cancer. Recent studies have demonstrated that miRNAs can be regulated by natural agents such as curcumin and resveratrol, resulting in the suppression of tumor growth, drug resistance, and metastasis (Fig. **3**). Here, in this chapter, natural products associated with miRNA regulation in tumorigenesis prevention have been discussed and their possible mechanisms of action have also been evaluated.

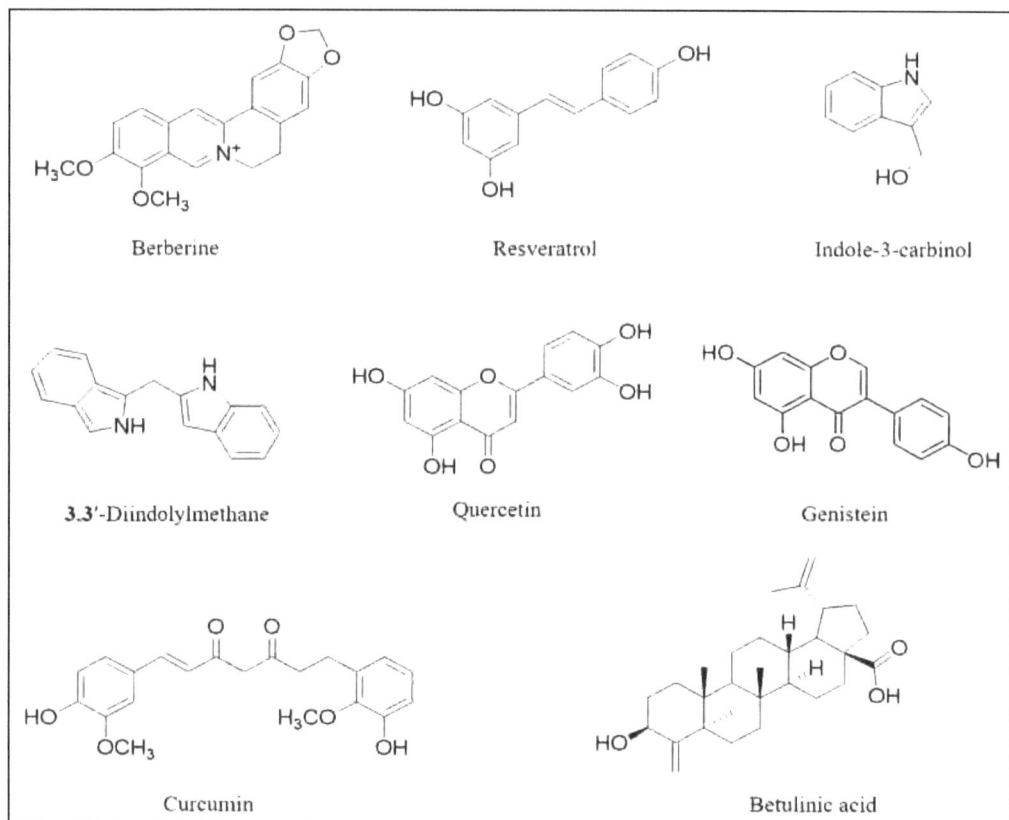

**Fig. (3).** Structures of some natural phytochemicals which modulate miRNAs (All the structures are drawn from Chemdraw pro 8.0 software).

## Resveratrol

Resveratrol (3,4',5-trihydroxystilbene) is a natural flavonoid or phytoextract derived from various plants such as mulberry, grapes, red wine, peanut, *etc.*, which shows several potential biological activities including, hepatoprotective anti-tumor, anti-cancer, and antioxidant activities [20, 21]. In MCF-7 and MDA-MB-231 breast cancer cell lines, carvacrol treatment showed a dose-dependent down-regulation of anti-apoptotic proteins [Bcl-2 and X-linked inhibitor of apoptosis protein (XIAP)] by key tumor-suppressive miRNAs miR-125b-5p, miR-200c-3p, miR-409-3p, miR-122-5p and miR-542-3p. This induction of resveratrol-mediated tumor suppressor miRNAs diminishes CDKs, X-linked inhibitor of anti-apoptosis protein (*XIAP*), and B-cell lymphoma 2 (Bcl-2) and caspase activation [22]. Triacetyl resveratrol (TCRV) inhibited epithelial-mesenchymal transition (EMT) in pancreatic cancer cells *via* the upregulation of miR-200a, miR-200b, and miR-200c, and the inhibition of Zeb1 expression on EMT is presumably exerted through the suppression of the Shh pathway and the upregulation of miR-200 [23]. Resveratrol reduces the tumor growth of glioblastoma cells by the downregulation of oncomirs (miR-19, miR-21, and miR-30a-5p) and restores the expression of tumor suppressor miRNAs [24]. Resveratrol exhibits an anti-tumor mechanism by enhancing the expression of tumor suppressors miR-34a, miR-424, and miR-503 in breast cancer cells, modifying the p53 signaling pathway and suppressing heterogeneous nuclear ribonucleoprotein A1 (HNRNPA1) by inducing miR-424 and miR-503 to prevent breast cancer tumorigenesis [25]. An experiment on breast cancer by downregulating miR-17 resveratrol suppressed c-Myc expression, which inhibited the transcription of the miR-17-92 cluster. MiR-17 expression inversely promoted MICA and MICB expression [26]. Resveratrol has the ability to prevent cell invasion and migration through the suppression of ROS/miR-21-mediated activation and glycolysis in pancreatic stellate cells [27]. By moderating tumor suppressor miR-200c, resveratrol decreases colorectal cancer cell viability, invasion, epithelial-mesenchymal transition and have the ability to induce cell death [28]. It was also found that resveratrol can inhibit the miR-221 regulating NF-κB activity and leading to a converse effect on TGF by miR-22,1 which is a tumor suppressor gene in melanoma [29]. In acute lymphoblastic leukemia, it was found that resveratrol decreased the overexpression of miR-196b/miR-1290 and can elevate IGFBP3 expression thereby exerting antitumor effects by inhibiting proliferation, cell cycle arrest, apoptosis, and migration inhibition [30].

## Berberine

Berberine is one of the main alkaloids, which has been widely used in China due to its extensive biological activities, such as anti-inflammation, antioxidative, and anti-diabetic effects. In addition, berberine also shows antitumor activity by interfering in tumor development [31]. From the study of Lu *et al.*, by interfering with the miR-21 expression and promoting protein ITGβ4 and PDCD4 expression in the human colon cancer cell lines, berberine can suppress cell viability, induce apoptosis and increase caspase-3 activity leading to apoptosis in HCT-116 cells [32]. Berberine has the ability to upregulate miR-373 *via* EGR1 activation that can inhibit AKT1-mTOR-S6K in hepatocytes, which was critical in the development of hepatosteatosis [33]. In ovarian cancer cells (SKOV3 and 3AO), berberine has the ability to inhibit proliferation, migration, and invasion by promoting miR-145 expression and decreasing MMP16 expression [34]. In human multiple myeloma cells, berberine suppresses NF-κB nuclear translocation *via* Set9-mediated lysine methylation, by dose-dependent downregulation of miR-21, which induces apoptosis [35]. Berberine treatment increases the expression level of miR-21-3p in the HepG2 human hepatoma cell line. The overexpression of miR-21-3p increased the S-adenosylmethionine (SAM) contents in cells, which causes growth disadvantages for hepatoma cells. The overexpression of miR-2--3p suppresses growth and induces apoptosis in HepG2 cells by targeting methionine adenosyltransferase (MAT) MAT2A and MAT2B [36].

## Indole-3-Carbinol (I3C)

The indole-3-carbinol (I3C), a natural glucosinolate, is found in *Brassica* vegetables such as cauliflower, cabbage, radish, broccoli, turnip, kale, and brussels sprouts. 3,3'-diindolylmethane (DIM) is a noticeable product found when I3C goes through condensation reactions in the stomach [37]. It is reported that both I3C and DIM modulate many regulatory genes of the cell cycle, signal transduction, cell proliferation, apoptosis, and other cellular processes [38]. Treatment of indole-3-carbinol (I3C) can repress the AKT pathway by enhancing the expression of phosphatase and PTEN in hepatocellular carcinoma by reducing the expression of miR-21 and miR-221&222 both *in vitro* and *in vivo* [39]. Vinyl carbamate-treated mice were given Indole-3-Carbamate in the diet, and the expressions of miR-31, miR-130a, miR-146b, miR-377, and miR-21 were reduced. Without I3C, the mir-31, miR-130a, miR-146b, miR-377, and miR-21 were upregulated and miR-1 and miR-143 were downregulated in lung tumors [40]. I3C enhances the cytotoxicity of gemcitabine-resistant human pancreatic cancer cells by downregulation of miR-21, which in turn increases the expression of PDCD4 thereby indicating apoptosis [41].

## Quercetin

Quercetin is a kind of flavonoid compound present in apples, onions, red wine, and tea and is widely used in the daily diet. From previous research works, it has been found that quercetin exhibits many biological effects including anti-inflammatory, anti-oxidation, and anti-cancer. Quercetin can enhance the tumor suppressor miR-143 by autophagy targeting Gamma-aminobutyric acid receptor-associated *protein*-like 1 (GABARAPL1) in gastric cancer [42]. Quercetin diminishes the cell viability and abrogates tumor cellular invasion, migration and MMP-9, and MMP-2 by upregulating miR-16 and HOXA10 in oral cancer cells [43]. In this study, quercetin exhibited an excellent effect on inhibiting human breast cancer cell proliferation by up-regulating miR-146a expression. miR-146a can induce apoptosis through cleaved caspase-3 activation and mitochondrial-dependent pathways, and by inhibiting invasion through down-regulating the expression of EGFR [44]. Quercetin has the ability to upregulate the let-7c miRNA expression in pancreatic ductal carcinoma (PDA) cells by inducing NUMB-like endocytic adaptor protein (Numbl) expression, which abrogates the Notch signaling pathway that prevents pancreatic tumorigenesis [45]. Anti-tumor mechanism of quercetin in liver cancer was identified through the p53-related pathway. In this pathway, the miR-34a is an element of a feedback loop of p53 and SIRT1, which will greatly improve the p53-related apoptosis signaling pathway [46]. Quercetin induces apoptosis in ovarian cancer cells (SKOV-3) by upregulating miR-145 expression [47].

### Epigallocatechin-3-Gallate (EGCG)

Epigallocatechin-3-gallate is the major polyphenol found in green tea (*Camellia sinensis*), which shows anti-proliferative, anti-inflammatory, anti-mutagenic, anti-oxidative as well as anticancer activities [48, 49]. EGCG is one of the most widely used natural compounds to identify the regulation of miRNA expression. EGCG has the ability to up-regulate the miRNA-let-7b expression through activating laminin receptor signaling(67LR) in melanoma cells. EGCG inducing up-regulation of let-7b expression can cause the 67LR-dependent cAMP or protein kinase A (PKA) or protein phosphatase 2A [50]. EGCG has the ability to induce miRNA-mediated regulation in NNK-induced mouse lung cancer. By upregulating miR-210, EGCG plays a critical role in lung cancer inhibition *in vivo* [51]. Another report published that EGCG can suppress growth by upregulating tumor suppressor miRNAs (miR-29a, miR-125b, miR-210, and miR-203) in human cervical cancer cells (HeLa, CaSki, SiHa, and C33A) infected with different types of human papillomavirus [52]. EGCG sensitizes cisplatin-mediated resistance and reduces CSC-like phenotypic features in NSCLC by upregulating and downregulating the expression of miR-485 and CD44, respectively [53]. From these studies, it was found that EGCG exhibits promising anti-tumor potential by modulating miRNAs. EGCG can downregulate miR-25 expression that leads to induce apoptosis and disruption in the cell cycle at the G2/M phase and increase PARP, pro-caspase-3, and pro-caspase-9, leading to apoptosis. Furthermore, the refurbishment of miR-25 inhibited EGCG-induced cell death [54].

### Curcumin

One of the important natural products having a high medicinal value compound is curcumin (diferuloylmethane), an important phytochemical from the rhizomes of turmeric (*Curcuma longa*). Curcumin has numerous health benefits as well as shows anti-tumor, anti-inflammatory, and antioxidant properties [55, 56]. Curcumin modifies the expression of a series of miRNAs. In metastatic breast cancer cells, miR181b down-modulates CXCL1 by binding to 3′-UTR. Curcumin can up-regulate miR181b and down-regulate inflammatory cytokines CXCL1 and -2 in breast cancer cells [57]. By NF-κB signaling, curcumin with the drug temozolomide induced miR-146a, which inhibited glioblastoma cell growth and survival [58]. By upregulating tumor suppressor miR-34a in prostate cancer cells, curcumin has the ability to inhibit β-catenin and cell cycle-associated regulatory proteins (cyclin D1, PCNA, and p21). As a result, curcumin can potentially cause cell cycle arrest and apoptosis [59]. Curcumin combined with radiation in bladder cancer cells (T24 and HT-1376) modifies 17 different miRNA expressions, including downregulating miR-1246 expression which reduces the cell viability and clonogenic property and causes cell cycle arrest at the G0/G1 phase. MicroRNA-1246 regulates the radio-sensitizing effect of curcumin in bladder cancer cells *via* activating P53 [60]. Curcumin exhibits an anti-cancer effect on a schwannoma cell line (RT4) by targeting miRNA 344a-3p which inhibits BCL-2, an anti-apoptotic protein [61]. By negatively targeting the miR-21 and decreasing phosphorylation of Akt and also by upregulating tumor suppressor protein PTEN curcumin triggers cell apoptosis in gastric carcinoma cells (MGC-803). Curcumin negatively regulates cell viability, and abrogates tumor cell invasion and migration by upregulating tumor suppressor miR-99a in gastric cancer cells [62]. By downregulating the expression of miR-27a, curcumin inhibits the growth and motility capability of thymic carcinoma cells and also retracts Notch and mTOR signaling pathways [63].

## Genistein

Genistein is a natural product compound of the isoflavone group extracted in large quantities from numerous plants, including fava beans, lupins, and soybeans. Genistein suppresses the appearance of many oncomirs and also helps in the appearance of miRNAs, which can suppress tumors. Genistein upregulates the appearance of let-7d, a tumor suppressor, and by regulating its 3'-UTR, it drastically decreases the appearance of stellar cell fibrosis marker thrombospondin 1 (THBS1). Through this process, it develops fibrosis, a pancreatic carcinogenesis marker [64]. In resistant ovarian cancer cells, Genistein analog breaks down their resistance mechanism by downregulating PI3K/AKT signaling, and by augmenting miR-7d, it suppresses nuclear c-Myc appearance [65]. Propofol and genistein or alone genistein can pause the cell division or proliferation in human gliosarcoma cells (U251). Its anti-proliferative activity enhances mediated cell death by apoptosis due to miRNA-218. The overexpressed miRNA-218 sets off the number of proteins that are associated with programmed cell death like the Bax gene and Bad gene and at the same time reduces the inflammatory cytokines like TNF-α, 1L-6, and IL-1β proteins [66]. Mcl-1 has oncogenic properties and plays a key role in laryngeal cancer formation. Genistein treatment always increases miR-1469, because it increases the production of tumor suppressive protein p53. This miR-1469 surge promotes apoptosis and inhibits Mcl-1 expression, as a result, it decreases the probability of cancer cell survival and proliferation [67]. When the drug Genistein and oxidized-LDL are applied in combination, this decreases the production of reactive oxygen species significantly and assists in reversing oxidative damage in HUVECs. This arrangement upregulates the catalase and superoxide dismutase production through miR-34a/sirtuin-1 axis regulating, which in turn supports epigenetic modulation and translocation, like deacetylation of forkhead box 03A (FOXO3A) [68]. The treatment of genistein induces programmed cell death of human retinoblastoma cells (Y79) and also decreases clonogenic ability, cell survival, and proliferation. Genistein promotes the modification of ATP binding cassette subfamily E member 1 (ABCE1) after translation, which is assisted by miR-145 and exerts a suppressed effect on cellular growth [69]. Gemcitabine-resistant (GR) pancreatic cancer cells became sensible to chemotherapy due to a dual drug combination of miR-223 inhibitor and genistein, which helps to decrease miR-223 formation. As a result, cell migration and invasion properties of EMT cells are decreased [70]. In breast cancer cells, its multidrug resistance property is encountered by escalating the production of ABCG2 and ABCC1 at the translation level. Interestingly, genistein promotes the production of ABC transporters by decreasing the miR-181a expression, which interferes with the production of ABC drug transporters [71]. Due to the application of genistein in breast cancer cells, miR-155 production is downregulated. This assists in developing pro-apoptotic genes p21, FOXO3, and PTEN and at the same time, promotes the reduction in cell viability which all together helps induce apoptosis [72]. In multiple myeloma (MM) cells, U266 miR-29b expression is promoted by genistein as it decreases the NF-κB signaling pathway. In cell apoptosis, caspase-3 is a very important protein, as its population is increased by miR-29b, and it leads to cell apoptosis and decreases cell viability. These studies prove genistein as a promising anti-cancer agent as it targets the regulation of miRNAs and interferes with different signaling pathways [73].

## Paclitaxel

Paclitaxel is a diterpenoid type of plant alkaloid derived from yew tree bark for its anti-neoplastic effects. Paclitaxel-induced chemotherapy results in the apoptosis of tumor cells by diminishing tubulin function and inhibiting cell division [74]. Paclitaxel induces chemotherapeutic resistance in cancer patients, mainly in lung cancer patients. In paclitaxel-resistant lung cancer patients, (A549) up-regulated miR-421 reduces KEAP1 gene expression and enhances malignant cell metastasis, leading to colonization of lung cancer cells [75]. Paclitaxel-resistant NSCLCH460 cell analysis showed 43 modulated miRNAs, out of which, 28 miRNAs were suppressed and 15 miRNAs were overexpressed equated to normal

H460 cells. Further analysis has shown the dysregulation of miRNAs (miR-76--3p, miR-362-3p, miR-6507-3p) due to paclitaxel resistance by affecting MAPT in NSCLC (H460) cells [76]. In NSCLC cells, paclitaxel resistance property is headed by miR-4262 as it suppresses the formation of PTEN, a tumor suppressor protein. On the other hand, it activates the downstream PI3K/Akt pathway in NSCLC cells and ultimately helps in cell proliferation [77]. A bioinformatics study confirmed that the expression of tumor suppressor miR-5195-3p in paclitaxel-resistant triple negative TNBC cancer cells breaks their resistance property by targeting Eukaryotic translation initiation factor 4 alpha 2 (EIF4A2), and enhancing apoptosis, anti-proliferation effect, and inducing cell cycle arrest [78]. In breast cancer cells, paclitaxel resistance is overwhelmed by tumor suppressor miR-107. The accumulation of miR-107 targets TDP 52 and reduces their expression; as a result, in breast cancer cells, the expression of cyclin D1, Wnt1, and β-catenin is reduced and apoptosis is induced [79]. A persuasive experiment demonstrated that long intergenic-noncoding RNA 00511 (LINC00511) regulates paclitaxel-resistant breast cancer cells by positively regulating CDK 6 expression and inversely regulating miR-29c. Synchronized knockdown of LINC00511 and paclitaxel chemotherapy upregulates miR-29c and reduces paclitaxel resistance of cancer cells, where CDK 6 acts as a target of miR-29c [80]. miR-29c in nasopharyngeal cancer aims at integrin beta-1 (ITBG1), nullifies paclitaxel resistance, and starts apoptosis in nasopharyngeal cancer cells [81]. A combination of miR-34a and paclitaxel in CRC cells overpowers resistance, and induces tumor cell killing and cell cycle arrest [82]. miR-155-3p is dysregulated in breast cancer cells causing poor survival of breast cancer patients. However, the overexpression of miR-155-3p targets MYD88, and paclitaxel drug resistance modulates miRNA expression and various cell signaling pathways [83].

**Betulinic Acid (BA)**

Betulinic acid is a plant secondary metabolite extracted from various fruits, vegetables and plants, a pentacyclic triterpene in structure. Betulinic acid has a lot of pharmacological properties like hepatoprotective, anti-angiogenic anti-fibrotic, and immune-modulatory. Betulinic acid assists in the production of miR-21 and p66shc which have tumor-suppressive potential. In HCC cells, betulinic acid displays tumor suppressive potential as it upregulates the production of p53, which is assisted by miR-21. As soon as p53 is activated, it neutralizes ROS formation by unmasking pro-apoptotic proteins, as a result, it causes mitochondrial membrane depolarization. However, research demonstrated that N-nitrosodiethylamine/carbon tetrachloride (DEN/CCl4)-induced tumor growth is suppressed in mice by betulinic acid, which concealed Sod2 signaling in HCC cells [84]. On a different type of human cancer cell line, betulinic acid blocks cell division. Despite having cancer-protecting potential by regulating miRNAs, it could not destroy tumor cells through a conventional anti-cancer process like the initiation of programmed cell death, inhibition of cell migration, and invasion [85]. Furthermore, an investigation has suggested that a combination of miR-101 and miR-24-2 with betulinic acid performs an anti-tumor synergistic effect in pancreatic cancer cells (Mia PaCa-2, PANC-1) [86].

## Cucurbitacin B

Cucurbitacin B is a plant secondary metabolite found in cucumber, pumpkin, etc., which belongs to the tetracyclic triterpene group. Cucurbitacin B shows cancer-neutralizing potential in a wide range of cancer carcinomas. The expression of actin-filament-associated protein 1-antisense RNA 1 (AFAP1-ASI) is a key factor for cell proliferation in pancreatic cancer cells. Cucurbitacin B partially blocks the AFAP1-ASI formation; as a result, the cell cycle is paused at the G2 to M phase. Thus, pancreatic cancer cells lost their proliferative effect. According to a research report, cucurbitacin B positively regulates the appearance of miR-146b, which is well known for its tumor-suppressing activity. This can oppose any tumorigenic effect of pancreatic cancer cells in both *in vitro* and *in vivo* models as they target EGFR and AFAP1-AS1 and block cell proliferation [87]. Cucurbitacin increases cell survival, assisting in significant anticancer properties through programmed cell death type I (apoptosis) and initiating cell cycle blocking at the G1 to S phase by positively regulating miR-34a, miR-145, and miR-143. It continues this by upregulating the expressions of protein p21, and p27 and suppressing the protein, CDK4, pRb, E6, Rb, and cyclin D1 [88]. Other observations revealed that long non-coding RNA (lncRNA) GACAT3 has a great role in the proliferation of gastric cancer. In most cancers, GACAT3 basically acts as an oncogene as it is reported to act as a miRNA suppressor for high mobility group A1 (HMGA1). However, the appearance of GACAT3 suppresses the cucurbitacin-mediated programmed cell death in gastric cancer [89].

## Oleanolic Acid

Oleanolic acid is a plant secondary metabolite of the pentacyclic triterpenoid group. It has a significant tumor resistance activity. It enhanced the activity of tumor inhibitor miR-122 in *in vitro* and *in vivo* models. Myocyte enhancer factor 2D (MEF2D) helped in the transition from G2 to M as well as cell proliferation, and miR-122 interferes with the production of MEF2D at the translation level and prevents cancer cell growth. miR-122 corrupts the mRNA, which produces Cyclin G1 protein, a cell cycle enhancer. As a result, lung carcinoma cell division is arrested at the G2 to M phase and apoptosis is initiated [90]. Both these combined actions encounter the cell proliferation, drug resistance, and anti-cancer properties of cancer cells.

## Camptothecin

Camptothecin, is a pentacyclic quinoline alkaloid obtained from the Chinese tree, *Camptotheca acuminate*. It has been acknowledged as a potential anticancer drug inhibiting the topoisomerase I activity. It displays antitumor activity in various experimental tumor models [91]. Camptothecin can induce apoptosis in different human cancer cell lines by miR-125b-mediated mitochondrial pathway. MicroRNA-125b is downregulated by camptothecin. MicroRNA-125b targets the Bak1, Mcl1, and p53 expression after binding with 3'UTR regions of multiple genes linked with apoptosis [92]. Camptothecin inhibited HIF-1$\alpha$ by enhancing miR-155, miR-17-5p, and miR-18a in HeLa cells [93].

## Vincristine

Vincristine (VCR) is a common vinca-alkaloid chemotherapeutic drug synthesized from *Catharanthus roseus*. It is an antimitotic compound, and by disrupting microtubule dynamics, it arrests the cell cycle. Vincristine significantly modulated 24 miRNAs associated with drug resistance in HCT-8 cells. Among 24 miRNAs, 17 and 7 miRNAs were upregulated and downregulated, respectively [94]. Vincristine up-regulated the expression of miR-155. Vincristine sensitizes drug-resistant diffusion of large B-cell lymphoma (DLBCL) to programmed cell death [95].

## CONCLUSION

In the last few decades, it has been proven that miRNAs have the ability to do epigenetic modifications. The miRNA can bind to the 3' UTR region of a specific gene thereby causing upregulation or downregulation of the specific mRNA. As a result, they are involved in various diseases including cancer. The present review highlights the importance of miRNAs, and their capabilities in epigenetic modifications and in carcinogenesis, and focuses on how natural product compounds modulate miRNAs expression in cancer for chemo-preventive therapeutic purposes. Having different biological actions, natural products with their chemical complexity can modify the miRNAs' expression leading to the upregulation or downregulation of specific pathways involved in carcinogenesis. miRNAs have the ability to interfere in between the cellular pathways including apoptosis, cell cycle, inflammation, *etc.* The main purpose is to enhance the use of phytochemicals in cancer therapeutics through the modification of miRNA. There are many limitations or disadvantages to using raw phytochemicals. Nowadays, different strategies have been used for the modifications or in the delivery system for cell-specific transport of the miRNAs, which will be a great benefit for future drug development in modern medical science.

# LIST OF ABBREVIATIONS

| | |
|---|---|
| **Bcl-2** | B-cell lymphoma 2 |
| **CDK** | Cyclin Dependent Kinase |
| **c-Myc** | Cellular myelocytomatosis oncogene |
| **CXCL1C-X-C** | Motif Chemokine Ligand 1 |
| **DGCR8** | DiGeorge Syndrome Critical Region 8 |
| **EGFR** | Epidermal Growth Factor Receptor |
| **EMT** | Epithelial-Mesenchymal Transition |
| **EXP-5** | Exportin5 |
| **FOXO3** | The Forkhead Box O |
| **GACAT3** | Gastric *Cancer* Associated Transcript 3 |
| **HIF-1α** | Hypoxia-inducible Factor-1α |
| **HNRNPA1** | Heterogeneous Nuclear Ribonucleoprotein A1 |
| **IGFBP3** | Insulin-like Growth Factor Binding Protein 3 |
| **MAPT** | Microtubule-Associated Protein Tau |
| **MAT** | Methionine Adenosyltransferase |
| **MCF-7** | Michigan Cancer Foundation-7- A Breast Cancer Cell Line |
| **MDA-MB-231** | Human Mammary Carcinoma (triple Negative Breast Cancer Cell Line) |
| **MICA** | Major Histocompatibility Complex (mhc) Class I Chain-related Protein A |
| **MICB** | MHC Class I Chain-related Protein B |
| **miRNA** | Micro Ribonucleic Acid |
| **MMP** | Matrix Metalloproteinases |
| **mRNA** | Messenger Ribonucleic Acid |
| **NF-Kb** | Nuclear Factor Kappa |
| **PDCD4** | Programmed Cell Death 4 |
| **PI3K** | Phosphatidylinositol-3-kinase |
| **PTEN** | Phosphatase and Tensin Homolog |
| **Rb** | Retinoblastoma |
| **RISC** | RNA-induced Silencing Complex |
| **RLC** | RISC-Loading Complex |
| **RNA pol-II** | RNA Polymerase II |
| **RNA** | Ribonucleic Acid |
| **RNAi** | RNA Interference |
| **ROS** | Reactive Oxygen Species |
| **SAM** | S-adenosylmethionine |

| | |
|---|---|
| **TRBP** | Transactivating Response (tar) Rna-binding Protein |
| **UTR** | Untranslated Region |
| **XIAP** | X-linked Inhibitor of Apoptosis Protein |
| **Zeb1** | Zinc Finger E-box-binding Homeobox 1 |

# REFERENCES

[1]   Siegel RL, Miller KD, Jemal A. Cancer statistics, 2018. CA Cancer J Clin 2018; 68(1): 7-30.
[http://dx.doi.org/10.3322/caac.21442] [PMID: 29313949]

[2]   Esquela-Kerscher A, Slack FJ. Oncomirs — microRNAs with a role in cancer. Nat Rev Cancer 2006; 6(4): 259-69.
[http://dx.doi.org/10.1038/nrc1840] [PMID: 16557279]

[3]   Bartel DP. MicroRNAs: genomics, biogenesis, mechanism, and function. Cell. 2004, 23; 116(2): 281-97.
[http://dx.doi.org/10.1016/s0092-8674(04)00045-5]

[4]   Iorio MV, Croce CM. MicroRNAs in cancer: small molecules with a huge impact. J Clin Oncol 2009; 27(34): 5848-56.
[http://dx.doi.org/10.1200/JCO.2009.24.0317] [PMID: 19884536]

[5]   Maher SG, Bibby BA, Moody HL, Reid G. MicroRNAs and cancer. In: Therapy EC, Ed. Elsevier. 2015; pp. 67-90.

[6]   Gong A, Ge N, Yao W, Lu L, Liang H. RETRACTED ARTICLE: Aplysin enhances temozolomide sensitivity in glioma cells by increasing miR-181 level. Cancer Chemother Pharmacol 2014; 74(3): 531-8.
[http://dx.doi.org/10.1007/s00280-014-2534-5] [PMID: 25047724]

[7]   Iorio MV, Croce CM. MicroRNAs in cancer: small molecules with a huge impact. J Clin Oncol 2009; 27(34): 5848.
[PMID: 19884536]

[8]   Rodriguez A, Griffiths-Jones S, Ashurst JL, Bradley A. Identification of mammalian microRNA host genes and transcription units. Genome Res 2004; 14(10a): 1902-10.
[http://dx.doi.org/10.1101/gr.2722704] [PMID: 15364901]

[9]   Ha M, Kim VN. Regulation of microRNA biogenesis. Nat Rev Mol Cell Biol 2014; 15(8): 509-24.
[http://dx.doi.org/10.1038/nrm3838] [PMID: 25027649]

[10]   Treiber T, Treiber N, Meister G. Regulation of microRNA biogenesis and its crosstalk with other cellular pathways. Nat Rev Mol Cell Biol 2019; 20(1): 5-20.
[http://dx.doi.org/10.1038/s41580-018-0059-1] [PMID: 30228348]

[11]   Iorio MV, Ferracin M, Liu CG, *et al.* MicroRNA gene expression deregulation in human breast cancer. Cancer Res 2005; 65(16): 7065-70.
[http://dx.doi.org/10.1158/0008-5472.CAN-05-1783] [PMID: 16103053]

[12]   Chendrimada TP, Gregory RI, Kumaraswamy E, *et al.* TRBP recruits the Dicer complex to Ago2 for microRNA processing and gene silencing. Nature 2005; 436(7051): 740-4.
[http://dx.doi.org/10.1038/nature03868] [PMID: 15973356]

[13]   Cheloufi S, Dos Santos CO, Chong MMW, Hannon GJ. A dicer-independent miRNA biogenesis pathway that requires Ago catalysis. Nature 2010; 465(7298): 584-9.
[http://dx.doi.org/10.1038/nature09092] [PMID: 20424607]

[14]   O'Carroll D, Schaefer A. General principals of miRNA biogenesis and regulation in the brain. Neuropsychopharmacology 2013; 38(1): 39-54.

[http://dx.doi.org/10.1038/npp.2012.87] [PMID: 22669168]

[15]   Iqbal MA, Arora S, Prakasam G, Calin GA, Syed MA. MicroRNA in lung cancer: role, mechanisms, pathways and therapeutic relevance. Mol Aspects Med 2019; 70: 3-20.
[http://dx.doi.org/10.1016/j.mam.2018.07.003] [PMID: 30102929]

[16]   Mendell JT. miRiad roles for the miR-17-92 cluster in development and disease. Cell 2008; 133(2): 217-22.
[http://dx.doi.org/10.1016/j.cell.2008.04.001] [PMID: 18423194]

[17]   Efferth T, Saeed MEM, Kadioglu O, *et al.* Collateral sensitivity of natural products in drug-resistant cancer cells. Biotechnol Adv 2020; 38: 107342.
[http://dx.doi.org/10.1016/j.biotechadv.2019.01.009] [PMID: 30708024]

[18]   Rah B, Nayak D, Rasool R, *et al.* Reprogramming of molecular switching events in upr driven er stress: Scope for development of anticancer therapeutics. Curr Mol Med 2016; 16(8): 690-701.
[http://dx.doi.org/10.2174/1566524016666160829152658] [PMID: 27573195]

[19]   Li S, Kuo HCD, Yin R, *et al.* Epigenetics/epigenomics of triterpenoids in cancer prevention and in health. Biochem Pharmacol 2020; 175: 113890.
[http://dx.doi.org/10.1016/j.bcp.2020.113890] [PMID: 32119837]

[20]   Stagos D, Amoutzias GD, Matakos A, Spyrou A, Tsatsakis AM, Kouretas D. Chemoprevention of liver cancer by plant polyphenols. Food Chem Toxicol 2012; 50(6): 2155-70.
[http://dx.doi.org/10.1016/j.fct.2012.04.002] [PMID: 22521445]

[21]   Carter LG, D'Orazio JA, Pearson KJ. Resveratrol and cancer: focus on *in vivo* evidence. Endocr Relat Cancer 2014; 21(3): R209-25.
[http://dx.doi.org/10.1530/ERC-13-0171] [PMID: 24500760]

[22]   Venkatadri R, Muni T, Iyer AKV, Yakisich JS, Azad N. Role of apoptosis-related miRNAs in resveratrol-induced breast cancer cell death. Cell Death Dis 2016; 7(2): e2104.
[http://dx.doi.org/10.1038/cddis.2016.6] [PMID: 26890143]

[23]   Fu J, Shrivastava A, Shrivastava S, Srivastava R, Shankar S. Triacetyl resveratrol upregulates miRNA-200 and suppresses the Shh pathway in pancreatic cancer: A potential therapeutic agent. Int J Oncol 2019; 54(4): 1306-16.
[http://dx.doi.org/10.3892/ijo.2019.4700] [PMID: 30720134]

[24]   Wang G, Dai F, Yu K, *et al.* Resveratrol inhibits glioma cell growth *via* targeting oncogenic microRNAs and multiple signaling pathways. Int J Oncol 2015; 46(4): 1739-47.
[http://dx.doi.org/10.3892/ijo.2015.2863] [PMID: 25646654]

[25]   Otsuka K, Yamamoto Y, Ochiya T. Regulatory role of resveratrol, a microRNA-controlling compound, in *HNRNPA1* expression, which is associated with poor prognosis in breast cancer. Oncotarget 2018; 9(37): 24718-30.
[http://dx.doi.org/10.18632/oncotarget.25339] [PMID: 29872500]

[26]   Pan J, Shen J, Si W, *et al.* Resveratrol promotes MICA/B expression and natural killer cell lysis of breast cancer cells by suppressing c-Myc/miR-17 pathway. Oncotarget 2017; 8(39): 65743-58.
[http://dx.doi.org/10.18632/oncotarget.19445] [PMID: 29029468]

[27]   Yan B, Cheng L, Jiang Z, *et al.* Resveratrol inhibits ROS-promoted activation and glycolysis of pancreatic stellate cells *via* suppression of miR-21. Oxid Med Cell Longev. 2018:2018:1346958.
[http://dx.doi.org/10.1155/2018/1346958]

[28]   Karimi Dermani F, Saidijam M, Amini R, Mahdavinezhad A, Heydari K, Najafi R. Resveratrol inhibits proliferation, invasion, and epithelial–mesenchymal transition by increasing miR-200c expression in HCT-116 colorectal cancer cells. J Cell Biochem 2017; 118(6): 1547-55.
[http://dx.doi.org/10.1002/jcb.25816] [PMID: 27918105]

[29]   Wu F, Cui L. Resveratrol suppresses melanoma by inhibiting NF-κB/miR-221 and inducing TFG expression. Arch Dermatol Res 2017; 309(10): 823-31.

[http://dx.doi.org/10.1007/s00403-017-1784-6] [PMID: 28936555]

[30]     Zhou W, Wang S, Ying Y, Zhou R, Mao P. miR-196b/miR-1290 participate in the antitumor effect of resveratrol *via* regulation of IGFBP3 expression in acute lymphoblastic leukemia. Oncol Rep 2017; 37(2): 1075-83.
[http://dx.doi.org/10.3892/or.2016.5321] [PMID: 28000876]

[31]     Refaat A, Abdelhamed S, Saiki I, Sakurai H. Inhibition of p38 mitogen-activated protein kinase potentiates the apoptotic effect of berberine/tumor necrosis factor-related apoptosis-inducing ligand combination therapy. Oncol Lett 2015; 10(3): 1907-11.
[http://dx.doi.org/10.3892/ol.2015.3494] [PMID: 26622773]

[32]     Lü Y, Han B, Yu H, Cui Z, Li Z, Wang J. Berberine regulates the microRNA-21-ITGB4-PDCD4 axis and inhibits colon cancer viability. Oncol Lett 2018; 15(4): 5971-6.
[PMID: 29564000]

[33]     Li CH, Tang SC, Wong CH, Wang Y, Jiang J, Chen Y. Berberine induces miR-373 expression in hepatocytes to inactivate hepatic steatosis associated AKT-S6 kinase pathway. Eur J Pharmacol 2018; 825: 107-18.
[http://dx.doi.org/10.1016/j.ejphar.2018.02.035] [PMID: 29477657]

[34]     Li J, Zhang S, Wu L, Pei M, Jiang Y. Berberine inhibited metastasis through miR-145/MMP16 axis *in vitro*. J Ovarian Res 2021; 14(1): 4.
[http://dx.doi.org/10.1186/s13048-020-00752-2] [PMID: 33407764]

[35]     Hu H, Li K, Wang X, *et al.* Set9, NF-κB, and microRNA-21 mediate berberine-induced apoptosis of human multiple myeloma cells. Acta Pharmacol Sin 2013; 34(1): 157-66.
[http://dx.doi.org/10.1038/aps.2012.161] [PMID: 23247593]

[36]     Lo TF, Tsai WC, Chen ST. MicroRNA-21-3p, a berberine-induced miRNA, directly down-regulates human methionine adenosyltransferases 2A and 2B and inhibits hepatoma cell growth. PLoS One 2013; 8(9): e75628.
[http://dx.doi.org/10.1371/journal.pone.0075628] [PMID: 24098708]

[37]     Anderton MJ, Manson MM, Verschoyle RD, *et al.* Pharmacokinetics and tissue disposition of indole-3-carbinol and its acid condensation products after oral administration to mice. Clin Cancer Res 2004; 10(15): 5233-41.
[http://dx.doi.org/10.1158/1078-0432.CCR-04-0163] [PMID: 15297427]

[38]     Sarkar FH, Li Y. Indole-3-carbinol and prostate cancer. J Nutr 2004; 134(12) (Suppl.): 3493S-8S.
[http://dx.doi.org/10.1093/jn/134.12.3493S] [PMID: 15570059]

[39]     Wang X, He H, Lu Y, *et al.* Indole-3-carbinol inhibits tumorigenicity of hepatocellular carcinoma cells *via* suppression of microRNA-21 and upregulation of phosphatase and tensin homolog. Biochim Biophys Acta Mol Cell Res 2015; 1853(1): 244-53.
[http://dx.doi.org/10.1016/j.bbamcr.2014.10.017] [PMID: 25447674]

[40]     Melkamu T, Zhang X, Tan J, Zeng Y, Kassie F. Alteration of microRNA expression in vinyl carbamate-induced mouse lung tumors and modulation by the chemopreventive agent indole--carbinol. Carcinogenesis 2010; 31(2): 252-8.
[http://dx.doi.org/10.1093/carcin/bgp208] [PMID: 19748927]

[41]     Paik WH, Kim HR, Park JK, Song BJ, Lee SH, Hwang JH. Chemosensitivity induced by down-regulation of microRNA-21 in gemcitabine-resistant pancreatic cancer cells by indole-3-carbinol. Anticancer Res 2013; 33(4): 1473-81.
[PMID: 23564788]

[42]     Du F, Feng Y, Fang J, Yang M. MicroRNA-143 enhances chemosensitivity of Quercetin through autophagy inhibition *via* target GABARAPL1 in gastric cancer cells. Biomed Pharmacother 2015; 74: 169-77.
[http://dx.doi.org/10.1016/j.biopha.2015.08.005] [PMID: 26349981]

[43]    Zhao J, Fang Z, Zha Z, *et al*. Quercetin inhibits cell viability, migration and invasion by regulating miR-16/HOXA10 axis in oral cancer. Eur J Pharmacol 2019; 847: 11-8.
[http://dx.doi.org/10.1016/j.ejphar.2019.01.006] [PMID: 30639311]

[44]    Tao S, He H, Chen Q. Quercetin inhibits proliferation and invasion acts by up-regulating miR-146a in human breast cancer cells. Mol Cell Biochem 2015; 402(1-2): 93-100.
[http://dx.doi.org/10.1007/s11010-014-2317-7] [PMID: 25596948]

[45]    Nwaeburu CC, Bauer N, Zhao Z, *et al*. Up-regulation of microRNA let-7c by quercetin inhibits pancreatic cancer progression by activation of Numbl. Oncotarget 2016; 7(36): 58367-80.
[http://dx.doi.org/10.18632/oncotarget.11122] [PMID: 27521217]

[46]    Lou G, Liu Y, Wu S, *et al*. The p53/miR-34a/SIRT1 positive feedback loop in quercetin-induced apoptosis. Cell Physiol Biochem 2015; 35(6): 2192-202.
[http://dx.doi.org/10.1159/000374024] [PMID: 25896587]

[47]    Zhou J, Gong J, Ding C, Chen G. Quercetin induces the apoptosis of human ovarian carcinoma cells by upregulating the expression of microRNA-145. Mol Med Rep 2015; 12(2): 3127-31.
[http://dx.doi.org/10.3892/mmr.2015.3679] [PMID: 25937243]

[48]    Roy M, Chakrabarty S, Sinha D, Bhattacharya RK, Siddiqi M. Anticlastogenic, antigenotoxic and apoptotic activity of epigallocatechin gallate: a green tea polyphenol. Mutat Res 2003; 523-524: 33-41.
[http://dx.doi.org/10.1016/S0027-5107(02)00319-6] [PMID: 12628501]

[49]    Yamane T, Nakatani H, Kikuoka N, *et al*. Inhibitory effects and toxicity of green tea polyphenols for gastrointestinal carcinogenesis. Cancer 1996; 77(8) (Suppl.): 1662-7.
[http://dx.doi.org/10.1002/(SICI)1097-0142(19960415)77:8<1662::AID-CNCR36>3.0.CO;2-W] [PMID: 8608559]

[50]    Yamada S, Tsukamoto S, Huang Y, *et al*. Epigallocatechin-3-O-gallate up-regulates microRNA-let-7b expression by activating 67-kDa laminin receptor signaling in melanoma cells. Sci Rep 2016; 6(1): 19225.
[http://dx.doi.org/10.1038/srep19225] [PMID: 26754091]

[51]    Zhou H, Chen JX, Yang CS, Yang MQ, Deng Y, Wang H. Gene regulation mediated by microRNAs in response to green tea polyphenol EGCG in mouse lung cancer. BMC Genomics 2014; 15(S11) (Suppl. 11): S3.
[http://dx.doi.org/10.1186/1471-2164-15-S11-S3] [PMID: 25559244]

[52]    Zhu Y, Huang Y, Liu M, *et al*. Epigallocatechin gallate inhibits cell growth and regulates miRNA expression in cervical carcinoma cell lines infected with different high-risk human papillomavirus subtypes. Exp Ther Med 2019; 17(3): 1742-8.
[PMID: 30783443]

[53]    Jiang P, Xu C, Chen L, *et al*. EGCG inhibits CSC-like properties through targeting miR-485/CD44 axis in A549-cisplatin resistant cells. Mol Carcinog 2018; 57(12): 1835-44.
[http://dx.doi.org/10.1002/mc.22901] [PMID: 30182373]

[54]    Zan L, Chen Q, Zhang L, Li X. Epigallocatechin gallate (EGCG) suppresses growth and tumorigenicity in breast cancer cells by downregulation of miR-25. Bioengineered 2019; 10(1): 374-82.
[http://dx.doi.org/10.1080/21655979.2019.1657327] [PMID: 31431131]

[55]    Wal P, Saraswat N, Pal RS, Wal A, Chaubey M. A detailed insight of the anti-inflammatory effects of curcumin with the assessment of parameters, sources of ROS and associated mechanisms. Open Med J 2019; 6(1): 64-76.
[http://dx.doi.org/10.2174/1874220301906010064]

[56]    Menon VP, Sudheer AR. Antioxidant and anti-inflammatory properties of curcumin. The molecular targets and therapeutic uses of curcumin in health and disease. 2007: 105-25.
[http://dx.doi.org/10.1007/978-0-387-46401-5_3]

[57] Kronski E, Fiori ME, Barbieri O, *et al.* miR181b is induced by the chemopreventive polyphenol curcumin and inhibits breast cancer metastasis *via* down-regulation of the inflammatory cytokines CXCL1 and -2. Mol Oncol 2014; 8(3): 581-95.
[http://dx.doi.org/10.1016/j.molonc.2014.01.005] [PMID: 24484937]

[58] Wu H, Liu Q, Cai T, Chen YD, Wang ZF. Induction of microRNA-146a is involved in curcumin-mediated enhancement of temozolomide cytotoxicity against human glioblastoma. Mol Med Rep 2015; 12(4): 5461-6.
[http://dx.doi.org/10.3892/mmr.2015.4087] [PMID: 26239619]

[59] Zhu M, Zheng Z, Huang J, *et al.* Modulation of miR-34a in curcumin-induced antiproliferation of prostate cancer cells. J Cell Biochem 2019; 120(9): 15616-24.
[http://dx.doi.org/10.1002/jcb.28828] [PMID: 31042325]

[60] Xu R, Li H, Wu S, *et al.* MicroRNA-1246 regulates the radio-sensitizing effect of curcumin in bladder cancer cells *via* activating P53. Int Urol Nephrol 2019; 51(10): 1771-9.
[http://dx.doi.org/10.1007/s11255-019-02210-5] [PMID: 31236854]

[61] Sohn EJ, Bak K, Nam Y, Park HT. Upregulation of microRNA 344a-3p is involved in curcumin induced apoptosis in RT4 schwannoma cells. Cancer Cell Int 2018; 18(1): 199.
[http://dx.doi.org/10.1186/s12935-018-0693-x] [PMID: 30534000]

[62] Qiang Z, Meng L, Yi C, Yu L, Chen W, Sha W. Curcumin regulates the miR-21/PTEN/Akt pathway and acts in synergy with PD98059 to induce apoptosis of human gastric cancer MGC-803 cells. J Int Med Res 2019; 47(3): 1288-97.
[http://dx.doi.org/10.1177/0300060518822213] [PMID: 30727807]

[63] Han Z, Zhang J, Zhang K, Zhao Y. Curcumin inhibits cell viability, migration, and invasion of thymic carcinoma cells *via* downregulation of microRNA-27a. Phytother Res 2020; 34(7): 1629-37.
[http://dx.doi.org/10.1002/ptr.6629] [PMID: 32067269]

[64] Asama H, Suzuki R, Hikichi T, Takagi T, Masamune A, Ohira H. MicroRNA let-7d targets thrombospondin-1 and inhibits the activation of human pancreatic stellate cells. Pancreatology 2019; 19(1): 196-203.
[http://dx.doi.org/10.1016/j.pan.2018.10.012] [PMID: 30393009]

[65] Ning YX, Luo X, Xu M, Feng X, Wang J. Let-7d increases ovarian cancer cell sensitivity to a genistein analog by targeting c-Myc. Oncotarget 2017; 8(43): 74836-45.
[http://dx.doi.org/10.18632/oncotarget.20413] [PMID: 29088827]

[66] Zheng Y, Liu H, Liang Y. Genistein exerts potent antitumour effects alongside anaesthetic, propofol, by suppressing cell proliferation and nuclear factor-κB-mediated signalling and through upregulating microRNA-218 expression in an intracranial rat brain tumour model. J Pharm Pharmacol 2017; 69(11): 1565-77.
[http://dx.doi.org/10.1111/jphp.12781] [PMID: 28776680]

[67] Ma C, Zhang Y, Tang L, *et al.* MicroRNA-1469, a p53-responsive microRNA promotes Genistein induced apoptosis by targeting Mcl1 in human laryngeal cancer cells. Biomed Pharmacother 2018; 106: 665-71.
[http://dx.doi.org/10.1016/j.biopha.2018.07.005] [PMID: 29990856]

[68] Zhang H, Zhao Z, Pang X, *et al.* MiR-34a/sirtuin-1/foxo3a is involved in genistein protecting against ox-LDL-induced oxidative damage in HUVECs. Toxicol Lett 2017; 277: 115-22.
[http://dx.doi.org/10.1016/j.toxlet.2017.07.216] [PMID: 28688900]

[69] Wei D, Yang L, Lv B, Chen L. Genistein suppresses retinoblastoma cell viability and growth and induces apoptosis by upregulating miR-145 and inhibiting its target ABCE1. Mol Vis 2017; 23: 385-94.
[PMID: 28706438]

[70] Wei D, Yang L, Lv B, Chen L. Genistein suppresses retinoblastoma cell viability and growth and

induces apoptosis by upregulating miR-145 and inhibiting its target ABCE1. Mol Vis 2017; 23: 385-94.
[PMID: 28706438]

[71]  Rigalli JP, Tocchetti GN, Arana MR, *et al.* The phytoestrogen genistein enhances multidrug resistance in breast cancer cell lines by translational regulation of ABC transporters. Cancer Lett 2016; 376(1): 165-72.
[http://dx.doi.org/10.1016/j.canlet.2016.03.040] [PMID: 27033456]

[72]  de la Parra C, Castillo-Pichardo L, Cruz-Collazo A, *et al.* Soy isoflavone genistein-mediated downregulation of miR-155 contributes to the anticancer effects of genistein. Nutr Cancer 2016; 68(1): 154-64.
[http://dx.doi.org/10.1080/01635581.2016.1115104] [PMID: 26771440]

[73]  Xie J, Wang J, Zhu B. Genistein inhibits the proliferation of human multiple myeloma cells through suppression of nuclear factor-κB and upregulation of microRNA-29b. Mol Med Rep 2016; 13(2): 1627-32.
[http://dx.doi.org/10.3892/mmr.2015.4740] [PMID: 26718793]

[74]  Abu Samaan TM, Samec M, Liskova A, Kubatka P, Büsselberg D. Paclitaxel's mechanistic and clinical effects on breast cancer. Biomolecules 2019; 9(12): 789.
[http://dx.doi.org/10.3390/biom9120789] [PMID: 31783552]

[75]  Duan FG, Wang MF, Cao YB, *et al.* MicroRNA-421 confers paclitaxel resistance by binding to the KEAP1 3′UTR and predicts poor survival in non-small cell lung cancer. Cell Death Dis 2019; 10(11): 821.
[http://dx.doi.org/10.1038/s41419-019-2031-1] [PMID: 31659154]

[76]  Cai Y, Jia R, Xiong H, *et al.* Integrative gene expression profiling reveals that dysregulated triple microRNAs confer paclitaxel resistance in non-small cell lung cancer *via* co-targeting MAPT. Cancer Manag Res 2019; 11: 7391-404.
[http://dx.doi.org/10.2147/CMAR.S215427] [PMID: 31496800]

[77]  Sun H, Zhou X, Bao Y, Xiong G, Cui Y, Zhou H. RETRACTED: Involvement of miR-4262 in paclitaxel resistance through the regulation of PTEN in non-small cell lung cancer. Open Biol 2019; 9(7): 180227.
[http://dx.doi.org/10.1098/rsob.180227] [PMID: 31337279]

[78]  Lu C, Wang D, Feng Y, Feng L, Li Z. miR-720 Regulates Insulin Secretion by Targeting Rab35. BioMed Res Int 2021; 2021: 1-9.
[http://dx.doi.org/10.1155/2021/6662612] [PMID: 33880375]

[79]  Wang G, Ma C, Shi X, Guo W, Niu J. miR-107 enhances the sensitivity of breast cancer cells to paclitaxel. Open Med (Wars) 2019; 14(1): 456-66.
[http://dx.doi.org/10.1515/med-2018-0069] [PMID: 31206033]

[80]  Zhang H, Zhao B, Wang X, Zhang F, Yu W. LINC00511 knockdown enhances paclitaxel cytotoxicity in breast cancer *via* regulating miR-29c/CDK6 axis. Life Sci 2019; 228: 135-44.
[http://dx.doi.org/10.1016/j.lfs.2019.04.063] [PMID: 31047896]

[81]  Huang L, Hu C, Chao H, *et al.* miR-29c regulates resistance to paclitaxel in nasopharyngeal cancer by targeting ITGB1. Exp Cell Res 2019; 378(1): 1-10.
[http://dx.doi.org/10.1016/j.yexcr.2019.02.012] [PMID: 30779921]

[82]  Irani S, Soleimani M, Soltani-Sedeh H, Mirfakhraie R. Potential using of microRNA-34A in combination with paclitaxel in colorectal cancer cells. J Cancer Res Ther 2019; 15(1): 32-7.
[http://dx.doi.org/10.4103/jcrt.JCRT_267_17] [PMID: 30880751]

[83]  Zhang L, Chen T, Yan L, *et al.* MiR-155-3p acts as a tumor suppressor and reverses paclitaxel resistance *via* negative regulation of MYD88 in human breast cancer. Gene 2019; 700: 85-95.
[http://dx.doi.org/10.1016/j.gene.2019.02.066] [PMID: 30878390]

[84]    Kumar P, Bhadauria AS, Singh AK, Saha S. Betulinic acid as apoptosis activator: Molecular mechanisms, mathematical modeling and chemical modifications. Life Sci 2018; 209: 24-33.
[http://dx.doi.org/10.1016/j.lfs.2018.07.056] [PMID: 30076920]

[85]    Pandita A, Manvati S, Singh SK, Vaishnavi S, Bamezai RNK. Combined effect of microRNA, nutraceuticals and drug on pancreatic cancer cell lines. Chem Biol Interact 2015; 233: 56-64.
[http://dx.doi.org/10.1016/j.cbi.2015.03.018] [PMID: 25841339]

[86]    Zhao X, Liu M, Li D. Oleanolic acid suppresses the proliferation of lung carcinoma cells by miR-122/Cyclin G1/MEF2D axis. Mol Cell Biochem 2015; 400(1-2): 1-7.
[http://dx.doi.org/10.1007/s11010-014-2228-7] [PMID: 25472877]

[87]    Zhou J, Liu M, Chen Y, Xu S, Guo Y, Zhao L. Cucurbitacin B suppresses proliferation of pancreatic cancer cells by ceRNA: Effect of miR-146b-5p and lncRNA-AFAP1-AS1. J Cell Physiol 2019; 234(4): 4655-67.
[http://dx.doi.org/10.1002/jcp.27264] [PMID: 30206930]

[88]    Sikander M, Hafeez BB, Malik S, *et al.* Cucurbitacin D exhibits potent anti-cancer activity in cervical cancer. Sci Rep 2016; 6(1): 36594.
[http://dx.doi.org/10.1038/srep36594] [PMID: 27824155]

[89]    Lin Y, Li J, Ye S, *et al.* LncRNA GACAT3 acts as a competing endogenous RNA of HMGA1 and alleviates cucurbitacin B-induced apoptosis of gastric cancer cells. Gene 2018; 678: 164-71.
[http://dx.doi.org/10.1016/j.gene.2018.08.037] [PMID: 30098426]

[90]    Zhao X, Liu M, Li D. Oleanolic acid suppresses the proliferation of lung carcinoma cells by miR-122/Cyclin G1/MEF2D axis. Mol Cell Biochem 2015; 400(1-2): 1-7.
[http://dx.doi.org/10.1007/s11010-014-2228-7] [PMID: 25472877]

[91]    Wall ME, Wani MC, Nicholas AW, *et al.* Plant antitumor agents. 30. Synthesis and structure activity of novel camptothecin analogs. J Med Chem 1993; 36(18): 2689-700.
[http://dx.doi.org/10.1021/jm00070a013] [PMID: 8410981]

[92]    Zeng CW, Zhang XJ, Lin KY, *et al.* Camptothecin induces apoptosis in cancer cells *via* microRNA-125b-mediated mitochondrial pathways. Mol Pharmacol 2012; 81(4): 578-86.
[http://dx.doi.org/10.1124/mol.111.076794] [PMID: 22252650]

[93]    Bertozzi D, Marinello J, Manzo SG, Fornari F, Gramantieri L, Capranico G. The natural inhibitor of DNA topoisomerase I, camptothecin, modulates HIF-1α activity by changing miR expression patterns in human cancer cells. Mol Cancer Ther 2014; 13(1): 239-48.
[http://dx.doi.org/10.1158/1535-7163.MCT-13-0729] [PMID: 24252850]

[94]    Dong WH, Li Q, Zhang XY, Guo Q, Li H, Wang TY. Deep sequencing identifies deregulation of microRNAs involved with vincristine drug-resistance of colon cancer cells. Int J Clin Exp Pathol 2015; 8(9): 11524-30.
[PMID: 26617885]

[95]    Due H, Schönherz AA, Ryø L, *et al.* MicroRNA-155 controls vincristine sensitivity and predicts superior clinical outcome in diffuse large B-cell lymphoma. Blood Adv 2019; 3(7): 1185-96.
[http://dx.doi.org/10.1182/bloodadvances.2018029660] [PMID: 30967394]

# CHAPTER 11

# Understanding the Mechanism of Targeted Therapy- The Next Generation for Cancer Treatment

**K.R. Padma**[1,*], **K.R. Don**[2] and **P. Josthna**[1]

[1] *Department of Biotechnology, Sri Padmavati Mahila Visvavidyalayam (Women's University), Tirupati, AP, India*

[2] *Department of Oral Pathology and Microbiology, Sree Balaji Dental College and Hospital, Bharath Institute of Higher Education and Research (BIHER) Bharath University, Chennai, Tamil Nadu, India*

**Abstract:** In recent years, there has been significant progress in understanding the cellular, molecular, and systemic factors that contribute to the development and spread of cancer. This has been made possible by advancements in sequencing methods and data analysis, which have allowed for the identification of various genomic alterations in tumors. While there are currently several specific therapies available, there is a growing focus on target-specific treatments that show better results in cancer treatment. Cancer is widely recognized as the second deadliest disease in the world. For many years, the main forms of treatment for cancer have been chemotherapy and radiotherapy for advanced stages. However, recent advancements in science and technology have led to the discovery of new chemotherapeutic drugs. Additionally, repurposing existing drugs has proven to be a cost-effective strategy for discovering new treatments that target specific cancer regimens and inhibit the growth of cancer cells. The next generation of cancer treatment is largely focused on targeting specific factors that contribute to the development and spread of cancer. This includes therapies that target hypoxia, p53, ERK, and specific proteins through the use of monoclonal antibodies. These treatments have shown promising results in inhibiting the growth of cancer cells and have been effective against various types of cancer. In this article, we will primarily focus on the mechanisms of next-generation therapies and the significance of repurposing drugs. We will also discuss the biology behind targeted cancer treatments and how they work to inhibit the growth of cancer cells.

**Keywords:** Cancer, Chemotherapy, Next-generation therapy, Radiotherapy, Targeted therapy.

*\* **Corresponding author K.R. Padma:** Department of Biotechnology, Sri Padmavati Mahila Visvavidyalayam (Women's University), Tirupati, AP, India; E-mail: thulasipadi@gmail.com*

**Ashok Kumar Pandurangan (Ed.)**

## INTRODUCTION

The most common maladies are cancer and regarded as a chief communal health issue worldwide. In accordance with GLOBOCAN estimates, approximately several million new cancer cases as well as deaths happened worldwide. Cancer is regarded as a deadly disease and one of the primary reasons for death globally [1, 2]. Discovery of new drugs with support of advancing technology helps in the mitigation of cancerous cell growth [3, 4]. However, new drug introduction requires clinical trials before releasing into the market. Approximately 13 years of research and clinical testing are necessary before the entry of drugs into the market [5, 6].

At present, understanding the molecular mechanism of the progression of cancerous cells to metastatic state needs to be analyzed for the identification of genomic modifications within tumor cells [7 - 11]. For decades, chemotherapy has been used to prevent the progression and intensification of tumor cells. The major drawback of chemotherapy is the incapability to differentiate between cancerous and regular cells. Nonetheless, with the progression of recent advancements, remarkable alteration has been seen in tumor therapy from a wide-continuum of cytotoxic agents to targeted drugs [12]. In contrast to conventional chemotherapeutic drugs, targeted drugs can particularly target cancerous cells and spare normal cells. In 2001, the Food and Drug Administration (FDA) [13] have permitted the expansion of targeted agents for cancer therapy. For precise comprehension of targeted therapy, recognition of tumor immunology is essential [14]. Therefore, our current article provides a clear understanding of targeted drug treatment for cancer disease and prognosis of patients [15]. In this article, our primary focus is on the mechanism of action of anticancer drugs on tumor resistance along with the mechanism of targeted therapy on proliferating cells and how further tumor resistance can be improved. Further, we also focusedon the drawbacks of chemotherapy as well as radiotherapy and diverse classes of targeted therapies as recent advancements. Thus, for an effective understanding of targeted treatment, *in-silico* approaches play a key role in exploiting potentially effective drugs with higher efficacy, and further, those oncological drugs after clinical trials might significantly reduce mortality in the populace suffering from cancer diseases.

## ROLE OF NATURAL PRODUCTS IN CHEMOTHERAPY

Although, for decades natural products have been playing a prominent role in the treatment of several diseases. The bioactive compounds present in plant parts provide relief to many. However, approximately 60 percent of present anticancer agents were obtained in one way or another from natural resources [16]. Table **1** shows the latest chemotherapeutic agents obtained from natural products such as fruits and vegetables [17] and the Mediterranean diet [18, 19]. However, several literature studies have reported on the significance of nutritional substances such as beta carotene from carrots, the bioactive agent lycopene present in tomatoes, catechins from green tea, anthocyanins from blueberries, and curcumin from turmeric. Nonetheless, with the help of *in-silico* approaches, it is possible to screen the drugs binding to receptors [20, 21] and regarded as a mainstay for chemotherapy.

**Table 1. Natural products used as chemotherapeutic compounds against proliferating cancerous cells.**

| Structure of Bioactive Compound | Mechanism of Action | Study Type | Target Gene | References |
|---|---|---|---|---|
| Lycopene | Through oxidative and non-oxidative mechanisms, it reduces chronic maladies like cancer. | *In-vitro* | Bax & Bcl2 | [22] |
| β-Carotenoid | The chief anti-oxidant alleviates oxidative stress and oxidative damage to DNA. | *In-vitro* | The epidermal growth factor (EPGF) receptor and NF-kB | [23, 24] |
| | Mitochondria within cancer cells control metastasis by altering reactive oxygen species (ROS) production. | *In-vitro* | transforming growth factor β (TGF-β) signaling. | [25, 26] |

| Structure of Bioactive Compound | Mechanism of Action | Study Type | Target Gene | References |
|---|---|---|---|---|
| | Curcumin and its analogues have been reported with enhanced antitumor effect. | *In-vitro* | NF-κB & TNF-α | [27] |
| | They satiate ROS formation and end the chain reaction that is accountable for the oxidative stress | - | Induce apoptosis through intrinsic mitochondrial pathway and TNF-α pathway. | [28 - 32] |

## NEW CANCER THERAPIES BASED ON BIO-TARGETS

The novel approach to chemotherapeutics can be classified into two types depending on their sources. 1) Conventionally plant-derived products [33, 34] or of synthetic resources [35 - 37]; 2) Monoclonal antibody targeted therapy. Nevertheless, based on the mode of activity, they are, in turn, classified into anti-metabolites, alkylating agents, mitotic spindle inhibitors, inhibitors of topoisomerase, *etc.*, (Fig. **1**) [38, 39]. Conventional chemotherapy chiefly works by refraining from the division of cells. Natural products are targeted at the site of cancer cells to inhibit proliferation and tumour growth. B cells produce monoclonal antibodies, which are regarded as specific target antigens. In 1975, Kohler & Milstein [40] instituted the hybridoma technique to make large amounts of pure mAbs to augment the fundamental research and possibility for their clinical usage. However, globally more than five hundred and seventy therapeutic mAbs have been investigated through clinical trials by various profitable corporations [41]. Moreover, the US Food & Drug Administration (US FDA) has permitted 79 therapeutic mAbs into the market [42] involving more than 30 monoclonal antibodies for the therapy of tumor (Table **2**).

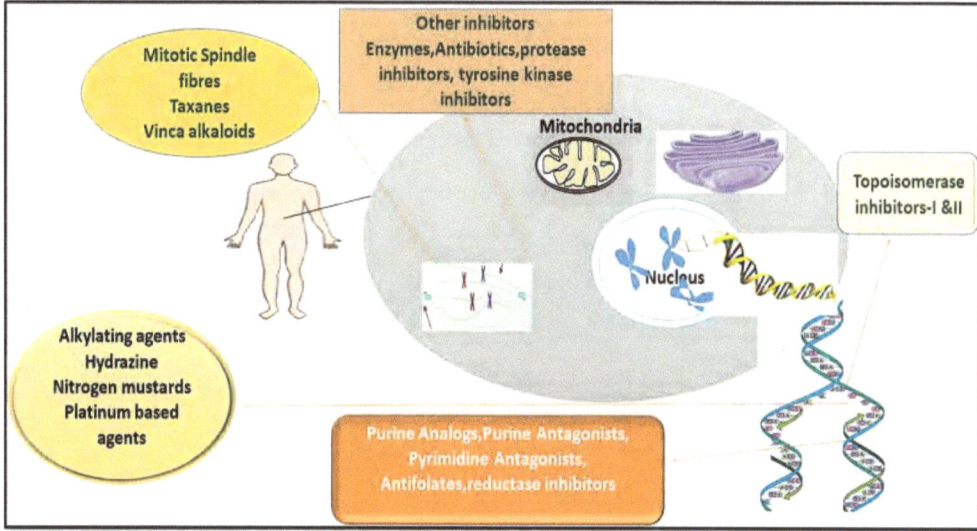

**Fig. (1).** Conventional drugs targeted biologics and their mode of action in improving the efficacy of drugs.

**Table 2. Therapeutic monoclonal antibodies approved by united states food and drug administration (US FDA).**

| USFDA Approval | Brand Name | Monoclonal Antibody | Target | Format | Methodology | Treatment of Disease | Company |
|---|---|---|---|---|---|---|---|
| 2017 | Besponsa | Ozogamicin & Inotuzumab | Cluster of Differentiation CD-22 | Humanized IgG4 | Hybridoma | Acute lymphoblastic leukemia (ALL) | Wyeth Pharmaceuticals/Pfizer |
| 2017 | Tremfya | Guselkumab | Interleukin-23 tumor suppressing protein (p19) | Human Immunoglobulin-G1 | Phage display | psoriasis & Plaque | MorphoSys/Janssen Biotech Inc. |
| 2017 | Kevzara | Sarilumab | Interleukin-6R | Human IgG1 | Transgenic mice | Rheumatoid arthritis | Regeneron Pharmaceuticals Inc./ Sanofi |
| 2003 | Xolair | Omalizumab | IgE | Humanized IgG1 | Hybridoma | Asthma | Roche, F. Hoffmann-La Roche, Ltd./ Genentech Inc./Novartis Pharmaceuticals Corp./Tanox Inc. |
| 2004 | Avastin | Bevacizumab | VEGF-A | Humanized IgG1 | Hybridoma | Colorectal cancer | Roche, F. Hoffmann-La Roche, Ltd./ Genentech Inc. |
| 1986 | Orthoclone OKT3 | Muromonab-CD3 | Cluster of Differentiation-3 | Murine Immunoglobulin G-2a | Janssen/ Hybridoma Biotech, Inc | Kidney transplant rejection | Centocor Ortho Biotech Products LP. |
| 2004 | Tysabri | Natalizumab | ITGA4 | Humanized IgG4 | Hybridoma | Multiple sclerosis | Biogen Inc./Elan Pharmaceuticals International, Ltd. |

*(Table 2) cont.....*

| USFDA Approval | Brand Name | Monoclonal Antibody | Target | Format | Methodology | Treatment of Disease | Company |
|---|---|---|---|---|---|---|---|
| 1994 | Reopro | Abciximab | GPIIb/IIIa | Chimeric IgG1 Fab | Hybridoma | Preclusion of blood clots in angioplasty | Centocor Inc./Eli Lilly/Janssen Biotech Inc. |
| 2011 | Yervoy | Ipilimumab | CTLA-4 | Human IgG1 | Transgenic | Metastatic melanoma | Bristol-Myers Squibb/Medarex |
| 2011 | Adcetris | vedotin Brentuximab | Cluster of Differentiation - 30 | Chimeric IgG1; ADC | Hybridoma | Systemic anaplastic large cell lymphoma and Hodgkin lymphoma, | Seattle genetics Inc./Takeda Pharmaceutical Co., Ltd. |
| 2011 | Benlysta | Belimumab | BLyS | Human IgG1 | Phage display | Systemic lupus erythematosus | GlaxoSmithKline /Human Genome Sciences Inc. |
| 2009 | Ilaris | Canakinumab | IL-1β | Human IgG1 | Transgenic mice | Muckle-Wells syndrome | Novartis Pharmaceuticals Corp. |
| 2010 | Xgeva, Prolia | Denosumab | RANKL | Human IgG2 | Transgenic mice | Bone loss | Amgen |
| 1998 | Herceptin | Trastuzumab | HER2 | Humanized IgG1 | Hybridoma | Cancer in breast | Roche, F. Hoffmann-La Roche, Ltd./Genentech Inc. |
| 1998 | Synagis | Palivizumab | RSV | Humanized IgG1 | Hybridoma | Prevention of respiratory syncytial virus infection | MedImmune/AbbVie Inc. |
| 1997 | MabThera, Rituxan | Rituximab | CD20 | Chimeric IgG1 | Hybridoma | Non-Hodgkin lymphoma | Biogen Inc./Roche, F. Hoffmann-La Roche Ltd./Genentech Inc. |
| 2001 | Campath, Lemtrada | Alemtuzumab | CD52 | Humanized IgG1 | Hybridoma | Chronic myeloid leukemia | Berlex Inc./Genzyme Corp./ Millennium Pharmaceuticals Inc |
| 1998 | Remicade | Infliximab | TNFα | Chimeric IgG1 | Hybridoma | Crohn's disease | Janssen Biotech Inc. |
| 2002 | Humira | Adalimumab | TNFα | Human IgG1 | Phage display | Rheumatoid arthritis | AbbVie Inc. |
| 2004 | Erbitux | Cetuximab | EGFR | Chimeric IgG1 | Hybridoma | Colo-rectal tumorr | Squibb/Merck & Co. Inc./Eli Lilly/ImClone Systems Inc Bristol-Myers |
| 2002 | Zevalin | Ibritumomab tiuxetan | CD20 | Murine IgG1 | Hybridoma | Non-Hodgkin lymphoma | Biogen Inc./Schering AG/Spectrum Pharmaceuticals Inc. |
| 2006 | Vectibix | Panitumumab | Epithelial Growth Factor Receptor | Human Immunoglobulin-G2 | Transgenic mice | Colorectal cancer | Amgen |
| 2009 | Simponi | Golimumab | TNFα | Human IgG1 | Transgenic mice | Rheumatoid and psoriatic arthritis, ankylosing spondylitis | Centocor Ortho Biotech Inc./ Janssen Biotech Inc. |

*(Table 2) cont.....*

| USFDA Approval | Brand Name | Monoclonal Antibody | Target | Format | Methodology | Treatment of Disease | Company |
|---|---|---|---|---|---|---|---|
| 2006 | Lucentis | Ranibizumab | Vascular Epithelial Growth Factor-A | Humanized IgG1 Fab | Hybridoma | Macular degeneration | Roche, F. Hoffmann-La Roche Ltd./ Genentech Inc./Novartis Pharmaceuticals Corp. |
| 2007 | Soliris | Eculizumab | C5 | Humanized IgG2/4 | Hybridoma | Paroxysmal nocturnal hemoglobinuria | Alexion Pharmaceuticals Inc. |
| 2010 | RoActemra, Actemra | Tocilizumab | IL-6R | Humanized IgG1 | Hybridoma | Rheumatoid arthritis | Chugai Pharmaceutical Co., Ltd./ Roche, F. Hoffmann-La Roche. Ltd./ Genentech Inc. |
| 2009 | Stelara | Ustekinumab | IL-12/23 | Human IgG1 | Transgenic mice | Psoriasis | Medarex/Centocor Ortho Biotech Inc./Janssen Biotech Inc. |
| 2009 | Arzerra | Ofatumumab | CD20 | Human IgG1 | Transgenic mice | Chronic lymphocytic leukemia | Genmab A/S /GlaxoSmithKline /Novartis |
| 2008 | Cimzia | Certolizumab pegol | TNFα | Humanized Fab, pegylated | Hybridoma | Crohn's disease | Celltech, UCB. |
| 2012 | Perjeta | Pertuzumab | HER2 | Humanized IgG1 | Hybridoma | Breast Cancer | Roche, F. Hoffmann-La Roche, Ltd./ Genentech Inc. |
| 2018 | Poteligeo | Mogamulizumab | CCR4 | Humanized IgG1 | Hybridoma | Mycosis fungoides or Sézary syndrome | Kyowa Hakko Kirin |
| 2018 | Ajovy | Fremanezumab | CGRP | Humanized IgG2 | Hybridoma | Migraine prevention | Teva Pharmaceutical Industries, Ltd. |
| 2019 | Evenity | Romosozumab | Sclerostin | Humanized IgG2 | Hybridoma | Osteoporosis in postmenopausal women at increased risk of fracture | Amgen/UCB |
| 2019 | Adakveo | Crizanlizumab | P-selectin | Humanized IgG2 | Hybridoma | Sickle cell anemia | Novartis Pharmaceuticals Corp. |

## UNDERSTANDING THE MECHANISM OF REPURPOSED DRUGS IN THE TREATMENT OF CANCER

Increasing focus is now directed to precision medicine, which permits medical care to skillfully modify genes and proteins based on each individual's molecular profiling in substitution to drug fit model presently utilized. Multi-omics initiatives are employed for the systematic analysis of genes and proteins for cancer treatment [37, 43, 44]. However, the repurposing of drugs can form targets for cancer-interlinked proteins [45, 46]. The major confrontation in drug discovery for cancer relies on exploiting the biochemical or phenotypic approaches to enhance clinical efficacy and augment the management of maladies [47, 48]. Comprehension of mono or multi-targeting drugs provides better opportunities for inhibiting cancer cell proliferation [49 - 51]. Fig. (2) summarizes non-oncology agents and differentiates between those compounds appropriate for monotherapy or multidrug combinations.

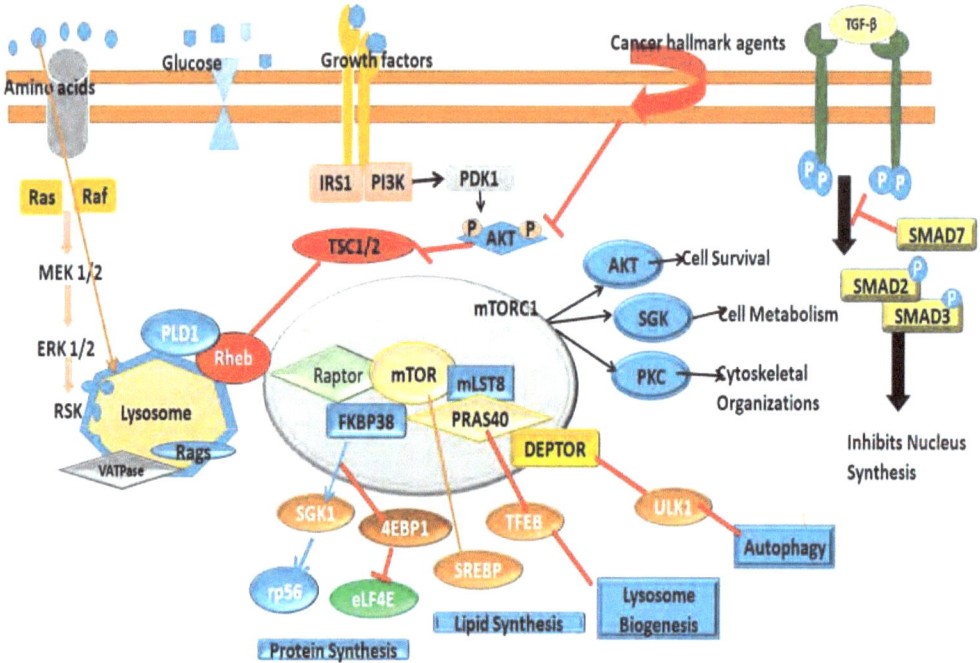

**Fig. (2).** mTOR complex signalling mechanism and its activation of Ras/Raf-MEK-ERK (MAPK) or the IRS1/PI3K-PDK1-PKB alleyways. Red lines indicate inhibitors/cancer hallmark agents.

The mammalian or mechanistic target of rapamycin (mTOR) is a protein kinase complex which results in the formation of two main distinctive multiprotein complexes, characterized as mTOR complexes 1 & 2 (mTORC1 & mTORC2). Both complexes play a specific role in the regulation of cells [52, 53]. The mTORC1 influences multiple constructive metabolism pathways involving the production of ribosomes, synthesis of proteins, synthesis of lipids, and nucleotide synthesis all of which are significant for the growth of cells as well as tissues. mTORC1 signaling modifies various oncogenic pathways such as Ras/MEK/ERK/AKT and PI3K [54]. An important negative upstream regulator of mTORC1 protein complex involves TSC1 and TSC2, which is named as tuberous sclerosis complex (TSC), which is characterized by benign tumors [55]. In particular, eIF4E-binding proteins are small phosphoproteins required for protein synthesis and anticancer agents inhibit their activation, which in turn refrains tumorigenesis [56 - 59] and Table **3** depicts cancer hallmark agents.

**Table 3. Drug candidates targeting the hallmarks of cancer employing repurposed drugs.**

| Hallmark | Therapy | Targeting |
|---|---|---|
| **Sustaining Proliferative signalling** | **Monotherapy Rapamycin Prazosin Indomethacin** | **EGFR inhibitors / mTOR and associated signaling networks** |
| **Defy Cell Death** | Monotherapy Artemisinin Chloroquine | Pro-apoptotic mimetics |
| **Evading Growth Suppressors** | Combinatorial therapy Quinacrine Ritonavir | Cyclin-dependent kinase inhibitors/ AKT-E2F-1 |
| **Instigating Invasion & Metastasis** | Berberine Niclosamide Combinatorial therapy | Inhibitors of HGF/c-Met |
| **Reprogramming Energy Metabolism** | Monotherapy Metformin Disulfiram | Instigates the PI3K-mTOR signaling pathway, directing to proliferative refrainment of those cancers with insulin receptor expression. |
| **Tumor-encouraging Inflammation** | Aspirin Thiocolchicoside Combinatorial therapy | Selective anti-inflammatory drugs/ NF–κB |

## IMMUNOGENICITY OF MONOCLONAL ANTIBODIES

The vital biophysical characteristics of mAbs include higher stability, greater antigen binding actions and lower immunogenicity [60]. Immunogenicity of antibodies indicates the extent of host immune action, which identifies and reacts to remedial agents. The antidrug antibodies (ADA) are triggered from immune system and possess the potential to neutralize therapeutic agents along with the mitigation of the efficacy of drugs [61]. However, ADA causes unfavorable effects on the host system such as rashes due to systematic inflammatory response, which considerably raises questions on its safety and duration of antibody drugs [62]. Nonetheless, immunogenicity is persuaded by various factors like drug dosage, route of administration, contamination, and Ab/Ag binding complex. Although, therapeutic monoclonal antibodies are generally classified into two types. In the beginning, naked type antibody is precisely employed for malady treatment. The treatment of tumor is mediated through the ADCC/CDC pathway, which instigates direct apoptosis/ targeting immune checkpoints/tumor microenvironment. Currently, the latest technological advancements are made to augment the remedial effectiveness of ADCC/CDC through point mutation of Fc antibody [63 - 65] or alteration through glycosylation [66 - 70], which significantly enhances cancer cell killing potentiality. Furthermore, new antibody-based therapy will greatly improve the efficacy as well as specificity of antibody-drug conjugates against human maladies.

## CUTTING-EDGE IN CANCER THERAPY

The finding of the latest drugs in oncology is a persistently emerging field and every year various novel methods are proposed. However, after World War II, there has been a robust expansion in the number of drugs obtained from genetic, molecular, and biological disciplines. Correspondingly it enhances the figures of available drugs and, in turn, enhances the value of drugs, which subsequently leads to momentous progression in the existence and characteristic features of a patient's life. Furthermore, clinical trials are ongoing for the development of the latest drugs and therapeutic methods in the treatment of various tumors. Various literature reports have revealed the results of clinical trials on chronic lymphocytic leukemia (CLL), and acute lymphoblastic leukemia (ALL). However, patients treated with Kymriah revealed potential and long-lasting antitumor efficacy [71]. Even therapy with tisagenlecleucel is related to a series of unfavorable consequences, among which the predominant significance is the release of cytokine for the treatment of specialized neurological centers [72]. Many studies are trying to develop the latest therapeutic methods, based on genomic editing using CRISPR/Cas9 technology to fix genetic aberrations conscientious for neoplastic transformation [73]. At last, in current years, the main focus is on anticancer vaccines, which trigger the immune system.

## CONCLUSION

Proteins become deregulated during the formation of cancerous cells. The latest therapy involves the use of monoclonal antibodies, which are small inhibitor/immunotoxin molecules that specifically target the deregulated protein and prevent its progression. These targeted therapies not only block the deregulated protein in the extracellular compartment, but they can also enter the cytosol and trigger apoptosis. This approach aims to alter tumor growth and minimize side effects on normal tissues. However, in order for targeted cancer therapies to be effective, it is important to have a proper understanding of the mechanisms of resistance. Therefore, our article provides comprehensive insights into targeted therapy as a cutting-edge method, and in the near future, this will provide researchers with a better understanding to conduct clinical trials and ultimately win the battle against this deadly disease.

## CONTRIBUTIONS

KRP and KRD contributed to writing, and drawing figures and tables in this review article. KRP solely drafted this article.

# REFERENCES

[1]     Bray F, Ferlay J, Soerjomataram I, Siegel RL, Torre LA, Jemal A. Global cancer statistics 2018: GLOBOCAN estimates of incidence and mortality worldwide for 36 cancers in 185 countries. CA Cancer J Clin 2018; 68(6): 394-424.
[http://dx.doi.org/10.3322/caac.21492] [PMID: 30207593]

[2]     Torre LA, Bray F, Siegel RL, Ferlay J, Lortet-Tieulent J, Jemal A. Global cancer statistics, 2012. CA Cancer J Clin 2015; 65(2): 87-108.
[http://dx.doi.org/10.3322/caac.21262] [PMID: 25651787]

[3]     Kirsch J, Siltanen C, Zhou Q, Revzin A, Simonian A. Biosensor technology: recent advances in threat agent detection and medicine. Chem Soc Rev 2013; 42(22): 8733-68.
[http://dx.doi.org/10.1039/c3cs60141b] [PMID: 23852443]

[4]     Shaked Y. The pro-tumorigenic host response to cancer therapies. Nat Rev Cancer 2019; 19(12): 667-85.
[http://dx.doi.org/10.1038/s41568-019-0209-6] [PMID: 31645711]

[5]     Eder J, Sedrani R, Wiesmann C. The discovery of first-in-class drugs: origins and evolution. Nat Rev Drug Discov 2014; 13(8): 577-87.
[http://dx.doi.org/10.1038/nrd4336] [PMID: 25033734]

[6]     Munos B. Lessons from 60 years of pharmaceutical innovation. Nat Rev Drug Discov 2009; 8(12): 959-68.
[http://dx.doi.org/10.1038/nrd2961] [PMID: 19949401]

[7]     Cancer Genome Atlas N. Comprehensive molecular characterization of human colon and rectal cancer. Nature 2012; 487(7407): 330-7.
[http://dx.doi.org/10.1038/nature11252] [PMID: 22810696]

[8]     Curtis C, Shah SP, Chin SF, *et al.* The genomic and transcriptomic architecture of 2,000 breast tumours reveals novel subgroups. Nature 2012; 486(7403): 346-52.
[http://dx.doi.org/10.1038/nature10983] [PMID: 22522925]

[9]     Lawrence MS, Stojanov P, Polak P, *et al.* Mutational heterogeneity in cancer and the search for new cancer-associated genes. Nature 2013; 499(7457): 214-8.
[http://dx.doi.org/10.1038/nature12213] [PMID: 23770567]

[10]    Shah SP, Roth A, Goya R, *et al.* The clonal and mutational evolution spectrum of primary triple-negative breast cancers. Nature 2012; 486(7403): 395-9.
[http://dx.doi.org/10.1038/nature10933] [PMID: 22495314]

[11]    Stephens PJ, Tarpey PS, Davies H, *et al.* The landscape of cancer genes and mutational processes in breast cancer. Nature 2012; 486(7403): 400-4.
[http://dx.doi.org/10.1038/nature11017] [PMID: 22722201]

[12]    Bedard PL, Hyman DM, Davids MS, Siu LL. Small molecules, big impact: 20 years of targeted therapy in oncology. Lancet 2020; 395(10229): 1078-88.
[http://dx.doi.org/10.1016/S0140-6736(20)30164-1] [PMID: 32222192]

[13]    Savage DG, Antman KH. Imatinib mesylate--a new oral targeted therapy. N Engl J Med 2002; 346(9): 683-93.
[http://dx.doi.org/10.1056/NEJMra013339] [PMID: 11870247]

[14]    González-Cao M, Karachaliou N, Viteri S, *et al.* Targeting PD-1/PD-L1 in lung cancer: current perspectives. Lung Cancer (Auckl) 2015; 6: 55-70.
[PMID: 28210151]

[15]    Longley DB, Johnston PG. Molecular mechanisms of drug resistance. J Pathol 2005; 205(2): 275-92.
[http://dx.doi.org/10.1002/path.1706] [PMID: 15641020]

[16]    Newman DJ, Cragg GM. Natural products as sources of new drugs over the 30 years from 1981 to

2010. J Nat Prod 2012; 75(3): 311-35.
[http://dx.doi.org/10.1021/np200906s] [PMID: 22316239]

[17]  Block G, Patterson B, Subar A. Fruit, vegetables, and cancer prevention: A review of the epidemiological evidence. Nutr Cancer 1992; 18(1): 1-29.
[http://dx.doi.org/10.1080/01635589209514201] [PMID: 1408943]

[18]  Pauwels EKJ. The protective effect of the Mediterranean diet: focus on cancer and cardiovascular risk. Med Princ Pract 2011; 20(2): 103-11.
[http://dx.doi.org/10.1159/000321197] [PMID: 21252562]

[19]  Key TJ. Fruit and vegetables and cancer risk. Br J Cancer 2011; 104(1): 6-11.
[http://dx.doi.org/10.1038/sj.bjc.6606032] [PMID: 21119663]

[20]  Maude SL, Frey N, Shaw PA, *et al.* Chimeric antigen receptor T cells for sustained remissions in leukemia. N Engl J Med 2014; 371(16): 1507-17.
[http://dx.doi.org/10.1056/NEJMoa1407222] [PMID: 25317870]

[21]  Steele VE, Lubet RA, Moon RC. 2005.

[22]  Ascenso A. Pinho S, Eleutério C, *et al.* Lycopene from Tomatoes: Vesicular Nanocarrier Formulations for Dermal Delivery. J Agric Food Chem 2013; 61: 7284-93.
[http://dx.doi.org/10.1021/jf401368w] [PMID: 23826819]

[23]  Chen QH, Wu BK, Pan D, Sang LX, Chang B. Beta-carotene and its protective effect on gastric cancer. World J Clin Cases 2021; 9(23): 6591-607.
[http://dx.doi.org/10.12998/wjcc.v9.i23.6591] [PMID: 34447808]

[24]  Molaei F, Forghanifard MM, Fahim Y, Abbaszadegan MR. Molecular signaling in tumorigenesis of gastric cancer. Iran Biomed J 2018; 22(4): 217-30.
[http://dx.doi.org/10.29252/ibj.22.4.217] [PMID: 29706061]

[25]  Yang CS, Maliakal P, Meng X. Inhibition of carcinogenesis by tea. Annu Rev Pharmacol Toxicol 2002; 42(1): 25-54.
[http://dx.doi.org/10.1146/annurev.pharmtox.42.082101.154309] [PMID: 11807163]

[26]  Yang CS, Wang X, Lu G, Picinich SC. Cancer prevention by tea: animal studies, molecular mechanisms and human relevance. Nat Rev Cancer 2009; 9(6): 429-39.
[http://dx.doi.org/10.1038/nrc2641] [PMID: 19472429]

[27]  Nelson KM, Dahlin JL. Bisson, Graham, J., Paulin G. F., and Walters, M. A. Curcumin May (Not) Defy Science. ACS Med Chem Lett 2017; 8: 467-70.
[http://dx.doi.org/10.1021/acsmedchemlett.7b00139] [PMID: 28523093]

[28]  Reddivari L, Vanamala J, Chintharlapalli S, Safe SH, Miller JC Jr. Anthocyanin fraction from potato extracts is cytotoxic to prostate cancer cells through activation of caspase-dependent and caspase-independent pathways. Carcinogenesis 2007; 28(10): 2227-35.
[http://dx.doi.org/10.1093/carcin/bgm117] [PMID: 17522067]

[29]  Chang Y, Huang H, Hsu J, Yang S, Wang C. anthocyanins rich extract-induced apoptotic cell death in human promyelocytic leukemia cells. Toxicol Appl Pharmacol 2005; 205(3): 201-12.
[http://dx.doi.org/10.1016/j.taap.2004.10.014] [PMID: 15922006]

[30]  Hientz K, Mohr A, Bhakta-Guha D, Efferth T. The role of p53 in cancer drug resistance and targeted chemotherapy. Oncotarget 2017; 8(5): 8921-46.
[http://dx.doi.org/10.18632/oncotarget.13475] [PMID: 27888811]

[31]  Bagchi D, Sen CK, Bagchi M, Atalay M. Anti-angiogenic, antioxidant, and anti-carcinogenic properties of a novel anthocyanin-rich berry extract formula. Biochemistry. Biokhimiia. 2004; 69:75-80.
[http://dx.doi.org/10.1023/B:BIRY.0000016355.19999.93]

[32]  Lamy S, Lafleur R, Bédard V, *et al.* Anthocyanidins inhibit migration of glioblastoma cells: Structure-

activity relationship and involvement of the plasminolytic system. J Cell Biochem 2007; 100(1): 100-11.
[http://dx.doi.org/10.1002/jcb.21023] [PMID: 16823770]

[33]  Kikuchi H, Yuan B, Hu X, Okazaki M. Chemopreventive and anticancer activity of flavonoids and its possibility for clinical use by combining with conventional chemotherapeutic agents. Am J Cancer Res 2019; 9(8): 1517-35.
[PMID: 31497340]

[34]  Lichota A, Gwozdzinski K. Anticancer activity of natural compounds from plant and marine environment. Int J Mol Sci 2018; 19(11): 3533.
[http://dx.doi.org/10.3390/ijms19113533] [PMID: 30423952]

[35]  Marchi E, O'Connor OA. Safety and efficacy of pralatrexate in the treatment of patients with relapsed or refractory peripheral T-cell lymphoma. Ther Adv Hematol 2012; 3(4): 227-35.
[http://dx.doi.org/10.1177/2040620712445330] [PMID: 23606933]

[36]  Peng X, Li L, Ren Y, *et al.* Synthesis of $N$ -carbonyl acridanes as highly potent inhibitors of tubulin polymerization *via* one-pot copper-catalyzed dual arylation of nitriles with cyclic diphenyl iodoniums. Adv Synth Catal 2020; 362(10): 2030-8.
[http://dx.doi.org/10.1002/adsc.201901460]

[37]  Aguirre AJ, Nowak JA, Camarda ND, *et al.* Real-time genomic characterization of advanced pancreatic cancer to enable precision medicine. Cancer Discov 2018; 8(9): 1096-111.
[http://dx.doi.org/10.1158/2159-8290.CD-18-0275] [PMID: 29903880]

[38]  Le T, Bhushan V, Sochat M, Chavda Y. First Aid for the USMLE Step 1. 1st ed. New York, NY, USA: McGraw-Hill Education 2017; pp. 416-9.

[39]  Nussbaumer S, Bonnabry P, Veuthey JL, Fleury-Souverain S. Analysis of anticancer drugs: A review. Talanta 2011; 85(5): 2265-89.
[http://dx.doi.org/10.1016/j.talanta.2011.08.034] [PMID: 21962644]

[40]  Köhler G, Milstein C. Continuous cultures of fused cells secreting antibody of predefined specificity. Nature 1975; 256(5517): 495-7.
[http://dx.doi.org/10.1038/256495a0] [PMID: 1172191]

[41]  Kaplon H, Reichert JM. Antibodies to watch in 2019. MAbs 2019; 11(2): 219-38.
[http://dx.doi.org/10.1080/19420862.2018.1556465] [PMID: 30516432]

[42]  The Antibody Society. In: Approved antibodies. Jun 27, 2019. Available from: https://www.antibodysociety.org/ Accessed 15 Jul 2019.

[43]  Li T, Kung HJ, Mack PC, Gandara DR. Genotyping and genomic profiling of non-small-cell lung cancer: implications for current and future therapies. J Clin Oncol 2013; 31(8): 1039-49.
[http://dx.doi.org/10.1200/JCO.2012.45.3753] [PMID: 23401433]

[44]  Pauli C, Hopkins BD, Prandi D, *et al.* Personalized *in vitro* and *in vivo* cancer models to guide precision medicine. Cancer Discov 2017; 7(5): 462-77.
[http://dx.doi.org/10.1158/2159-8290.CD-16-1154] [PMID: 28331002]

[45]  Rubio-Perez C, Tamborero D, Schroeder MP, *et al. In silico* prescription of anticancer drugs to cohorts of 28 tumor types reveals targeting opportunities. Cancer Cell 2015; 27(3): 382-96.
[http://dx.doi.org/10.1016/j.ccell.2015.02.007] [PMID: 25759023]

[46]  Cheng F, Lu W, Liu C, *et al.* A genome-wide positioning systems network algorithm for *in silico* drug repurposing. Nat Commun 2019; 10(1): 3476.
[http://dx.doi.org/10.1038/s41467-019-10744-6] [PMID: 31375661]

[47]  Kim M, Mun H, Sung CO, *et al.* Patient-derived lung cancer organoids as *in vitro* cancer models for therapeutic screening. Nat Commun 2019; 10(1): 3991.
[http://dx.doi.org/10.1038/s41467-019-11867-6] [PMID: 31488816]

[48]    Huang L, Holtzinger A, Jagan I, *et al.* Ductal pancreatic cancer modeling and drug screening using human pluripotent stem cell– and patient-derived tumor organoids. Nat Med 2015; 21(11): 1364-71.
[http://dx.doi.org/10.1038/nm.3973] [PMID: 26501191]

[49]    Katsnelson A. Drug development: Target practice. Nature 2013; 498(7455): S8-9.
[http://dx.doi.org/10.1038/498S8a] [PMID: 23803950]

[50]    Flavahan WA, Gaskell E, Bernstein BE. Epigenetic plasticity and the hallmarks of cancer. Science 2017; 357(6348): eaal2380.
[http://dx.doi.org/10.1126/science.aal2380] [PMID: 28729483]

[51]    Sarmento-Ribeiro AB, Scorilas A, Gonçalves AC, Efferth T, Trougakos IP. The emergence of drug resistance to targeted cancer therapies: Clinical evidence. Drug Resist Updat 2019; 47: 100646.
[http://dx.doi.org/10.1016/j.drup.2019.100646] [PMID: 31733611]

[52]    Kennedy BK, Lamming DW. The mechanistic target of rapamycin: the grand conductor of metabolism and aging. Cell Metab 2016; 23(6): 990-1003.
[http://dx.doi.org/10.1016/j.cmet.2016.05.009] [PMID: 27304501]

[53]    Shimobayashi M, Hall MN. Making new contacts: the mTOR network in metabolism and signalling crosstalk. Nat Rev Mol Cell Biol 2014; 15(3): 155-62.
[http://dx.doi.org/10.1038/nrm3757] [PMID: 24556838]

[54]    Kim YC, Guan KL. mTOR: a pharmacologic target for autophagy regulation. J Clin Invest 2015; 125(1): 25-32.
[http://dx.doi.org/10.1172/JCI73939] [PMID: 25654547]

[55]    Henske EP, Jóźwiak S, Kingswood JC, Sampson JR, Thiele EA. Tuberous sclerosis complex. Nat Rev Dis Primers 2016; 2(1): 16035.
[http://dx.doi.org/10.1038/nrdp.2016.35] [PMID: 27226234]

[56]    Brunn GJ, Hudson CC, Sekulić A, *et al.* Phosphorylation of the translational repressor PHAS-I by the mammalian target of rapamycin. Science 1997; 277(5322): 99-101.
[http://dx.doi.org/10.1126/science.277.5322.99] [PMID: 9204908]

[57]    Siddiqui N, Sonenberg N. Signalling to eIF4E in cancer. Biochem Soc Trans 2015; 43(5): 763-72.
[http://dx.doi.org/10.1042/BST20150126] [PMID: 26517881]

[58]    Huo Y, Iadevaia V, Proud CG. Differing effects of rapamycin and mTOR kinase inhibitors on protein synthesis. Biochem Soc Trans 2011; 39(2): 446-50.
[http://dx.doi.org/10.1042/BST0390446] [PMID: 21428917]

[59]    Iadevaia V, Huo Y, Zhang Z, Foster LJ, Proud CG. Roles of the mammalian target of rapamycin, mTOR, in controlling ribosome biogenesis and protein synthesis. Biochem Soc Trans 2012; 40(1): 168-72.
[http://dx.doi.org/10.1042/BST20110682] [PMID: 22260684]

[60]    Ducancel F, Muller BH. Molecular engineering of antibodies for therapeutic and diagnostic purposes. MAbs 2012; 4(4): 445-57.
[http://dx.doi.org/10.4161/mabs.20776] [PMID: 22684311]

[61]    Harding FA, Stickler MM, Razo J, DuBridge R. The immunogenicity of humanized and fully human antibodies. MAbs 2010; 2(3): 256-65.
[http://dx.doi.org/10.4161/mabs.2.3.11641] [PMID: 20400861]

[62]    Hansel TT, Kropshofer H, Singer T, Mitchell JA, George AJT. The safety and side effects of monoclonal antibodies. Nat Rev Drug Discov 2010; 9(4): 325-38.
[http://dx.doi.org/10.1038/nrd3003] [PMID: 20305665]

[63]    Saunders KO. Conceptual approaches to modulating antibody effector functions and circulation half-life. Front Immunol 2019; 10: 1296.
[http://dx.doi.org/10.3389/fimmu.2019.01296] [PMID: 31231397]

[64]    Kelley RF, Meng YG. Methods to engineer and identify IgG1 variants with improved FcRn binding or effector function. Methods Mol Biol 2012; 901: 277-93.
[http://dx.doi.org/10.1007/978-1-61779-931-0_18] [PMID: 22723108]

[65]    Liu Z, Gunasekaran K, Wang W, *et al.* Asymmetrical Fc engineering greatly enhances antibody-dependent cellular cytotoxicity (ADCC) effector function and stability of the modified antibodies. J Biol Chem 2014; 289(6): 3571-90.
[http://dx.doi.org/10.1074/jbc.M113.513366] [PMID: 24311787]

[66]    Monnet C, Jorieux S, Souyris N, *et al.* Combined glyco- and protein-Fc engineering simultaneously enhance cytotoxicity and half-life of a therapeutic antibody. MAbs 2014; 6(2): 422-36.
[http://dx.doi.org/10.4161/mabs.27854] [PMID: 24492301]

[67]    Mimura Y, Katoh T, Saldova R, *et al.* Glycosylation engineering of therapeutic IgG antibodies: challenges for the safety, functionality and efficacy. Protein Cell 2018; 9(1): 47-62.
[http://dx.doi.org/10.1007/s13238-017-0433-3] [PMID: 28597152]

[68]    Li T, DiLillo DJ, Bournazos S, Giddens JP, Ravetch JV, Wang LX. Modulating IgG effector function by Fc glycan engineering. Proc Natl Acad Sci USA 2017; 114(13): 3485-90.
[http://dx.doi.org/10.1073/pnas.1702173114] [PMID: 28289219]

[69]    Chen CL, Hsu JC, Lin CW, *et al.* Crystal structure of a homogeneous igg-fc glycoform with the n-glycan designed to maximize the antibody dependent cellular cytotoxicity. ACS Chem Biol 2017; 12(5): 1335-45.
[http://dx.doi.org/10.1021/acschembio.7b00140] [PMID: 28318221]

[70]    Lin CW, Tsai MH, Li ST, *et al.* A common glycan structure on immunoglobulin G for enhancement of effector functions. Proc Natl Acad Sci USA 2015; 112(34): 10611-6.
[http://dx.doi.org/10.1073/pnas.1513456112] [PMID: 26253764]

[71]    Mueller KT, Maude SL, Porter DL, *et al.* Cellular kinetics of CTL019 in relapsed/refractory B-cell acute lymphoblastic leukemia and chronic lymphocytic leukemia. Blood 2017; 130(21): 2317-25.
[http://dx.doi.org/10.1182/blood-2017-06-786129] [PMID: 28935694]

[72]    Badieyan ZS, Hoseini SS. Adverse effects associated with clinical applications of CAR engineered T cells. Arch Immunol Ther Exp (Warsz) 2018; 66(4): 283-8.
[http://dx.doi.org/10.1007/s00005-018-0507-9] [PMID: 29427174]

[73]    Zhan T, Rindtorff N, Betge J, Ebert MP, Boutros M. CRISPR/Cas9 for cancer research and therapy. Semin Cancer Biol 2019; 55: 106-19.
[http://dx.doi.org/110.1016/j.semcancer.2018.04.001]

# Cell Death Apoptotic Pathways and Targeted Therapeutic Research in Cancer

**Jutishna Bora**[1,#], **Richismita Hazra**[2,#] and **Sumira Malik**[1,*]

[1] *Amity Institute of Biotechnology, Amity University, Jharkhand, Ranchi, Jharkhand-834002, India*

[2] *Amity Institute of Biotechnology, Amity University Kolkata, Kolkata, West Bengal-700135, India*

**Abstract:** Apoptosis or programmed cell death refers to a form of death in cells critical to physiological homeostasis occurring in almost every organ system and is characterized by distinct morphological features and a cascade of energy-dependent biochemical processes. This modulation ability of cells is recognised for its immense therapeutic potential. Cancer being the outcome of a spectrum of genetic alterations transforms a healthy body into a cancerous one. Oncologists have been targeting newer therapies for the elimination of cancer cells by apoptosis. Understanding the underlying mechanism of the ordered and orchestrated cellular mechanism plays a pivotal role in disease pathogenesis. There are two major pathways for the induction of apoptosis in malignant cells: Intrinsic and Extrinsic pathways. In this chapter, we summarise the various treatment strategies and therapeutic classes for curbing the different tumor types. This chapter also highlights the utilization of plants and their bioactive compounds in medicine for the treatment of various types of cancer.

**Keywords:** Apoptotic pathways, Cancer, Tumours, Therapies.

## INTRODUCTION

Cell death is an inevitable fate or contrived consequence of cellular life. It is a condition in which biological cells lose their activity or cease to perform their functions. Numerous research over the past decades have revealed the involvement of a broad spectrum of genetically encrypted mechanisms for targeted elimination of excessive, irreversibly damaged, infected, and/or potentially harmful cells [1]. The phenomenon of cell death is crucial during the development, homeostasis, and immune regulation of multicellular organisms and is associated with morphological alterations, deregulation of which might lead to numerous pathologies. Morphologically cell death can be broadly classified as

* **Corresponding author Sumira Malik:** Amity Institute of Biotechnology, Amity University, Jharkhand, Ranchi, Jharkhand-834002, India; E-mail: smalik@rnc.amity.edu
# These authors are equallly contribed to this work.

Ashok Kumar Pandurangan (Ed.)

apoptosis, necrosis, autophagy, oncosis and pyroptosis. Apoptosis is associated with cell content shrinkage including the nuclei, mitochondria, and cytoplasm and the cell becomes encased in 'apoptotic bodies', which are surrounded by plasma membrane followed by cytomorphological events including membrane blebbing and chromatin condensation. The apoptotic bodies are engulfed by nearby phagocytic cells and get digested in the lysosomes. The apoptotic mechanisms are highly complex and involve a cascade of energy-dependent molecular events. This process is biochemically characterised by the involvement of cysteinyl-aspartate-specific proteases called caspases followed by internucleosomal fragmentation of DNA and phosphatidylserine externalization. This brings about alterations in the mitochondrial membrane permeability and this type of cell death is regulated by B-cell lymphoma 2 (Bcl-2) family proteins. Apoptotic pathways are majorly of three types namely intrinsic, extrinsic, and perforin/granzyme pathways that trigger a series of molecular events. Intrinsic pathway involves the activation of stimuli including DNA damage, oxidative stress, and lack of growth factor, and is directed by permeabilization of the outer membrane of mitochondria [2]. This permits the release of Cytochrome-C that induces Apaf-1. Apaf-1 is a protease-activating factor that stimulates caspase-9 activation to assemble the apoptosome. This apoptosome is involved in activating executioner caspases. At the same time, the extrinsic apoptotic pathway is associated with the involvement of external signals of death ligands including tumor necrosis factor (TNF) superfamily and TNF-related apoptosis-induced ligands (TRAIL) that activate membrane receptors [3]. This leads to the stimulation of death-inducing signalling complex (DISC) that activates caspase-8. Caspase-8 then activates executioner caspase-3, -6, or -7 performing the process of apoptosis. However, the functioning of Granzyme A is caspase-independent [4].

Necrosis is regarded as 'passive' cell death since it encompasses nonapoptotic, accidental cell death. This uncontrolled cell death mechanism occurs due to severe insult resulting in the spillage of cellular contents into surrounding or nearby tissues. Regardless of the pre-lethal process, necrosis is the sum total of all changes that occur within a cell after its death [5]. Oncosis refers to a prelethal pathway that leads to cell death followed by swelling, organelle swelling, blebbing, and elevated membrane permeability [6]. Oncosis might occur due to the interference of toxic agents with ATP generation or might also occur due to conditions that cause uncontrolled consumption of cellular energy. Ultimately cellular energy stores get depleted and ionic pumps fail in the plasma membrane. Pyroptosis cell death is induced by infection with *Salmonella* and *Shigella* species [7]. This inherently pro-inflammatory cell death pathway relies on caspase-1. Caspase-1, which is not involved in apoptosis, processes the pro-forms of inflammatory cytokines, IL-1beta, and IL-18 to their activated form. Hence, this is an inflammatory and programmed cell death mechanism that is likely to be involved in antimicrobial response [8]. Autophagy is regarded as an evolutionarily conserved cellular process that involves the engulfing of cytoplasm by autophagic vesicles or lysosomal degradation of intracellular macromolecular components. Three major types of autophagy are microautophagy, macroautophagy, and chaperone-mediated autophagy. The autophagic cellular machinery is encoded by Autophagy-related genes (ATG), which contribute to the activation of various signalling complexes *via* 19 core Atg proteins. It involves the engulfing of the cytoplasm by autophagic vesicles [9].

For over three decades, clinical oncologists have aimed at the development of therapies for the effective elimination of cancer cells by apoptosis. Cancer biology and cancer genetics involve dynamic interactions between cancer cells and their tissue microenvironments. Bypassing the apoptotic pathway to instigate cancer cell death is considered to be a potential approach to overcoming this deadly complication. This is because the programmed cell death mechanism acts as a natural blockade that defends against cancer development [10]. Research has suggested that certain oncogenic alterations promote apoptosis instead of suppressing it and that anticancer agents induce apoptosis. Induction of apoptotic cell death by anticancer agents hints upon cellular responses after drug-target interaction could potentially affect drug-induced cell death. In the early days, viral and cellular oncogenes, cell proliferation, and transformation were the main parameters for anticancer therapeutic approaches. However, in the 1980s, the advent of apoptosis as a realistic anticancer therapeutic approach came to the forefront. BCL2 [11] and Bu2L1 [12] were anti-apoptotic oncogenes that exhibited powerful mechanisms for tumor growth [13] and drug resistance [14].

Cancer is a serious metabolic syndrome that is one of the principal causes of mortality and morbidity across the world [15]. Despite the advancements in tools for diagnosing, treating, and preventing this frightful disease, the number of cases is elevating constantly and it is estimated to reach 21 million by 2030 [16]. Cancer is a critical condition in which genetic instabilities and alterations occur within a cell caused by the uncontrolled proliferation of normal cells leading to the transformation of the normal cells into cancerous ones. Malignancy can occur due to various external factors including smoking, tobacco, radiation, intake of contaminated substances (water, food, air, chemicals), and infectious agents as well as internal factors including gene mutation, improper immunity, and hormonal disorder [17]. Around 60% of the drugs useful for treating cancer have been obtained from natural products with plant kingdom as the major source. Plants and their bioactive compounds have been utilized in medicine for ages and these have served as nature's blessing to mankind to help them pursue improved health. Although the plant kingdom embodies 250,000 plants, only 10% of these have been studied for medical practices. Phytochemicals and their derivatives perform numerous pharmacological activities and are potentially present in various parts of the plant including the flower and its parts, pericarp, sprouts, stem, leaf, embryo, roots, rhizomes, seeds, fruits, and bark. Although there are other potential methods for cancer treatment like tumor surgery, radiotherapy, immunotherapy, chemotherapy, vaccinations, photodynamic therapy, and stem cell transformations, these are often accompanied by severe side effects including toxicity, limited bioavailability, non-specificity, fast clearance, and metastatic restrictions [18]. Primary metabolites, secondary metabolites, and phytochemicals like alkaloids, flavonoids, lignans, glycosides, gums, oils, saponins, terpenes, taxanes, vitamins, minerals, and biomolecules inhibit malignant cells by either activating DNA repair mechanisms or by hindering cancer cell activating proteins, enzymes, and signalling pathways. Hence, researchers have confirmed that plant-derived compounds possess remarkably promising properties for enhanced and less toxic cancer treatment [19].

## MECHANISM OF CELL DEATH

The process of apoptosis is triggered by multi-signal pathways, which are regulated by various complex extrinsic and intrinsic ligands. Extrinsic and intrinsic pathways are the two major basic pathways that a cell undergoes for executing the process of programmed cell death or apoptosis. This pathway involves the presence of a cascade of caspases including caspase-8, caspase-9, caspase-12, caspase-7, and caspase-3 along with a variety of receptors including death receptor TNF-alpha, FasL, and TLR. The series of mechanisms begins with the activation of Caspase-8 through the death complex followed by the activation of Bcl-2 protein, which induces mitochondria membrane change that further stimulates Cytochrome-C. Upon infection in a cell, immune cells like cytotoxic T cells or natural killer cells come into its vicinity, which expresses FasL (Fas Ligand), and the target cell exhibits receptors for the FasL. FADD (Fas Associated protein with death domain) is an adapter protein that binds to the receptor which recognises the death domain of the receptor. This recruits caspase-8 and the complex hence formed is known as DISC (Death-inducing silencing complex). This is a brief outline of the extrinsic apoptotic pathway. On the other hand, the intrinsic pathway or the intracellular pathway is triggered by DNA damage or mitochondrial damage. Mitochondria upon damage releases Cytochrome C, which binds with Apaf-1 (Apoptosis protease activating factor) leading to the recruitment of caspase-9 in its procaspase form. The combination of Cytochrome C, Apaf-1, and procaspase-9 is referred to as apoptosome. Thereafter procaspase-9 activates caspase-9, which activates caspase-3 for executing the process of apoptosis [20, 21]. Fig. (**1**) represents a crosstalk between cell death pathways- ZBP1 in its activated form recruits RIPK3, FADD, and Caspase-8.

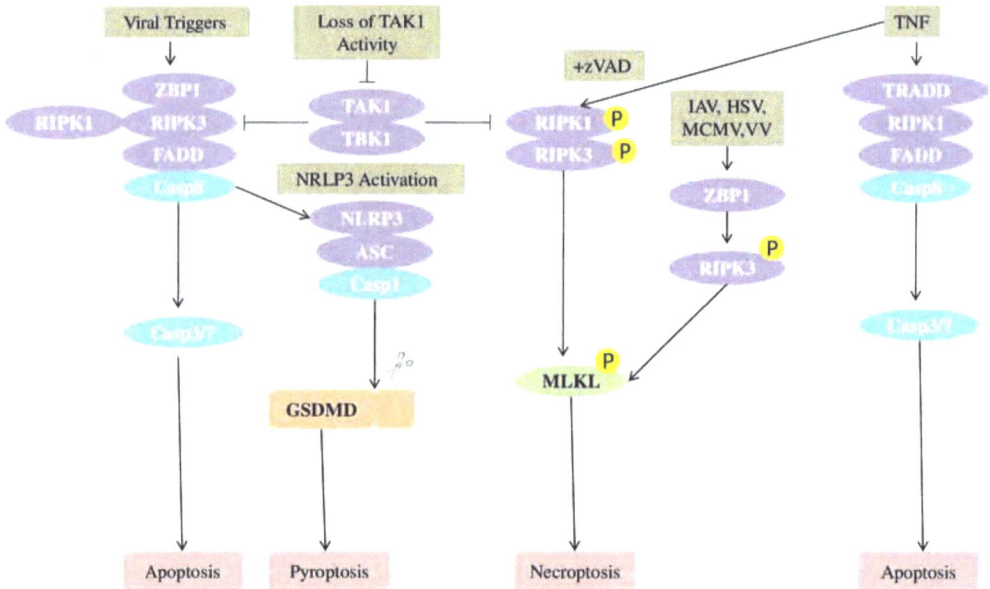

**Fig. (1).** Crosstalk between cell death pathways- ZBP1 in its activated form recruits RIPK3, FADD, and Caspase-8. This drives a parallel cell death pathway of apoptosis and pyroptosis. NLRP3 in its activated form leads to ASC and Caspase-1 inflammasome assembly and cleavage of GSDMD. TNF-mediated cell death induces apoptosis *via* TRADD, RIPK1, RIPK3, caspase-8, caspase-3, and caspase-7. When caspase-8 (by zVAD) is inhibited, TNF drives RIPK1, RIPK3, and MLKL phosphorylation resulting in necroptotic cell death. The nucleic acid binding protein ZBP1 can be directly activated with the help of viral infection (influenza A virus [IAV], HSV, mouse cytomegalovirus [MCMV], and vaccinia virus [VV]) for inducing cell death through parallel pathways of necroptosis, apoptosis, and pyroptosis.

## APOPTOSIS AND CANCER

Cancer can be seen as the outcome of a series of genetic alterations that transform a healthy cell into a cancerous one. Evading apoptosis or resisting cell death is one of the critical changes that lead to oncogenesis [22]. One of the major roles of apoptosis is to prevent cancer. Various cancer cells, however, acquire strategies to escape this firmly controlled cell death pathway by the overexpression of some anti-apoptotic molecules or by halting pathways that promote apoptosis [23]. Cancer cells employ a variety of mechanisms to suppress apoptosis and evade cell death. This can be done either by the disruption of intrinsic, extrinsic, or convergence signaling pathways [24].

Carcinogenesis is aided by a change in the balance of anti-apoptotic and pro-apoptotic molecules. For instance, the survival of tumor cells is enhanced by the lack of balance between pro- and anti-apoptotic members of the Bcl-2 family as well as their genetic and epigenetic modifications. Overexpression of some anti-apoptotic proteins and/or under-expression of some pro-apoptotic proteins contribute to the dysregulation of apoptosis in cancer cells. The suppression of apoptosis by the overexpression of Bcl-2 in neuroblastoma, glioblastoma, prostate, and breast tumor cells has been reported by several studies [25, 26]. Downregulation of BAX is another mechanism through which cancer cells try to evade cell death. In approximately half of all cancer cases, frameshift mutation contributes to the inactivation of BAX [27].

In many malignancies, abnormality in the expression of Inhibitors of Apoptosis (IAPs) is often observed. Survivin, an IAP generally confined to embryonic cells, but identified in a range of tumor forms, is perhaps the most prominent example of IAP overexpression in malignancies [28]. Overexpression of survivin has been correlated with reduced vulnerability to apoptosis in cancer cells *in vitro* [29]. It has also been confirmed by several patient investigations that survivin overexpression in tumors is associated with a poorer prognosis, as well as greater rates of therapeutic failure and recurrence [30].

Reduced caspase activity is another pro-survival mechanism through which cancer cells evade apoptosis [31]. Caspases are required for the proper execution of apoptosis, making them ideal candidates for studying the mechanism of suppression of apoptosis by cancer cells. Generally, under-expression of executioner caspases is observed in cancer cells. Furthermore, in a variety of malignancies, caspase gene deletions or inactivation has also been found [32].

## APOPTOSIS AND CANCER THERAPY

Controlling or potentially terminating the uncontrolled proliferation of tumor cells is one of the methods of treating cancers. It is indeed a massively effective strategy to kill cancer cells by using their natural cell death process. Furthermore, the most effective non-surgical way to treat cancers is by targeting their apoptotic cell death machinery either intrinsic or extrinsic pathways. Therapeutic approaches that can re-establish normalcy to apoptotic machinery have the capability to eradicate tumor cells that rely on these abnormalities to survive. Several recent and significant findings have paved the way for promising new classes of anticancer therapeutics. Anticancer agents that operate *via* targeting apoptotic pathways are listed in Table **1**.

## PLANT-DERIVED COMPOUNDS EXHIBITING ANTI-CANCEROUS ACTIVITY

The four major classes of plant-derived compounds exhibiting anti-cancer activities are vinca alkaloids that include vinblastine, vincristine, and vindesine, taxanes including paclitaxel and docetaxel, the epipodophyllotoxins like etoposide and teniposide and lastly camptothecin derivatives including camptothecin and irinotecan [58]. Vincristine is useful for the treatment of acute leukemia, Hodgkin lymphoma, and lung cancer. Vinblastine is effective against Hodgkin lymphoma, lung cancer, bladder cancer, and other cancer types as well. Vinorelbine treats breast cancer and non-small cell lung cancer. Eribulin is helpful for treating breast cancer and sarcoma. The mechanism of action of vinca alkaloids involves the binding of beta-tubulin that inhibits microtubule assembly and mitotic spindle formation. Cell death occurs by microtubule assembly and tubulin self-association [59]. Taxanes are a class of anticancer drugs that are natural cytostatic agents isolated from the bark of the Yew tree. They are widely used in treating solid tumors including breast, lung, and ovarian cancer and Kaposi sarcoma. The mechanism behind the activity of taxanes is its effect on microtubules, which is an essential part of mitotic spindles. Paclitaxel functions by the disruption of microtubule assembly, which has toxic effects on chick, rat, and rabbit embryos when applied during organogenesis. Docetaxel is a semisynthetic analog [60 - 62]. Etoposide, an Epipodophyllotoxin, is derived from the roots of the mayapple or mandrake plant which aids in the stabilization of DNA strand breaks created by Topoisomerase II at the time of coiling and supercoiling of DNA during the process of mitosis. It acts in the late S and early G2 phases of the cell cycle. Etoposide is used with drugs to treat small cell lung, testicular, bladder, prostate, stomach, and uterine cancers [63]. *Camptotheca acuminata, Chonemorpha grandiflora,* and *Nothapodytes nimmoniana* are trees native to China that possess compounds responsible for antitumor activities. A tryptophan-derived quinoline alkaloid with a specific pentacyclic ring structure, Camptothecin, obtained from these trees was found to be active in the life prolongation of mice that were treated with leukemia cells (L1210). The compound showed activity in inhibiting solid tumors that were at an early stage. Camptothecin affects topoisomerase I, which induces DNA cleavage and inhibits subsequent ligation leading to DNA strand breaks [64]. Colchicine, extracted from *Colchicum autumnale,* is a bioactive compound that is useful for the treatment of crystal arthritis, cirrhosis, gout, *etc.* This compound binds to tubulin and stabilizes microtubule formation. This arrests the cell cycle at various phases and promotes apoptosis [65]. However, the action mechanism of colchicine is nonspecific since it acts upon rapidly dividing normal cells thereby arresting its cell cycle. However, colchicinamide and deacetylcolchicine are the semisynthetic derivatives and are useful for treating colorectal cancer, chronic granulocytic leukemia, melanoma, and breast cancers [66]. Berberine is obtained from the roots and rhizome of *Tinospora cordifolia, Berberis vulgaris, Berberis aquifolium,* and *Rhizoma coptidis* [67]. This phytochemical is useful for the treatment of breast, prostate, and colorectal cancer. Berberine promotes apoptosis and cell cycle arrest in certain forms of cancer.

**Table 1. Anticancer agents that operate *via* apoptosis (*FDA Approved).**

| Treatment Strategy | Therapeutic Class | Agent | Tumor Type | References |
|---|---|---|---|---|
| Targeting the Bcl-2 family of proteins | Histone deacetylase inhibitors | Vorinostat* | Cutaneous T-cell Lymphoma | [33] |
| | | Romidepsin* | Cutaneous T-cell Lymphoma, Peripheral T-cell Lymphoma | [34] |
| | | Belinostat* | Relapsed or Refractory Peripheral T-cell Lymphoma | [35] |
| | | Panabiostat* | Relapsed Multiple Myeloma | [36, 37] |
| | Antisense Oligonucleotides | Oblimersen | Malignant Melanoma, Chronic Lymphocytic Leukemia, Acute Myeloid Leukemia, Multiple Myeloma | [38] |
| | BH3-mimetics | Venetoclax* | Chronic Myeloid Leukemia, Acute Myeloid Leukemia | [39] |
| | | Gossypol | Colon cancer, Breast Cancer | [40] |
| | | Obatoclax mesylate | Several types of Leukemia and Lymphoma, Myelofibrosis | [41] |
| | | Navitoclax | Small cell lung cancer, Acute Lymphocytic Leukemia | [42] |
| | | Apogossypolone | Nasopharyngeal carcinoma | [43] |
| | | Sabutoclax | Breast cancer, Prostate cancer | [44, 45] |
| | | Maritoclax | Acute Myeloid Leukemia | [46] |
| Targeting p53 | MDM2 inhibitors | Nutlin-3 | Nasopharyngeal carcinoma | [47] |
| | | RG7112 | Osteosarcooma, Leukemia | [48, 49] |
| | | AMG-232 (KRT-232) | Multiple Myeloma, Advanced p53-wild type solid tumors | [50] |
| | | APG-115 | Acute Myeloid Leukemia | [51] |
| | | Milademetan | Solid Tumors | [52] |
| | Restoring mutant p53 | Gendicine* | Head and Neck cancer | [53] |
| | | Eprenetapopt* | Myelodysplastic Syndromes | [54] |
| | | COTI-2 | Head and Neck Squamous cell carcinoma, Gynecological malignancies | [55] |
| Targeting IAPs | SMAC mimetics | Smac mimetic Compound A | Triple-Negative Breast Cancer | [56] |
| - | - | LCL161, GDC-0152 | Osteosarcoma | [57] |

Flavonoids, tannins, curcumin, resveratrol, and gallacatechins (Table **2**) are phenolic compounds that potentially exhibit anticancer activities [68, 69]. These compounds contain at least one or more hydroxyl groups and their high potency to chelate metals contribute to their antioxidant action. Polyphenols being natural antioxidants not only improve health but also reduce the risk of cancer. These compounds are present in common food items including green tea (gallocatechin), peanuts, grapes, and red wine (resveratrol) so, the major source of phenolic antioxidants is dietary. Curcumin is a yellow-orange turmeric powder which is a polyphenolic compound obtained from *Curcuma longa* that is an effective chemo preventive agent. Research suggested that polyphenols possess apoptosis-inducing properties that exhibit anticancer activities as well. Polyphenols initiate apoptosis through the regulation of mobilization of copper ions bound to chromatin that bring about DNA degradation. Plant polyphenols can interact with proteins of cancerous cells that promote growth in these cells. Hence, the agents causing malignancy could particularly be affected or altered *via* the polyphenol regulating acetylation, methylation or phosphorylation by direct bonding mechanisms [70, 71]. Flavonoids are polyphenolic compounds constituting plant secondary metabolites with 10,000 known structures [72, 73]. These compounds including flavones, flavonols, and chalcones can be found in abundance in just a single plant structure like seed. The anticancerous nature of flavonoids, their cytotoxicity on cancer cells, and free radical scavenging ability in human lung cancer cells was found in fern species (Dryopteris erythrosora). Research suggests that flavonoids in the purified form demonstrate anticancer activity against hematoma (Hep-G2), cervical carcinoma (Hela) and breast cancer (MCF-7) [74]. Moreover, M'-Methoxy licoflavanone (MLF) and Alpinumi soflavone (AIF) extracted from the stem bark of *Erythrina suberosa* are flavonoids that have cytotoxic effects in human leukemia cells (HL-60 cells). These flavonoids induce apoptotic proteins that reduce the mitochondrial membrane potential as a result of the mitochondrial damage, the cancer cells fail to survive.

**Table 2. Different plant-derived compounds and their involvement in inducing apoptosis.**

| Compound | Source | Action Mechanism | References |
|---|---|---|---|
| Aloe-emodin | *Rheum palmatum* | Induces cytochrome release | [75] |
| Black cohosh | *Actaea racemosa* | Activates caspases | [76] |
| Curcumin | Turmeric | Inhibits BCL-2 and XIAP | [77] |
| Epigallocatechin-3-gallate | Green tea component | Activates cell death Receptus | [78] |
| Genistein | Soyabeans | Cell cycle arrest activation | [79] |
| Graviola | *Annona muricata* | Inhibits BCL-2 and activates BAX | [80] |
| Juglone | *Juglans mandshurica* | Increases caspase 9 cleavage | [81] |

*(Table 2) cont.....*

| Compound | Source | Action Mechanism | References |
|---|---|---|---|
| Quercetin | Bark of many plants | Modulating cell cycle regulators to arrest the cell cycle | [82] |

## CONCLUSION

With the rising population, the number of cancer affected victims has also risen and any solution to controlling the initiation and proliferation of malignancy is of paramount importance. The aim of various cytotoxic as well as molecular management approaches is not only to eradicate the affected cells but also to control the cancer phenotype. Attempts have been made to explore the effectiveness of bioactive and chemo-preventive compounds isolated from plants. Therefore, we can conclude that the complex mechanisms of apoptosis play vital roles in cancer treatment and have been a popular target of various treatment strategies. The field of apoptosis research continues to focus on the elucidation of cellular mechanisms and has been proliferating forward at an alarmingly rapid rate.

## ACKNOWLEDGEMENTS

The authors would like to acknowledge the Amity Institute of Biotechnology, Amity University Kolkata, and Jharkhand for their constant assistance in writing this review paper.

## REFERENCES

[1] Galluzzi L, Vitale I, Aaronson SA, *et al.* Molecular mechanisms of cell death: recommendations of the Nomenclature Committee on Cell Death 2018. Cell Death Differ 2018; 25(3): 486-541.
[http://dx.doi.org/10.1038/s41418-017-0012-4] [PMID: 29362479]

[2] D'Arcy MS. Cell death: a review of the major forms of apoptosis, necrosis and autophagy. Cell Biol Int 2019; 43(6): 582-92.
[http://dx.doi.org/10.1002/cbin.11137] [PMID: 30958602]

[3] Kashyap D, Garg VK, Goel N. Intrinsic and extrinsic pathways of apoptosis: Role in cancer development and prognosis. Adv Protein Chem Struct Biol 2021; 125: 73-120.
[http://dx.doi.org/10.1016/bs.apcsb.2021.01.003] [PMID: 33931145]

[4] Elmore S. Apoptosis: a review of programmed cell death. Toxicol Pathol 2007; 35(4): 495-516.
[http://dx.doi.org/10.1080/01926230701320337] [PMID: 17562483]

[5] Sethi JK, Hotamisligil GS. Metabolic Messengers: tumour necrosis factor. Nat Metab 2021; 3(10): 1302-12.
[http://dx.doi.org/10.1038/s42255-021-00470-z] [PMID: 34650277]

[6] Sun Y, Yu J, Liu X, *et al.* Oncosis-like cell death is induced by berberine through ERK1/2-mediated impairment of mitochondrial aerobic respiration in gliomas. Biomed Pharmacother 2018; 102: 699-710.
[http://dx.doi.org/10.1016/j.biopha.2018.03.132] [PMID: 29604589]

[7]     Kesavardhana S, Malireddi RKS, Kanneganti TD. Caspases in cell death, inflammation, and pyroptosis. Annu Rev Immunol 2020; 38(1): 567-95.
[http://dx.doi.org/10.1146/annurev-immunol-073119-095439] [PMID: 32017655]

[8]     Messer JS. The cellular autophagy/apoptosis checkpoint during inflammation. Cell Mol Life Sci 2017; 74(7): 1281-96.
[http://dx.doi.org/10.1007/s00018-016-2403-y] [PMID: 27837217]

[9]     Mohammadinejad R, Moosavi MA, Tavakol S, *et al.* Necrotic, apoptotic and autophagic cell fates triggered by nanoparticles. Autophagy 2019; 15(1): 4-33.
[http://dx.doi.org/10.1080/15548627.2018.1509171] [PMID: 30160607]

[10]    Hanahan D, Weinberg RA. Hallmarks of cancer: the next generation. Cell. 2011, 4; 144(5): 646-74.
[http://dx.doi.org/10.1016/j.cell.2011.02.013]

[11]    Montero J, Letai A. Why do BCL-2 inhibitors work and where should we use them in the clinic? Cell Death Differ 2018; 25(1): 56-64.
[http://dx.doi.org/10.1038/cdd.2017.183] [PMID: 29077093]

[12]    Boise LH, González-García M, Postema CE, *et al.* bcl-x, a bcl-2-related gene that functions as a dominant regulator of apoptotic cell death. cell. 1993, 27; 74(4): 597-608.
[http://dx.doi.org/10.1016/0092-8674(93)90508-N]

[13]    Fuchs Y, Steller H. Programmed cell death in animal development and disease. Cell 2011; 147(4): 742-58.
[http://dx.doi.org/10.1016/j.cell.2011.10.033] [PMID: 22078876]

[14]    Fulda S. Tumor resistance to apoptosis. Int J Cancer 2009; 124(3): 511-5.
[http://dx.doi.org/10.1002/ijc.24064] [PMID: 19003982]

[15]    Ferlay J, Colombet M, Soerjomataram I, *et al.* Cancer statistics for the year 2020: An overview. Int J Cancer 2021; 149(4): 778-89.
[http://dx.doi.org/10.1002/ijc.33588] [PMID: 33818764]

[16]    Society AC. Cancer facts & figures. American Cancer Society. 2016, 24.

[17]    Krishnamurthi K. Screening of natural products for anticancer and antidiabetic properties. Health Administrator. XX (1&2). 2000; 69: 2000.

[18]    Patra CR, Mukherjee S, Kotcherlakota R. Biosynthesized silver nanoparticles: a step forward for cancer theranostics? Nanomedicine (Lond) 2014; 9(10): 1445-8.
[http://dx.doi.org/10.2217/nnm.14.89] [PMID: 25253493]

[19]    Singh S, Sharma B, Kanwar SS, Kumar A. Lead phytochemicals for anticancer drug development. Front Plant Sci 2016; 7: 1667.
[http://dx.doi.org/10.3389/fpls.2016.01667] [PMID: 27877185]

[20]    Pfeffer C, Singh A. Apoptosis: a target for anticancer therapy. Int J Mol Sci 2018; 19(2): 448.
[http://dx.doi.org/10.3390/ijms19020448] [PMID: 29393886]

[21]    Jan R, Chaudhry GS. Understanding apoptosis and apoptotic pathways targeted cancer therapeutics. Adv Pharm Bull 2019; 9(2): 205-18.
[http://dx.doi.org/10.15171/apb.2019.024] [PMID: 31380246]

[22]    Wong RSY. Apoptosis in cancer: from pathogenesis to treatment. J Exp Clin Cancer Res 2011; 30(1): 87.
[http://dx.doi.org/10.1186/1756-9966-30-87] [PMID: 21943236]

[23]    Igney FH, Krammer PH. Death and anti-death: tumour resistance to apoptosis. Nat Rev Cancer 2002; 2(4): 277-88.
[http://dx.doi.org/10.1038/nrc776] [PMID: 12001989]

[24]    Hassan M, Watari H, AbuAlmaaty A, Ohba Y, Sakuragi N. Apoptosis and molecular targeting therapy

in cancer. BioMed research international. 2014; 2014.
[http://dx.doi.org/10.1155/2014/150845]

[25] Fulda S, Meyer E, Debatin KM. Overexpression of Bcl-2 inhibits TRAIL-induced apoptosis. Oncogene 2002; 21: 2283-94.
[http://dx.doi.org/10.1038/sj.onc.1205258] [PMID: 11948412]

[26] Karnak D, Xu L. Chemosensitization of prostate cancer by modulating Bcl-2 family proteins. Curr Drug Targets 2010; 11(6): 699-707.
[http://dx.doi.org/10.2174/138945010791170888] [PMID: 20298153]

[27] Rampino N, Yamamoto H, Ionov Y, *et al.* Somatic frameshift mutations in the BAX gene in colon cancers of the microsatellite mutator phenotype. Science 1997; 275(5302): 967-9.
[http://dx.doi.org/10.1126/science.275.5302.967] [PMID: 9020077]

[28] Mittal RD, Jaiswal PK, Goel A. Survivin: A molecular biomarker in cancer. Indian J Med Res 2015; 141(4): 389-97.
[http://dx.doi.org/10.4103/0971-5916.159250] [PMID: 26112839]

[29] Chu XY, Chen LB, Wang JH, *et al.* Overexpression of survivin is correlated with increased invasion and metastasis of colorectal cancer. J Surg Oncol 2012; 105(6): 520-8.
[http://dx.doi.org/10.1002/jso.22134] [PMID: 22065492]

[30] Xia H, Chen S, Huang H, Ma H. Survivin over-expression is correlated with a poor prognosis in esophageal cancer patients. Clin Chim Acta 2015; 446: 82-5.
[http://dx.doi.org/10.1016/j.cca.2015.04.009] [PMID: 25896962]

[31] Koff J, Ramachandiran S, Bernal-Mizrachi L. A time to kill: targeting apoptosis in cancer. Int J Mol Sci 2015; 16(2): 2942-55.
[http://dx.doi.org/10.3390/ijms16022942] [PMID: 25636036]

[32] Yip KW, Reed JC. Bcl-2 family proteins and cancer. Oncogene 2008; 27(50): 6398-406.
[http://dx.doi.org/10.1038/onc.2008.307] [PMID: 18955968]

[33] Mann BS, Johnson JR, Cohen MH, Justice R, Pazdur R. FDA approval summary: vorinostat for treatment of advanced primary cutaneous T-cell lymphoma. Oncologist 2007; 12(10): 1247-52.
[http://dx.doi.org/10.1634/theoncologist.12-10-1247] [PMID: 17962618]

[34] Barbarotta L, Hurley K. Romidepsin for the treatment of peripheral T-cell lymphoma. J Adv Pract Oncol 2015; 6(1): 22-36.
[PMID: 26413372]

[35] Grant C, Rahman F, Piekarz R, *et al.* Romidepsin: a new therapy for cutaneous T-cell lymphoma and a potential therapy for solid tumors. Expert Rev Anticancer Ther 2010; 10(7): 997-1008.
[http://dx.doi.org/10.1586/era.10.88] [PMID: 20645688]

[36] Lee HZ, Kwitkowski VE, Del Valle PL, *et al.* FDA approval: belinostat for the treatment of patients with relapsed or refractory peripheral T-cell lymphoma. Clin Cancer Res 2015; 21(12): 2666-70.
[http://dx.doi.org/10.1158/1078-0432.CCR-14-3119] [PMID: 25802282]

[37] Raedler LA. Farydak (Panobinostat): first HDAC inhibitor approved for patients with relapsed multiple myeloma. Am Health Drug Benefits 2016; 9(Spec Feature): 84-7.

[38] Oblimersen: Augmerosen, BCL-2 antisense oligonucleotide - Genta, G 3139, GC 3139, oblimersen sodium. Drugs R D 2007; 8(5): 321-43.
[http://dx.doi.org/10.2165/00126839-200708050-00006]

[39] Scheffold A, Jebaraj BM, Stilgenbauer S. Venetoclax: targeting BCL2 in hematological cancers. Recent Results Cancer Res 2018:212:215-242.
[http://dx.doi.org/10.1007/978-3-319-91439-8_11]

[40] Cao H, Sethumadhavan K, Cao F, Wang TTY. Gossypol decreased cell viability and down-regulated the expression of a number of genes in human colon cancer cells. Sci Rep 2021; 11(1): 5922.

[http://dx.doi.org/10.1038/s41598-021-84970-8] [PMID: 33723275]

[41] Goard CA, Schimmer A. An evidence-based review of obatoclax mesylate in the treatment of hematological malignancies. Core Evid 2013; 8: 15-26.
[http://dx.doi.org/10.2147/CE.S42568] [PMID: 23515850]

[42] Mohamad Anuar NN, Nor Hisam NS, Liew SL, Ugusman A. Clinical review: navitoclax as a pro-apoptotic and anti-fibrotic agent. Front Pharmacol 2020; 11: 564108.
[http://dx.doi.org/10.3389/fphar.2020.564108] [PMID: 33381025]

[43] Zheng R, Chen K, Zhang Y, *et al.* Apogossypolone induces apoptosis and autophagy in nasopharyngeal carcinoma cells in an *in vitro* and *in vivo* study. Oncol Lett 2017; 14(1): 751-7.
[http://dx.doi.org/10.3892/ol.2017.6176] [PMID: 28693230]

[44] Hu Y, Yagüe E, Zhao J, *et al.* Sabutoclax, pan-active BCL-2 protein family antagonist, overcomes drug resistance and eliminates cancer stem cells in breast cancer. Cancer Lett 2018; 423: 47-59.
[http://dx.doi.org/10.1016/j.canlet.2018.02.036] [PMID: 29496539]

[45] Jackson RS II, Placzek W, Fernandez A, *et al.* Sabutoclax, a Mcl-1 antagonist, inhibits tumorigenesis in transgenic mouse and human xenograft models of prostate cancer. Neoplasia 2012; 14(7): 656-IN24.
[http://dx.doi.org/10.1593/neo.12640] [PMID: 22904682]

[46] Doi K, Liu Q, Gowda K, *et al.* Maritoclax induces apoptosis in acute myeloid leukemia cells with elevated Mcl-1 expression. Cancer Biol Ther 2014; 15(8): 1077-86.
[http://dx.doi.org/10.4161/cbt.29186] [PMID: 24842334]

[47] Zhang WW, Li L, Li D, *et al.* The first approved gene therapy product for cancer Ad-p53 (Gendicine): 12 years in the clinic. Hum Gene Ther 2018; 29(2): 160-79.
[http://dx.doi.org/10.1089/hum.2017.218] [PMID: 29338444]

[48] Yee-Lin V, Pooi-Fong W, Soo-Beng AK. Nutlin-3, a p53-Mdm2 antagonist for nasopharyngeal carcinoma treatment. Mini Rev Med Chem 2018; 18(2): 173-83.
[PMID: 28714398]

[49] Tovar C, Graves B, Packman K, *et al.* MDM2 small-molecule antagonist RG7112 activates p53 signaling and regresses human tumors in preclinical cancer models. Cancer Res 2013; 73(8): 2587-97.
[http://dx.doi.org/10.1158/0008-5472.CAN-12-2807] [PMID: 23400593]

[50] Andreeff M, Kelly KR, Yee K, *et al.* Results of the phase I trial of RG7112, a small-molecule MDM2 antagonist in leukemia. Clin Cancer Res 2016; 22(4): 868-76.
[http://dx.doi.org/10.1158/1078-0432.CCR-15-0481] [PMID: 26459177]

[51] Gluck WL, Gounder MM, Frank R, *et al.* Phase 1 study of the MDM2 inhibitor AMG 232 in patients with advanced P53 wild-type solid tumors or multiple myeloma. Invest New Drugs 2020; 38(3): 831-43.
[http://dx.doi.org/10.1007/s10637-019-00840-1] [PMID: 31359240]

[52] Fang DD, Tang Q, Kong Y, *et al.* MDM2 inhibitor APG-115 exerts potent antitumor activity and synergizes with standard-of-care agents in preclinical acute myeloid leukemia models. Cell Death Discov 2021; 7(1): 90.
[http://dx.doi.org/10.1038/s41420-021-00465-5] [PMID: 33941774]

[53] Takahashi S, Fujiwara Y, Nakano K, *et al.* Safety and pharmacokinetics of milademetan, a MDM2 inhibitor, in Japanese patients with solid tumors: A phase I study. Cancer Sci 2021; 112(6): 2361-70.
[http://dx.doi.org/10.1111/cas.14875] [PMID: 33686772]

[54] Sallman DA, DeZern AE, Garcia-Manero G, *et al.* Eprenetapopt (APR-246) and azacitidine in TP53-mutant myelodysplastic syndromes. J Clin Oncol 2021; 39(14): 1584-94.
[http://dx.doi.org/10.1200/JCO.20.02341] [PMID: 33449813]

[55] Lindemann A, Patel AA, Silver NL, *et al.* COTI-2, a novel thiosemicarbazone derivative, exhibits antitumor activity in HNSCC through p53-dependent and -independent mechanisms. Clin Cancer Res

2019; 25(18): 5650-62.
[http://dx.doi.org/10.1158/1078-0432.CCR-19-0096] [PMID: 31308060]

[56]    Lalaoui N, Merino D, Giner G, *et al.* Targeting triple-negative breast cancers with the Smac-mimetic birinapant. Cell Death Differ 2020; 27(10): 2768-80.
[http://dx.doi.org/10.1038/s41418-020-0541-0] [PMID: 32341449]

[57]    Shekhar TM, Burvenich IJG, Harris MA, *et al.* Smac mimetics LCL161 and GDC-0152 inhibit osteosarcoma growth and metastasis in mice. BMC Cancer 2019; 19(1): 924.
[http://dx.doi.org/10.1186/s12885-019-6103-5] [PMID: 31521127]

[58]    Taneja SC, Qazi GN. Bioactive Molecues in Medicinal Plants: A perspective in their therapeutic action. Drug discovery and development. 2007 Feb 16; 1: 1-50.

[59]    Zhang D, Kanakkanthara A. Beyond the paclitaxel and vinca alkaloids: Next generation of plant-derived microtubule-targeting agents with potential anticancer activity. Cancers (Basel) 2020; 12(7): 1721.
[http://dx.doi.org/10.3390/cancers12071721] [PMID: 32610496]

[60]    Lynch CD, Lee MJ, Del Priore G. Chemotherapy in pregnancy. Clinical pharmacology during pregnancy. 2013, 1; 201.
[http://dx.doi.org/10.1016/B978-0-12-386007-1.00014-3]

[61]    Shahpar S, Mhatre PV, Oza S. Rehabilitation. InThe Breast 2018, 1, pp. 1031-1038. Elsevier.

[62]    Tsuji W, Plock JA. Breast cancer metastasis. InIntroduction to Cancer Metastasis, 2017,1 pp. 13-31. Academic Press.
[http://dx.doi.org/10.1016/B978-0-12-804003-4.00002-5]

[63]    Bookman MA. Principles of chemotherapy in gynecologic cancer. Principles and Practice of Gynecologic Oncology. 2009:381.

[64]    Nelson MR, Bryc K, King KS, *et al.* The Population Reference Sample, POPRES: a resource for population, disease, and pharmacological genetics research. Am J Hum Genet 2008; 83(3): 347-58.
[http://dx.doi.org/10.1016/j.ajhg.2008.08.005] [PMID: 18760391]

[65]    Negi AS, Gautam Y, Alam S, *et al.* Natural antitubulin agents: Importance of 3,4,5-trimethoxyphenyl fragment. Bioorg Med Chem 2015; 23(3): 373-89.
[http://dx.doi.org/10.1016/j.bmc.2014.12.027] [PMID: 25564377]

[66]    Lin X, Peng Z, Su C. Potential anti-cancer activities and mechanisms of costunolide and dehydrocostuslactone. Int J Mol Sci 2015; 16(5): 10888-906.
[http://dx.doi.org/10.3390/ijms160510888] [PMID: 25984608]

[67]    Mantena SK, Sharma SD, Katiyar SK. Berberine, a natural product, induces G1-phase cell cycle arrest and caspase-3-dependent apoptosis in human prostate carcinoma cells. Mol Cancer Ther 2006; 5(2): 296-308.
[http://dx.doi.org/10.1158/1535-7163.MCT-05-0448] [PMID: 16505103]

[68]    Teodor ED, Ungureanu O, Gatea F, Radu GL. The potential of flavonoids and tannins from medicinal plants as anticancer agents. Anti-cancer agents in medicinal chemistry (formerly current medicinal chemistry-anti-cancer agents). 2020, 1; 20(18): 2216-27.
[http://dx.doi.org/10.2174/1871520620666200516150829]

[69]    Bora J, Sahariah P, Patar AK, Syiem D, Bhan S. Attenuation of diabetic hepatopathy in alloxan-induced diabetic mice by methanolic flower extract of Phlogacanthus thyrsiflorus Nees. J Appl Pharm Sci 2018; 8(7): 114-20.
[http://dx.doi.org/10.7324/JAPS.2018.8718]

[70]    Gupta SC, Tyagi AK, Deshmukh-Taskar P, Hinojosa M, Prasad S, Aggarwal BB. Downregulation of tumor necrosis factor and other proinflammatory biomarkers by polyphenols. Arch Biochem Biophys 2014; 559: 91-9.
[http://dx.doi.org/10.1016/j.abb.2014.06.006] [PMID: 24946050]

[71]    Heo BG, Park YJ, Park YS, *et al.* Anticancer and antioxidant effects of extracts from different parts of indigo plant. Ind Crops Prod 2014; 56: 9-16.
[http://dx.doi.org/10.1016/j.indcrop.2014.02.023]

[72]    Cao J, Xia X, Chen X, Xiao J, Wang Q. Characterization of flavonoids from Dryopteris erythrosora and evaluation of their antioxidant, anticancer and acetylcholinesterase inhibition activities. Food Chem Toxicol 2013; 51: 242-50.
[http://dx.doi.org/10.1016/j.fct.2012.09.039] [PMID: 23063594]

[73]    Bora J, Syiem D, Bhan S. Methanolic flower extract of Phlogacanthus thyrsiflorus nees. Attenuates diabetic nephropathy in alloxan-induced diabetic mice. Asian J Pharm Clin Res 2018; 11(7): 113-6.
[http://dx.doi.org/10.22159/ajpcr.2018.v11i7.25393]

[74]    Wen L, Wu D, Jiang Y, *et al.* Identification of flavonoids in litchi (Litchi chinensis Sonn.) leaf and evaluation of anticancer activities. J Funct Foods 2014; 6: 555-63.
[http://dx.doi.org/10.1016/j.jff.2013.11.022]

[75]    Dalimi A, Delavari M, Ghaffarifar F, Sadraei J. *In vitro* and *in vivo* antileishmanial effects of aloe-emodin on Leishmania major. J Tradit Complement Med 2015; 5(2): 96-9.
[http://dx.doi.org/10.1016/j.jtcme.2014.11.004] [PMID: 26151018]

[76]    Grant P, Ramasamy S. An update on plant derived anti-androgens. Int J Endocrinol Metab 2012; 10(2): 497-502.
[http://dx.doi.org/10.5812/ijem.3644] [PMID: 23843810]

[77]    Willenbacher E, Khan S, Mujica S, *et al.* Curcumin: new insights into an ancient ingredient against cancer. Int J Mol Sci 2019; 20(8): 1808.
[http://dx.doi.org/10.3390/ijms20081808] [PMID: 31013694]

[78]    Irimie AI, Braicu C, Zanoaga O, *et al.* Epigallocatechin-3-gallate suppresses cell proliferation and promotes apoptosis and autophagy in oral cancer SSC-4 cells. OncoTargets Ther 2015; 8: 461-70.
[PMID: 25759589]

[79]    Tuli HS, Tuorkey MJ, Thakral F, *et al.* Molecular mechanisms of action of genistein in cancer: Recent advances. Front Pharmacol 2019; 10: 1336.
[http://dx.doi.org/10.3389/fphar.2019.01336] [PMID: 31866857]

[80]    Ioannis P, Anastasis S, Andreas Y. Graviola: A systematic review on its anticancer properties. Am J Cancer Prev 2015; 3(6): 128-31.
[http://dx.doi.org/10.12691/ajcp-3-6-5]

[81]    Wu J, Zhang H, Xu Y, *et al.* Juglone induces apoptosis of tumor stem-like cells through ROS-p38 pathway in glioblastoma. BMC Neurol 2017; 17(1): 70.
[http://dx.doi.org/10.1186/s12883-017-0843-0] [PMID: 28388894]

[82]    Vafadar A, Shabaninejad Z, Movahedpour A, *et al.* Quercetin and cancer: new insights into its therapeutic effects on ovarian cancer cells. Cell Biosci 2020; 10(1): 32.
[http://dx.doi.org/10.1186/s13578-020-00397-0] [PMID: 32175075]

# CHAPTER 13

# Apoptosis Defects in Cancer and its Therapeutic Implications

**Jutishna Bora[1,#], Sayak Banerjee[2,#], Indrani Barman[3], Sarvesh Rustagi[4], Richa Mishra[5] and Sumira Malik[1,*]**

[1] *Amity Institute of Biotechnology, Amity University, Jharkhand, Ranchi, Jharkhand-834002, India*

[2] *Amity Institute of Biotechnology, Amity University Kolkata, Kolkata, West Bengal-700135, India*

[3] *Program of Biotechnology, Faculty of Science, Assam Down Town University, Guwahati, Assam, India*

[4] *School of Applied and Life Sciences, Uttaranchal University, Dehradun, 248007 Uttarakhand, India*

[5] *Department of Computer Engineering, Parul University, Ta. Waghodia, Vadodara, Gujarat, 391760, India*

**Abstract:** Apoptosis is the programmed cell death that regulates the cell survival or cell death balance in animals. Defects in apoptosis can cause cancer or autoimmunity, while enhanced apoptosis may cause degenerative diseases. The apoptotic signals mostly contribute to protecting the genomic integrity whereas defective apoptosis might lead to carcinogenesis. The signals of carcinogenesis alter the central points of the apoptotic pathways, which include the FLICE-inhibitory protein (c-FLIP) and the inhibitor of apoptosis (IAP) proteins. The tumor cells trigger the expression of antiapoptotic proteins such as Bcl-2 or downregulate the proapoptotic proteins like BAX. Most of these changes lead to intrinsic resistance to the most common anticancer therapy, chemotherapy. Apoptosis-resistant cells and transduction pathways that inhibit apoptosis can stimulate non-apoptotic mechanisms of cell death and senescence; this preserves the antitumor effect of several anticancer agents. The development of some promising cancer treatment strategies has been discussed below, which target apoptotic inhibitors including Bcl-2 family proteins, IAPs, and c-FLIP for the induction of apoptosis.

**Keywords:** Apoptosis, Cell death, Cancer, Carcinogenesis, Therapies.

[*] **Corresponding author Sumira Malik:** Amity Institute of Biotechnology, Amity University, Jharkhand, Ranchi, Jharkhand-834002, India; E-mail: smalik@rnc.amity.edu
[#] These authors are equallly contribed to this work.

**Ashok Kumar Pandurangan (Ed.)**

## INTRODUCTION

Programmed cell death is a central component of many biological processes in animals. It plays a crucial role in the development of immunity, embryogenesis, and integrity of eukaryotic organisms [1]. This firmly coordinated event when subjected to dysregulation leads to an array of diseases such as immunodeficiency, autoimmune disease, developmental disorders, neurode-generation, and cancer [2]. Programmed cell death can be characterized into apoptotic and non-apoptotic cell death, conventionally called necrosis. Indisputably, apoptosis is the best-described and most evolutionary conserved form of programmed cell death. It not only involves homeostatic mechanisms of cell suicide for controlling the cell populations in tissues but also the defense mechanisms in immune reactions and disease pathogenesis [3]. Apoptosis is modulated by complex molecular signaling pathways and can be initiated by both external and internal stimuli. The stimuli can result from various DNA-damaging agents like chemotherapeutic agents and UV radiations giving rise to intracellular stresses such as oxidative stress, DNA damage, or oncogene activation. Extracellular signals include the death-inducing signaling complex (DISC), which comprises Fas ligand, TNF-α, FADD, TRADD, caspase-8 and -10 [4, 5]. On the contrary to apoptosis, non-apoptotic cell death or necrosis is an uncontrolled form of cell death mediated by different mechanisms from apoptosis leading to accidental cell death. Pathologists often use the term necrosis to classify the presence of dead cells or tissues. Irrespective of the processes occurring before cell death, it includes the overall changes that take place after cell death [6]. Necrotic cells are the dying cells that neither showed morphological traits of apoptotic nor any sign of autophagic cell death. Even though pathological traumas like ischemia and infection generally initiate necrosis, both death receptors as well as DNA damage can lead to necrosis [7].

## APOPTOTIC DEFECTS AND CANCER

There is a massive amount of different biochemical components in the various apoptotic pathways that still have ongoing research [8]. The normal functioning of a pathway is often deranged resulting in a compromise to normal apoptosis thus leading to disastrous effects such as disorders or diseases. Apoptotic defects are the genetic and epigenetic modifications that directly affect the expression of the specific machinery of the intrinsic and extrinsic apoptosis pathways. These modifications have been chiefly observed in primary adenocarcinoma.

### Defects in Caspase Signaling

Alterations in the gene encoding caspase proteases affect the expression of caspases in human tumors. These generally include mutation of initiator caspase-

8, caspase-9, and caspase-10, along with executioner caspase-3 and caspase-7. A mutant form of caspase-8 was observed in head and neck carcinoma as well as gastric and colorectal carcinoma specimens [9]. It leads to the decreased ability of the stimulation of apoptosis due to a frameshift mutation in the caspase-8 gene. Hyper methylation of this gene has been observed to have a loss of caspase-8 expression in neuroblastoma patients [10, 11]. It has also been observed in small-cell lung cancer (SCLC), hepatocellular carcinoma (HCC), and bladder cancer [12, 13]. Caspase-10 mutations have not only been observed in tumors but also in autoimmune disorders. Inactivating caspase-10 point mutations are the principal causes of the autoimmune lymphoproliferative syndrome (ALPS). Frameshift mutations give rise to the termination of premature caspase-10 in systemic juvenile idiopathic arthritis [14]. Multiple myeloma, hematopoietic carcinoma, and T-acute lymphoblastic leukemia also have been detected to have caspase-10 mutations. There is not much information on the mutation of caspase-3, caspase-7, and caspase-9.

The inhibitor of apoptosis (IAP) family of proteins, on the other hand, usually gets activated resulting in dysregulation of the intracellular activities of caspase-3, caspase-7, and caspase-9 [15]. X-linked IAP or XIAP acts directly to potentially inhibit these caspases, while cIAP or cellular IAP (cIAP1 and cIAP2) indirectly act upon the caspases to inhibit their activities. XIAP possesses baculovirus IAP repeat (BIR) domains, which have a high affinity for binding to caspase-3 and caspase-7. When the BIR1 and BIR2 domains are potentially bound to the active site of the caspases, access to the caspase substrate protein is prevented. The BIR3 domain binds to the monomeric form of caspase-9, thus inhibiting dimerization and enzyme activation [16, 17]. cIAP1 and cIAP2 involve two separate mechanisms, firstly, they can bind to the second mitochondria-derived activator of caspases (SMAC) and inhibit the action of SMAC protein by hindering XIAP from moving away from the bound caspases. Secondly, cIAP1 and cIAP2 subject the executioner caspases to ubiquitination leading to a gradual disintegration by the proteasome [18, 19]. Hematopoietic carcinoma and many other solid tumors have been detected to have an overexpression of IAPs, particularly XIAP. High levels of XIAP correlate with poor prognosis in adult acute myeloid leukemia (AML), childhood T-cell acute lymphoblastic leukemia, and diffuse large B-cell lymphomas (DLBCL) [Ibrahim AM *et al.* 2012, Hussain AR *et al.* 2010]. Both cIAP1 and cIAP2 including survivin have been observed to have reduced expression in various tumors with poor clinical outcomes. Overexpression of cIAP2 has been frequently detected in MALT lymphomas [20].

## Defects in Intrinsic Pathways

The intrinsic apoptosis pathway is highly coordinated by the members of the Bcl-

2 protein family. They share a similarity in the presence of conserved domains termed as Bcl-2 homology, or BH domains. There are two groups of proteins under the Bcl-2 family, namely "BH3 domain-only" proteins and "multiple-domain" proteins [21]. The multiple BH domains constitute Bak and Bax and the cells lacking them have shown to be resistant to the activation of the apoptosis pathway [22].

Increased expression of anti-apoptotic Bcl-2 has been observed in a wide range of hematopoietic malignancies such as DLBCL, AML, anaplastic large cell lymphoma (ALCL), chronic lymphocytic leukemia (CLL), multiple myeloma, and follicular B-cell lymphoma. The overexpression of Bcl-2 has been reported in solid tumors including SCLC, glioblastoma, melanoma, as well as colon cancer and prostate cancer [23, 24]. High levels of anti-apoptotic Bcl-$X_L$ have also been identified various in cancers like AML, squamous cell carcinoma of the head and neck (SCCHN), melanoma, multiple myeloma, along with breast, pancreatic, and bladder cancer [25]. There is very little evidence to date about the overexpression of anti-apoptotic Mcl-1 and Bcl-w in human tumors.

A complicated network of physical interactions has been discovered between anti-apoptotic members of the Bcl-2 family and proapoptotic members of the Bcl-2 protein family. Colorectal and hematopoietic carcinomas have been found to have an inactivated bax gene with a frameshift mutation whereas colon and gastric malignancies have been detected with bak gene mutations [26]. Homozygous deletion of the bim gene has been reported in mantle cell lymphomas (MCL) [27]. Promoter methylation also plays a significant role in dysregulating the expression of proapoptotic proteins in cancer. Hypermethylation of the puma gene takes place in Burkitt's lymphoma (BL), that of Noxa gene occurs in DLBCL, and that of the bik gene takes place in renal cell carcinomas [28].

## Defects in Extrinsic Pathways

Similar to the expression as well as the function of caspase-8 and caspase-10, autoimmune disease and malignant tumors also show modifications in the expression and function of the Fas death receptor. Human autoimmune lymphoproliferative syndrome (ALPS) is associated with somatic Fas mutations due to the loss of heterozygosity in the fas gene leading to an inactive Fas protein [29, 30]. In addition to that, Fas mutations have been observed in hematopoietic tumors such as MALT-type, non-Hodgkin, thyroid lymphomas, DLBC, and multiple myeloma [31]. Solid tumors associated with Fas mutation may include malignant melanoma, squamous cell carcinoma, stomach, testis, and bladder carcinoma [32]. The death ligand TRAIL that is involved in apoptosis is controlled by TRAIL-R1 and TRAIL-R2 (death receptors D4 and D5). Mutations in TRAIL-R1 and TRAIL-R2 are found in metastatic breast cancer, NSCLC, non-Hodgkin's, and gastric cancer. Hypermethylation of the TRAIL-R1 gene has been reported in glioma, SCLC, gastric, and ovarian cancer. TRAIL-R2 has been observed with loss of heterozygosity in NSCLC, gastric and colorectal cancers [33, 34].

The FADD (Fas-associated death domain) has an essential role in the Fas and TRAIL receptor-mediated activation of caspase-8 after being added to the DISC (death-inducing signaling complex). FADD mutations have been detected in ALS, NSCLC, and colon cancer [35]. IAPs and anti-apoptotic members of the Bcl-2 family are endogenous inhibitors of caspase expression and cytochrome c release respectively. Similarly, c-FLIP (cellular FLICE-inhibitory protein) proteins act as endogenous negative regulators of death receptor-mediated caspase-8/caspase-10 activation. Thus, the execution of the extrinsic apoptosis pathway is compromised due to the high levels of the c-FLIP proteins by inhibiting the activation of caspase-8/caspase-10. Overexpression of c-FLIP is reported in glioblastomas, NSCLCs, and melanomas, along with endometrial, ovarian, colon, breast and prostate cancers [36, 37].

## POTENTIAL LIMITED ROLE OF APOPTOTIC CELL DEATH

Although apoptosis is believed to be the major contributor causing cell death after treatment with anti-cancer drugs, an association between apoptotic and non-apoptotic pathways following therapy has also been indicated by various studies. In some studies, it was found that the treatment of carcinoma cell lines with TRAIL (Tumor Necrosis Factor-Related Apoptosis-Inducing Ligand) under normal oxygen concentrations led to the induction of apoptosis. But in hypoxic conditions, the apoptotic pathways were blocked by the inhibition of Bax and increased expression of some anti-apoptotic proteins including Bcl-XL, Bcl-2, and other IAP (Inhibitor of Apoptosis) proteins [38, 39]. However, non-apoptotic cell death is still stimulated by TRAIL under hypoxic or normoxic conditions [40]. Moreover, it has been found that non-apoptotic pathways like autophagy and necrosis play an important role in anticancer drug-stimulated cell deaths in some defective apoptotic models. In a p53-mutant model treated with anti-cancer drugs, no role of apoptosis in causing cell deaths was reported. However, some late-responsive non-apoptotic cell death pathways played significant roles in the killing of cancer cells [41]. This suggests that the non-apoptotic cell death pathways get activated in apoptosis-impaired cells, thus contributing to the comprehensive tumor response to anti-cancer drugs. The genotype of the cancer cell can also play an important role in determining sensitivity to some specific anti-cancer drugs. For example, in Akt and Bcl-2 overexpressing lymphoma cells with defective apoptosis, treatment with anti-cancer drugs Rapamycin and

Doxorubicin showed no effects. However, combined treatment with both these drugs led to the induction of cell death pathways in Akt-overexpressing lymphoma cells but remained ineffective in Bcl-2 overexpressing cells [42, 43]. Thus, combination treatment can be more effective in causing enhanced cell death by activation of diverse cell death pathways (Fig. **1**).

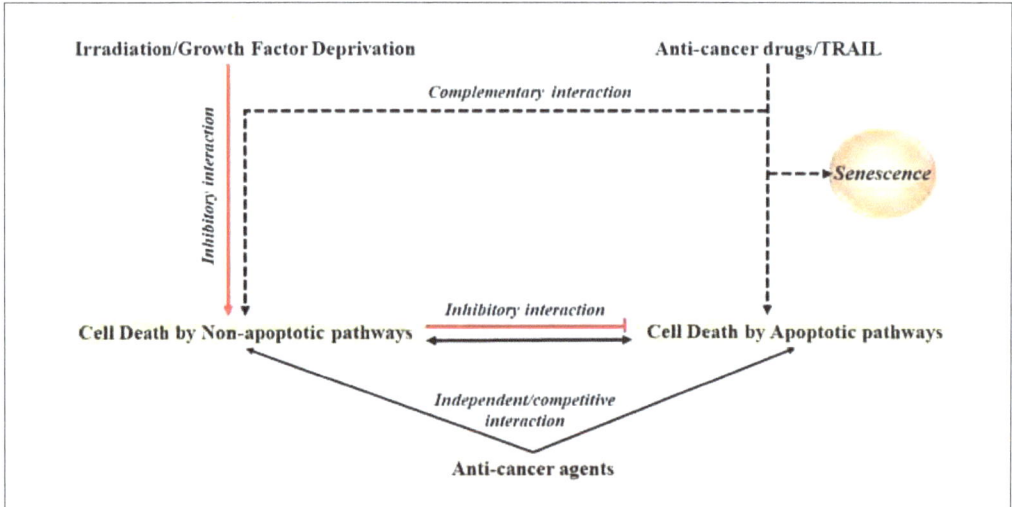

**Fig. (1).** Interaction between apoptotic and non-apoptotic pathways in cancer cell death triggered by anti-cancer agents and radiations.

Even though both apoptotic as well as non-apoptotic cell deaths are induced by anti-cancer agents and radiation, the interconnection between these two cell death pathways is not completely clear. Interconnection between different cell death pathways in response to anti-cancer agents or irradiations can be explained *via* three probable mechanisms. The first mechanism suggests the inhibition of one cell death pathway by another. Macroautophagy induced by depriving growth factors in IL-3-dependent Bax$^{-/-}$ Bak$^{-/-}$ cancer cells leads to the inhibition of the apoptotic pathways (Lum *et al.*, 2005). The second mechanism suggests that the upregulation of one pathway may lead to the inhibition of another. Although, both necrotic and apoptotic pathways are stimulated in case of cell death induced by TRAIL, enhanced necrosis leads to the inhibition of apoptosis by obstructing caspases [44]. Moreover, the inhibition of Caspase-8 also induces cell death similar to autophagy in RIP- (Receptor Interacting Proteins) and JNK- (c-Jun N-terminal Kinases) -activated cancer cells [45]. Thus, the role of autophagy in ensuring the survival of cancer cells under growth factor deprivation or irradiation is now well-established. However, when the cell damage surpasses the verge, autophagy is impeded, resulting in the promotion of cell death by apoptosis [46, 47]. Furthermore, the involvement of autophagy is narrowed in certain instances, resulting in the activation of apoptotic pathways. Thus, different mechanisms for the interplay between apoptotic and non-apoptotic cell death pathways must exist. The third mechanism suggests the independent functioning of apoptotic and non-apoptotic pathways. Many evidences support this mechanism. For example, in T-lymphoblastic lymphoma cells treated with TNF-α, the induction of autophagy is followed by the stimulation of apoptosis. However, apoptotic cell death pathways were not inhibited when autophagy was prevented by 3-MA [48]. In another study, it was found that the inhibition of apoptosis by etoposide in Bax$^{-/-}$/Bak$^{-/-}$ cancer cells does not affect non-apoptotic cell deaths [49].

Although apoptotic pathways are inhibited by overexpressing Bcl-2 and mutating the p53 gene, the proliferation of cancer cells is still not prevented, thus questioning the credibility of apoptosis in determining the results of an anti-cancerous agent in cancer patients. As suggested by various studies, the prognosis with or without therapy is not affected by mutation or overexpression of the p53 gene [50, 51]. Furthermore, anticancer agent-induced cell death is not affected by overexpression of Bcl-2, suggesting the replacement of apoptosis by other non-apoptotic cell death pathways [52]. Thus, these findings suggest the potential limited role of apoptosis in determining the efficiency and performance of an anti-cancer agent.

## TARGETED THERAPIES AND CANCER

### Targeting Anti-apoptotic Bcl-2 Family Members

Overexpression of Bcl-2 is observed in various types of malignancies and imparts therapeutic intractability to such tumors. Venetoclax, a highly selective inhibitor of Bcl-2, has been accepted for routine clinical practice. Venetoclax is a Bcl2-selective BH3-mimetic, and at the moment it is in use for the treatment of multiple myeloma T-cell prolymphocytic leukemia, ALL, and CLL. BH3-mimetics fall under the class of anticancer drugs that imitate the working of BH3-only proteins. These mimetics restrain their potential to bind to Bax or Bak by binding to prosurvival proteins such as Bcl-2 [53]. Hence, when cancer cells with overexpressed Bcl-2 proteins are treated with venetoclax *in vitro*, cancer cells undergo apoptosis. Mostly, venetoclax can be taken alone or in other ways like in combination with other drugs. Dexamethasone, azacitidine, ibrutinib, and srituximab can be used as a combination against different hematological tumors [54].

### Mcl-1 Inhibitors

Overexpression of Mcl-1 has been reported with drug resistance in both hematological as well as solid tumor malignancies against various therapeutic agents. There has been the development of many inhibitors that show potential anticancer properties in preclinical and clinical trials. It was observed that S63845 triggers apoptosis in SCLC cell lines *in vitro*, whereas when this molecule is administered in xenograft models, a considerable reduction in tumor volumes is detected. S63845 can be employed along with navitoclax, which can inhibit both Bcl-xL and Bcl-2 and this led to the reduction in cell viability of SCLC cells [55]. Moreover, because of its non-apoptotic association with DNA repair, Mcl-1 is a striking drug target in lung cancer. Mcl-1-mediated HR DNA repair is blocked by targeting Mcl-1 with a small molecule inhibitor named MI-233 which sensitizes cancer cells to treatment-induced replication stress. A strong synergism is observed when MI-233 is combined with olaparib in lung cancer models [56]. Tumor cell death can be triggered by another specific Mcl-1 inhibitor, VU661013, which might result in a synergistic decrease in tumor volume when used in combination with ABT-263 [57].

## XIAP Inhibitors

Several small molecules have been developed for targeting IAP proteins and one such class of molecules is called mimetics (SMs) .An XIAP inhibitor named BMT-062789 was found to inhibit both the caspase 3/7 and caspase 9 binding domains ofXIAP [58]. This inhibition was used against a panel of lymphoma cell lines and it demonstrated anticancer activity. BMT-062789 triggers apoptosis in rituximab-resistant cell line models Raji 4RH and RL 4RH when used along with etoposide. ASTX660 is another antagonist that selectively binds to and inhibits the action of XIAP and cIAP1 *via* potential pro-apoptotic and antineoplastic activities [59].

## Caspase Activators in Cancer Therapy

Small molecule activators can be used as an effective therapeutic strategy for pharmacological activation of caspases. These are used for killing cancer cells and have the capability to reverse drug resistance. Capase-3 is generally present in an inactive form by an intramolecular electrostatic interaction between aspartic acid residues. Apoptin, an essential caspase activating agent, is a protein that is rich in proline and has the potential to trigger apoptosis in cancer cells. It is extracted from the chicken anemia virus that causes tumor-specific apoptosis without disrupting the normal cells. Apoptin is regarded as a highly tumor-specific therapeutic agent [60, 61].

## CONCLUSION

Hence, on a concluding note, from various evidences, it can be stated that apoptotic defects play a significant part in the development of carcinoma.

Moreover, several treatment strategies targeting the apoptotic pathway have been a fascinating approach in the discovery of novel anticancer therapies. The drugs that have gained robust potential for their use as cancer therapeutics act either by inhibiting the action of antiapoptotic proteins or by blocking the transcription of siRNA, nevertheless, the hope to cure cancer is yet to be seen. Although many preclinical studies showed that resistance to apoptosis might lead to drug resistance, the exact association between apoptosis and tumor sensitivity is unclear. Future studies are required for understanding the specific compounds and their molecular mechanism that might be useful for cancer therapy as well as determining the relationship between various other cell death pathways for the limitation of tumor proliferation.

## ACKNOWLEDGEMENTS

The authors would like to acknowledge the Amity Institute of Biotechnology, Amity University Kolkata, and Jharkhand for their constant assistance in writing this review paper.

## REFERENCES

[1]    Tait SWG, Ichim G, Green DR. Die another way – non-apoptotic mechanisms of cell death. J Cell Sci 2014; 127(10): 2135-44.
[http://dx.doi.org/10.1242/jcs.093575] [PMID: 24833670]

[2]    Ameisen JC. On the origin, evolution, and nature of programmed cell death: a timeline of four billion years. Cell Death Differ 2002; 9(4): 367-93.
[http://dx.doi.org/10.1038/sj.cdd.4400950] [PMID: 11965491]

[3]    Norbury CJ, Hickson ID. Cellular responses to DNA damage. Annu Rev Pharmacol Toxicol 2001; 41(1): 367-401.
[http://dx.doi.org/10.1146/annurev.pharmtox.41.1.367] [PMID: 11264462]

[4]    Kischkel FC, Hellbardt S, Behrmann I, *et al.* Cytotoxicity-dependent APO-1 (Fas/CD95)-associated proteins form a death-inducing signaling complex (DISC) with the receptor. EMBO J 1995; 14(22): 5579-88.
[http://dx.doi.org/10.1002/j.1460-2075.1995.tb00245.x] [PMID: 8521815]

[5]    Nagata S. Apoptosis by death factor. Cell. 1997, 7; 88(3): 355-65.
[http://dx.doi.org/10.1016/s0092-8674(00)81874-7]

[6]    Vercammen D, Beyaert R, Denecker G, *et al.* Inhibition of caspases increases the sensitivity of L929 cells to necrosis mediated by tumor necrosis factor. J Exp Med 1998; 187(9): 1477-85.
[http://dx.doi.org/10.1084/jem.187.9.1477] [PMID: 9565639]

[7]    Levin S, Bucci TJ, Cohen SM, *et al.* The nomenclature of cell death: recommendations of an ad hoc Committee of the Society of Toxicologic Pathologists. Toxicol Pathol 1999; 27(4): 484-90.
[http://dx.doi.org/10.1177/019262339902700419] [PMID: 10485836]

[8]    Thompson CB. Apoptosis in the pathogenesis and treatment of disease. Science 1995; 267(5203): 1456-62.
[http://dx.doi.org/10.1126/science.7878464] [PMID: 7878464]

[9]    Soung YH, Lee JW, Kim SY, *et al.* CASPASE-8 gene is inactivated by somatic mutations in gastric carcinomas. Cancer Res 2005; 65(3): 815-21.
[http://dx.doi.org/10.1158/0008-5472.815.65.3] [PMID: 15705878]

[10] Kamimatsuse A, Matsuura K, Moriya S, *et al.* Detection of CpG island hypermethylation of caspase-8 in neuroblastoma using an oligonucleotide array. Pediatr Blood Cancer 2009; 52(7): 777-83.
[http://dx.doi.org/10.1002/pbc.21977] [PMID: 19260109]

[11] Banelli B, Casciano I, Croce M, *et al.* Expression and methylation of CASP8 in neuroblastoma: Identification of a promoter region. Nat Med 2002; 8(12): 1333-5.
[http://dx.doi.org/10.1038/nm1202-1333] [PMID: 12457155]

[12] Cho S, Lee JH, Cho SB, *et al.* Epigenetic methylation and expression of caspase 8 and survivin in hepatocellular carcinoma. Pathol Int 2010; 60(3): 203-11.
[http://dx.doi.org/10.1111/j.1440-1827.2009.02507.x] [PMID: 20403046]

[13] Shivapurkar N, Toyooka S, Eby MT, *et al.* Erratum: Differential inactivation of caspase-8 in lung cancers. Cancer Biol Ther 2002; 1(1): 65-9.
[http://dx.doi.org/10.4161/cbt.1.1.45]

[14] Tadaki H, Saitsu H, Kanegane H, *et al.* Exonic deletion of CASP10 in a patient presenting with systemic juvenile idiopathic arthritis, but not with autoimmune lymphoproliferative syndrome type IIa. Int J Immunogenet 2011; 38(4): 287-93.
[http://dx.doi.org/10.1111/j.1744-313X.2011.01005.x] [PMID: 21382177]

[15] Fulda S, Vucic D. Targeting IAP proteins for therapeutic intervention in cancer. Nat Rev Drug Discov 2012; 11(2): 109-24.
[http://dx.doi.org/10.1038/nrd3627] [PMID: 22293567]

[16] Scott FL, Denault JB, Riedl SJ, Shin H, Renatus M, Salvesen GS. XIAP inhibits caspase-3 and -7 using two binding sites: evolutionarily conserved mechanism of IAPs. EMBO J 2005; 24(3): 645-55.
[http://dx.doi.org/10.1038/sj.emboj.7600544] [PMID: 15650747]

[17] Shiozaki EN, Chai J, Rigotti DJ, *et al.* Mechanism of XIAP-mediated inhibition of caspase-9. Mol Cell 2003; 11(2): 519-27.
[http://dx.doi.org/10.1016/S1097-2765(03)00054-6] [PMID: 12620238]

[18] Schile AJ, García-Fernández M, Steller H. Regulation of apoptosis by XIAP ubiquitin-ligase activity. Genes Dev 2008; 22(16): 2256-66.
[http://dx.doi.org/10.1101/gad.1663108] [PMID: 18708583]

[19] Choi YE, Butterworth M, Malladi S, Duckett CS, Cohen GM, Bratton SB. The E3 ubiquitin ligase cIAP1 binds and ubiquitinates caspase-3 and -7 *via* unique mechanisms at distinct steps in their processing. J Biol Chem 2009; 284(19): 12772-82.
[http://dx.doi.org/10.1074/jbc.M807550200] [PMID: 19258326]

[20] Gyrd-Hansen M, Meier P. IAPs: from caspase inhibitors to modulators of NF-κB, inflammation and cancer. Nat Rev Cancer 2010; 10(8): 561-74.
[http://dx.doi.org/10.1038/nrc2889] [PMID: 20651737]

[21] Kelly GL, Strasser A. The essential role of evasion from cell death in cancer. Adv Cancer Res 2011; 111: 39-96.
[http://dx.doi.org/10.1016/B978-0-12-385524-4.00002-7] [PMID: 21704830]

[22] Wei MC, Zong WX, Cheng EHY, *et al.* Proapoptotic BAX and BAK: a requisite gateway to mitochondrial dysfunction and death. Science 2001; 292(5517): 727-30.
[http://dx.doi.org/10.1126/science.1059108] [PMID: 11326099]

[23] Reed JC. Bcl-2–family proteins and hematologic malignancies: history and future prospects. Blood 2008; 111(7): 3322-30.
[http://dx.doi.org/10.1182/blood-2007-09-078162] [PMID: 18362212]

[24] ten Berge RL, Meijer CJLM, Dukers DF, *et al.* Expression levels of apoptosis-related proteins predict clinical outcome in anaplastic large cell lymphoma. Blood 2002; 99(12): 4540-6.
[http://dx.doi.org/10.1182/blood.V99.12.4540] [PMID: 12036886]

[25] Shangary S, Johnson DE. Recent advances in the development of anticancer agents targeting cell death inhibitors in the Bcl-2 protein family. Leukemia 2003; 17(8): 1470-81.
[http://dx.doi.org/10.1038/sj.leu.2403029] [PMID: 12886234]

[26] Kondo S, Shinomura Y, Miyazaki Y, *et al.* Mutations of the bak gene in human gastric and colorectal cancers. Cancer Res 2000; 60(16): 4328-30.
[PMID: 10969770]

[27] Tagawa H, Karnan S, Suzuki R, *et al.* Genome-wide array-based CGH for mantle cell lymphoma: identification of homozygous deletions of the proapoptotic gene BIM. Oncogene 2005; 24(8): 1348-58.
[http://dx.doi.org/10.1038/sj.onc.1208300] [PMID: 15608680]

[28] Garrison SP, Jeffers JR, Yang C, *et al.* Selection against PUMA gene expression in Myc-driven B-cell lymphomagenesis. Mol Cell Biol 2008; 28(17): 5391-402.
[http://dx.doi.org/10.1128/MCB.00907-07] [PMID: 18573879]

[29] Hsu AP, Dowdell KC, Davis J, *et al.* Autoimmune lymphoproliferative syndrome due to FAS mutations outside the signal-transducing death domain: molecular mechanisms and clinical penetrance. Genet Med 2012; 14(1): 81-9.
[http://dx.doi.org/10.1038/gim.0b013e3182310b7d] [PMID: 22237435]

[30] Tauzin S, Debure L, Moreau JF, Legembre P. CD95-mediated cell signaling in cancer: mutations and post-translational modulations. Cell Mol Life Sci 2012; 69(8): 1261-77.
[http://dx.doi.org/10.1007/s00018-011-0866-4] [PMID: 22042271]

[31] Wohlfart S, Sebinger D, Gruber P, *et al.* FAS (CD95) mutations are rare in gastric MALT lymphoma but occur more frequently in primary gastric diffuse large B-cell lymphoma. Am J Pathol 2004; 164(3): 1081-9.
[http://dx.doi.org/10.1016/S0002-9440(10)63195-1] [PMID: 14982861]

[32] Watson CJ, O'Kane H, Maxwell P, *et al.* Identification of a methylation hotspot in the death receptor Fas/CD95 in bladder cancer. Int J Oncol 2012; 40(3): 645-54.
[PMID: 22076446]

[33] Park WS, Lee JH, Shin MS, *et al.* Inactivating mutations of KILLER/DR5 gene in gastric cancers. Gastroenterology 2001; 121(5): 1219-25.
[http://dx.doi.org/10.1053/gast.2001.28663] [PMID: 11677215]

[34] Elias A, Siegelin MD, Steinmüller A, *et al.* Epigenetic silencing of death receptor 4 mediates tumor necrosis factor-related apoptosis-inducing ligand resistance in gliomas. Clin Cancer Res 2009; 15(17): 5457-65.
[http://dx.doi.org/10.1158/1078-0432.CCR-09-1125] [PMID: 19706813]

[35] Elias A, Siegelin MD, Steinmüller A, *et al.* Epigenetic silencing of death receptor 4 mediates tumor necrosis factor-related apoptosis-inducing ligand resistance in gliomas. Clin Cancer Res 2009; 15(17): 5457-65.
[http://dx.doi.org/10.1158/1078-0432.CCR-09-1125] [PMID: 19706813]

[36] Safa A, Day T, Wu CH. Cellular FLICE-like inhibitory protein (C-FLIP): a novel target for cancer therapy. Curr Cancer Drug Targets 2008; 8(1): 37-46.
[http://dx.doi.org/10.2174/156800908783497087] [PMID: 18288942]

[37] Du X, Bao G, He X, *et al.* Expression and biological significance of c-FLIP in human hepatocellular carcinomas. J Exp Clin Cancer Res 2009; 28(1): 24.
[http://dx.doi.org/10.1186/1756-9966-28-24] [PMID: 19232089]

[38] Nagaraj NS, Vigneswaran N, Zacharias W. Hypoxia inhibits TRAIL-induced tumor cell apoptosis: Involvement of lysosomal cathepsins. Apoptosis 2007; 12(1): 125-39.
[http://dx.doi.org/10.1007/s10495-006-0490-1] [PMID: 17136492]

[39] Nagaraj NS, Vigneswaran N, Zacharias W. Hypoxia inhibits TRAIL-induced tumor cell apoptosis:

Involvement of lysosomal cathepsins. Apoptosis 2007; 12(1): 125-39.
[http://dx.doi.org/10.1007/s10495-006-0490-1] [PMID: 17136492]

[40]    Fulda S. The dark side of TRAIL signaling. Cell Death Differ 2013; 20(7): 845-6.
[http://dx.doi.org/10.1038/cdd.2013.36] [PMID: 23749177]

[41]    Brown JM, Wouters BG. Apoptosis, p53, and tumor cell sensitivity to anticancer agents. Cancer Res 1999; 59(7): 1391-9.
[PMID: 10197600]

[42]    Wendel HG, Stanchina E, Fridman JS, *et al.* Survival signalling by Akt and eIF4E in oncogenesis and cancer therapy. Nature 2004; 428(6980): 332-7.
[http://dx.doi.org/10.1038/nature02369] [PMID: 15029198]

[43]    Wendel HG, Lowe SW. Reversing drug resistance *in vivo*. Cell Cycle 2004; 3(7): 845-7.
[http://dx.doi.org/10.4161/cc.3.7.976] [PMID: 15190216]

[44]    Dai X, Zhang J, Arfuso F, *et al.* Targeting TNF-related apoptosis-inducing ligand (TRAIL) receptor by natural products as a potential therapeutic approach for cancer therapy. Exp Biol Med (Maywood) 2015; 240(6): 760-73.
[http://dx.doi.org/10.1177/1535370215579167] [PMID: 25854879]

[45]    Yu L, Alva A, Su H, *et al.* Regulation of an ATG7-beclin 1 program of autophagic cell death by caspase-8. Science 2004; 304(5676): 1500-2.
[http://dx.doi.org/10.1126/science.1096645] [PMID: 15131264]

[46]    Li Y, Luo P, Wang J, *et al.* Autophagy blockade sensitizes the anticancer activity of CA-4 *via* JNK-Bcl-2 pathway. Toxicol Appl Pharmacol 2014; 274(2): 319-27.
[http://dx.doi.org/10.1016/j.taap.2013.11.018] [PMID: 24321340]

[47]    Boya P, González-Polo RA, Casares N, *et al.* Inhibition of macroautophagy triggers apoptosis. Mol Cell Biol 2005; 25(3): 1025-40.
[http://dx.doi.org/10.1128/MCB.25.3.1025-1040.2005] [PMID: 15657430]

[48]    Djavaheri-Mergny M, Giuriato S, Tschan MP, Humbert M. Therapeutic modulation of autophagy in leukaemia and lymphoma. Cells 2019; 8(2): 103.
[http://dx.doi.org/10.3390/cells8020103] [PMID: 30704144]

[49]    Dai X, Wang D, Zhang J. Programmed cell death, redox imbalance, and cancer therapeutics. Apoptosis 2021; 26(7-8): 385-414.
[http://dx.doi.org/10.1007/s10495-021-01682-0] [PMID: 34236569]

[50]    Yu XY, Zhang XW, Wang F, *et al.* Correlation and prognostic significance of PD-L1 and P53 expression in resected primary pulmonary lymphoepithelioma-like carcinoma. J Thorac Dis 2018; 10(3): 1891-902.
[http://dx.doi.org/10.21037/jtd.2018.03.14] [PMID: 29707344]

[51]    Carnio S, Novello S, Papotti M, Loiacono M, Scagliotti GV. Prognostic and predictive biomarkers in early stage non-small cell lung cancer: tumor based approaches including gene signatures. Transl Lung Cancer Res 2013; 2(5): 372-81.
[PMID: 25806256]

[52]    Um HD. Bcl-2 family proteins as regulators of cancer cell invasion and metastasis: a review focusing on mitochondrial respiration and reactive oxygen species. Oncotarget 2016; 7(5): 5193-203.
[http://dx.doi.org/10.18632/oncotarget.6405] [PMID: 26621844]

[53]    Trisciuoglio D, Del Bufalo D. New insights into the roles of antiapoptotic members of the Bcl-2 family in melanoma progression and therapy. Drug Discov Today 2021; 26(5): 1126-35.
[http://dx.doi.org/10.1016/j.drudis.2021.01.027] [PMID: 33545382]

[54]    Suvarna V, Singh V, Murahari M. Current overview on the clinical update of Bcl-2 anti-apoptotic inhibitors for cancer therapy. Eur J Pharmacol 2019; 862: 172655.
[http://dx.doi.org/10.1016/j.ejphar.2019.172655] [PMID: 31494078]

[55]　Mattox TE, Chen X, Valiyaveettil J, *et al.* Novel RAS inhibitor, MCI-062, potently and selectively inhibits the growth of KRAS mutant pancreatic tumor cells by blocking GTP loading of RAS.

[56]　Cidado J, Boiko S, Proia T, *et al.* AZD4573 is a highly selective CDK9 inhibitor that suppresses MCL-1 and induces apoptosis in hematologic cancer cells. Clin Cancer Res 2020; 26(4): 922-34.
　　　[http://dx.doi.org/10.1158/1078-0432.CCR-19-1853] [PMID: 31699827]

[57]　Luedtke DA, Niu X, Pan Y, *et al.* Inhibition of Mcl-1 enhances cell death induced by the Bcl--selective inhibitor ABT-199 in acute myeloid leukemia cells. Signal Transduct Target Ther 2017; 2(1): 17012.
　　　[http://dx.doi.org/10.1038/sigtrans.2017.12] [PMID: 29263915]

[58]　Holcik M, Gibson H, Korneluk RG. XIAP: apoptotic brake and promising therapeutic target. Apoptosis 2001; 6(4): 253-61.
　　　[http://dx.doi.org/10.1023/A:1011379307472] [PMID: 11445667]

[59]　Schimmer AD, Dalili S, Batey RA, Riedl SJ. Targeting XIAP for the treatment of malignancy. Cell Death Differ 2006; 13(2): 179-88.
　　　[http://dx.doi.org/10.1038/sj.cdd.4401826] [PMID: 16322751]

[60]　Maddika S, Mendoza FJ, Hauff K, Zamzow CR, Paranjothy T, Los M. Cancer-selective therapy of the future: Apoptin and its mechanism of action. Cancer Biol Ther 2006; 5(1): 10-9.
　　　[http://dx.doi.org/10.4161/cbt.5.1.2400] [PMID: 16410718]

[61]　Los M, Panigrahi S, Rashedi I, *et al.* Apoptin, a tumor-selective killer. Biochim Biophys Acta 2009; 1793(8): 1335-42.
　　　[http://dx.doi.org/10.1016/j.bbamcr.2009.04.002]

# SUBJECT INDEX

## A

ABC 29, 30, 211
    drug transporters 211
    -mediated efflux 29
    transporter inhibitors 30
    transporter superfamily 29
Aberrant 33, 34, 67, 186, 197
    Hedgehog signaling 34
    STAT3 signaling 67
    Wnt signaling 33
    Hh pathway activation 186, 197
*Acalypha indica* 74
Acetylcholine receptor 11
Acid 6, 55, 96, 103, 104, 115, 123, 144, 161, 162, 208, 212, 213
    3,4,5-trimethoxybenzoic 104
    arachidonic 6
    betulinic 55, 212, 213
    corosolic 144
    lysophosphatidic 96
    phosphatidic 115
    targeting Gamma-aminobutyric 208
    ursodeoxycholic 123
    ursolic 103, 104
Acid ceramidase (AC) 118
Activated 143, 188, 191
    HSCs 143
    signalling pathway 191
    SMO 188
    YAP/TAZ 143
Acute 31, 51, 160, 169, 245, 255, 256
    myeloid leukemia 169, 245
    myelogenous leukaemia (AML) 31, 51, 160, 169, 255, 256
Adeno-associated viruses (AAVs) 14, 15, 16
Adenomatous polyposis 123
Advanced colorectal cancer 171
Alemtuzumab 228
*Allium cepa* 74
*Alpinia officinarum* 74
*Alpinumi soflavone* 246

Anaplastic large cell lymphoma (ALCL) 160, 165, 256
Anti-apoptotic 113, 117, 125, 242, 256, 257
    Bcl-XL 256
    Mcl-1 256
    members 242, 256, 257
    properties 113
    role 117
    signals 125
Anti-cancer 50, 55, 66, 80, 82
    cytokines 66
    lignans 80
    measures 82
    therapy 50
    traits 55
Antibodies 160, 163, 164, 165, 166
    humanized 165
    murine 160, 165, 166
    radiolabeled 163
    single-sphere 164
Antibody-drug conjugates (ADCs) 157, 159, 160, 161, 162, 165, 228, 231
Antibody target format methodology 227, 228, 229
*Antrodia cinnamomea* 146
*Antrodia cinnamomeahas* 146
Apoptosis 79, 80, 117, 119, 141, 143, 231, 253, 257
    bioflavonoid-induced 141
    ceramide-induced 117
    defective 253, 257
    developmental 141
    direct 119, 231
    doxorubicin-induced 143
    enhanced 253
    mitochondrial 79, 80
*Arctostaphylos uva-ursi* 74
*Argemone mexicana* 74
Arsenic Trioxide (ATO) 196
ATP 3, 29, 55, 101, 119, 239
    -binding cassette sub-family 119
    -binding cassette transporter A1 3

citrate lyase 55
generation 101, 239
hydrolysis 29
Autophagy 41, 49, 50, 120, 144, 240
　activating 120
　canonical 49, 50
　chaperone-mediated 240
　suppressed 144
　machinery 41
*Azadirachta indica* 74

# B

*Bacillus amyloliquefac* 167, 168
*Bacopa moneirra* 73
Basal cell nevus syndrome (BCNS) 190
Bayberry leaf proanthocyanidins (BLPs) 102
Bcl-2 56, 241, 253, 256, 257
　family proteins 253
　genes 56
　homology 256
　overexpressing lymphoma cells 257
　protein 241
　protein family 256
*Berberis* 74, 244
　*aquifolium* 244
　*aristata* 74
　*vulgaris* 74, 244
*Betula pendula* 74
Bioactive agent lycopene 22
Bovine milk 10, 12
BRAF genes 95
BRCA gene transformation 18
Burkitt's lymphoma (BL) 256
*Butea monosperma* 74

# C

*Camellia sinensis* 74, 209
*Camptotheca acuminata* 244
Cancer stem cell (CSCs) 7, 8, 27, 28, 29, 30, 31, 32, 33, 34, 35, 47, 94, 96, 97, 98, 100, 103, 121, 189
*Cannabis sativa* 74
*Capromab pendetide* 163
*Capsicum annuum* 73, 74
Cargo 9, 17
　complex 9
　exosome 9
　gene-editing 17

releasing 9
Caspase 54, 101, 102, 241, 254, 257
　activity 101, 102
　cascade 54, 241
　expression 254, 257
　signaling 254
*Catharanthus roseus* 214
Ceramide 49, 51, 113, 116, 117, 118, 119, 120, 122, 123, 124, 125
　converting 118
　role of 116, 120, 125
　activation 120
　digestion 123
　kinase 116
　levels 117, 123
Chemotherapy 30, 51, 95, 114, 115, 157, 161
　adjuvant 95
　cisplatin-containing 161
　platinum-based 95
　-induced peripheral neuropathy (CIPN) 115
　medications 157
　regimens 30
　resistance 114
　sensitivity 51
*Chonemorpha grandiflora* 244
*Cinnamomum camphora* 74
Colitis-associated cancer (CAC) 50, 120, 124
*Commiphora mukul* 75
*Corynebacterium diphtheria* 158
CRISPR 1, 4, 5, 7, 14, 15, 16, 17, 19, 20, 232
　-associated endonucleases 4
　-associated protein 1
　-based therapy 20
　/Cas9 delivery 19
　/Cas9 system 4, 5, 7, 14, 15, 16, 17
　/Cas9 technology 20, 232
*Cucurbita moschata* 167, 168
*Curcuma longa* 54, 209, 246
Cyclooxygenase 7

# D

Death-inducing signalling complex (DISC) 239, 241, 254, 257
Defy Cell Death 231
Demcizumab 35
Denileukin difititox 172
Desert Hedgehog (DHh) 184, 188
Dexamethasone 259

Diferuloylmethane 209
DNA 4, 8, 16, 17, 18, 28, 54, 96, 134, 161,
   203, 239, 241, 244, 246, 254
   donor 16
   plasmid 17
   repair 28
   -binding protein 134
   cleavage 161, 244
   damage 8, 239, 241, 254
   degradation 4, 246
   fragmentation 54
   impairment 18, 96
   integrity 4
   sequences 203
   strand breaks 244
*Dryopteris erythrosora* 246
Ductal Carcinoma *In Situ* (DCIS) 44

## E

Eculizumab 229
Eliglustat 118
Embryonic stem cells (ESCs) 33, 34, 96, 98,
   100
Enoticumab 35
Enzymes 7, 18, 113, 116, 117, 158, 204
   ceramidase 116
   critical 113, 117
   debranching 204
   metabolic 113
   nuclear 18
   potential target 113
   proteolytic 7
   ribosomal 158
Epithelialmesenchymal transition 201
Eprenetapopt 245
Erismodegib 196
*Erythrina droogmansiana* 73
*Erythrina suberosa* 246
Esophageal cancer lines 114
*Eucalyptus sieberi* 73, 76
Exosomes 4, 9, 10, 11, 12, 13, 105
   cell-derived 10, 12, 13, 105
   derived 10, 11, 12, 13
   iRGD-tagged 12, 13
   isolated 9
   line-derived 9
   macrophage-derived 4, 9
   plant-derived 4

## F

*Fagopyrum esculentum* 73
Famtrastuzumab 162
Flavonolignan 75
Focal adhesion kinase (FAK) 5, 6, 8, 99
Formation 51, 54, 96, 98, 100, 102, 103, 186,
   210, 226, 244
   gonadal 186
   large vacuole 54
   laryngeal cancer 210
   lipidated LC3 51
   microtubule 244
   mitotic spindle 244
   new blood vessel 96
   satiate ROS 226
   spheroid 98, 102, 103
   tumor sphere 102
   tumorsphere 100
*Fragaria ananassa* 74
Fresolimumab 35

## G

G-protein-coupled receptor (GPCR) 99
*Galega officinalis* 105
Galunisertib 35
Gaucher's disease 118
Gefitinib 69, 70
*Gelonium multiflorum* 167, 168
Gemcitabine-resistant (GR) 208, 211
Genistin 74
GLIoma 188, 192
   -associated oncogene 192
   transcription factors 188
Glucose transporters 3
Glucosylceramide 118, 122
GLUT1 stimulation 48
Glycine max 74
Golimumab 228
Gorlin syndrome 185, 186, 189, 190

## H

Hairy cell leukemia (HCL) 157, 172
Hedgehog 186, 187, 188, 189, 191, 193
   -GLI 186
   -interacting protein 191
   -Patched-Smoothened 186
   proteins 188

signaling pathways 187, 188, 193
signals 189
transcriptional program 189
Hepatic stellate cells (HSCs) 143
Hepatitis B virus (HBV) 143
Hepatocyte growth factor (HGF) 67
Hippo/YAP signaling pathways 146
Human papillomavirus 209
Humanized 227, 228, 229
    Fab 229
    IgG1 227, 228, 229
    IgG2 229
    IgG4 227
*Humulus lupulus* 73, 74, 76
*Hydrastis canadensis* 74

**I**

*Ibritumomab tiuxetan* 163, 228
Immunotoxin 169, 170, 171, 173
    LMB 171
    N901 bR 171
    RG 170
    targets 169
    therapy 170, 173
Indian Hedgehog (IHh) 184, 188
Inflammatory bowel disease (IBD) 10
Inhibitors of Apoptosis (IAPs) 140, 243, 253,
    255, 257
Internal Tandem Duplication (ITD) 51

**J**

Janus Kinase 69, 76
Jolkinolide B (JB) 56
Juvenile autosomal-recessive Parkinsonism 46

**K**

Kaposi sarcoma 244
KEGG pathway molecules RAS 105
Kinases 5, 8, 68, 69, 80, 99, 101, 136, 141,
    145
    cyclin-dependent 101
    epsilon 136
    extracellular-signal-regulated 69
    focal adhesion 5, 8, 99
    inhibiting 68
    novel 145
    pro-apoptotic 141

serine threonine 141
serine/threonine 68, 80
targeting 69
KRAS 11, 13, 48, 49, 95, 172
    altered 95
    mutated 95
    wild-type 172
    gene 48
    miRNA translation 13
    mutations 48, 49
    siRNA 11, 13

**L**

Lapatinib 69, 70
LC3 Interacting Region (LIR) 47, 49
Lenvatinib 146
Lestaurtinib 69, 70
Leukemia inhibitory factor (LIF) 67
Lucentis 229
Luteolin-7-*O*-glycoside 73

**M**

Macular degeneration 229
*Magnolia grandiflora* 80
*Mahonia aquifolium* 74
Malignant mesothelioma 31
*Malus domestica* 74
Mantle cell lymphomas (MCL) 143, 256
Manuka honey (MH) 75
Maritoclax Acute Myeloid Leukemia 245
*Mentha longifolia* 73
Mesenchymal Epithelial Transition 81
Metformin 105
Methoxy licoflavanone 246
Micro-RNAs 201, 202
Mitochondrial 42, 51, 52, 54, 100, 101
    depletion 51
    dynamics 100, 101
    fission 100
    fragmentation 101
    fusion process 54
    hyperpolarization 52
    mass 42, 52
Mitophagic 46, 50, 56
    dysfunction 50
    pathways 56
    removal 46
Mogamulizumab 229

*Momordica charantia* 73
Mono-ADP-ribosyltransferases 166, 167, 168
Mononuclear phagocyte system (MPS) 9
*Moxetumomab pasudotox* 172
Murine IgG 163
Myelodysplastic syndromes 245
Myelofibrosis 245
Myeloid leukemia 245

# N

Nanog protein 33
Nasopharyngeal cancer 31
Natalizumab 227
National Comprehensive Cancer Network
    (NCCN) 42
Natural killer (NK) 164
Necrotic cells 254
*Nelumbo nucifera* 53
Neoplastic meningitis 164
Nofetumomab merpentan 163
Non-Hodgkin lymphoma 228
*Nothapodytes nimmoniana* 244
Noxa gene 256

# O

Obatoclax mesylate 245
Oblimersen 245
Ofatumumab 229
*Olea europaea* 74
Oleanolic Acid 213
Omalizumab 227
Optic Atrophy Protein 54
*Oroxylum indicum* 73
Ovarian 95, 96, 97, 98, 99, 101, 103, 189
    cancer stem cells (OCSC) 96, 98, 101,
        103
    fibromas 189
    malignancies 95
    tissues 97, 99
    tumors 95
Oxaliplatin 115
Ozogamicin 161

# P

Paclitaxel 98, 211, 212, 244
    chemoresistance 98

drug resistance 212
    functions 244
    -induced chemotherapy 211
    resistance 212
Palivizumab 228
Pallister-Hall syndrome 189
Panitumumab 69, 70, 172, 228
Parkinson's disease 50
Patidegib 35, 197
Pedicellus Melo 55
Peroxisome proliferator-activated receptors
    (PPARs) 34
Pertuzumab 229
Pharynx Squamous Cell Carcinoma 13
Physalin 193, 195
Pinocembrin 73
Platelet-activating factors (PAF) 116, 124
Pleiotropic cytokine 105
Population Based Cancer Registries (PBCRs)
    44
Poteligeo 229
Poziotinib 104
Proxinium 164
*Prunus avium* 74
*Prunus persica* 74
*Pseudomonas aeruginosa* 159, 166, 167, 168
Purmorphamine 197

# R

Ranibizumab 229
Renal cell carcinoma 32, 256
Reticulocytes 3
Rheumatoid arthritis 227, 229
Rhinovirus 56
*Rhizoma coptidis* 244
Rhizomes 144, 209, 241, 244
*Ribes nigrum* 74
*Ricinus communis* 167, 168
Romosozumab 229
*Rubus fruticosus* 74
*Rubus idaeus* 74
Ruxolitinib 35, 69, 70

# S

*Saponaria officinalis* 167, 168
Sarilumab 227
Schwann cells 188
*Scutellaria baicalensis* 73

Sertoli-Leydig cell 95
Sézary syndrome 229
*Siegesbeckia glabrescens* 195
*Silybum marianum* 75
*Solanum lycopersicum* 74
Sphingomyelin 116, 122
    phosphodiesterase 122
    synthase 116
Sphingosine 113, 115, 116, 117, 119, 121,
    123, 124, 125
    kinase HK1 113
    kinase HK2 113
    kinase inhibitors 124
    -1-phosphate 113, 116
Systemic lupus erythematosus 228

## T

Teratocarcinoma 28
Theaflavin 74, 77
Theasaponin E1 102, 104
*Tinospora cordifolia* 244
Tocilizumab 229
Trabedersen 35
Transcription factors (TFs) 8, 32, 33, 66, 67,
    72, 134, 142, 188, 192, 194
Triacetyl resveratrol 207
Trimebutine maleate (TM) 102, 104
Tuberous sclerosis complex (TSC) 230
Tumor-initiating cells (TICs) 32, 33, 77, 100,
    101
Tumor suppressor 4, 80, 81
    LKB1 80
    phosphoprotein 4
    PTEN 81

## U

Ustekinumab 229

## V

Vantictumab 35
Vascular endothelial growth factor (VEGF)
    67, 76, 77, 96, 124, 192
Verrucarin 105
Vismodegib 35, 184, 185, 192, 193, 194

## W

Warburg hypothesis 45
Withaferin 53
*Withania somnifera* 53
Wnt signaling pathway 192
World Health Organization (WHO) 94, 156

## Y

YAP silencing 143
Yew tree 244
Yki phosphorylation 134

## Z

Zerumbone 196
Zevalin 163, 228
*Zingiber officinale* 74
Zynlonta 161

www.ingramcontent.com/pod-product-compliance
Lightning Source LLC
Chambersburg PA
CBHW050816220326
41598CB00006B/229